Radiosurgery and Pathological Fundamentals

Progress in Neurological Surgery

Vol. 20

Series Editor

L. Dade Lunsford, Pittsburgh, Pa.

Radiosurgery and Pathological Fundamentals

Volume Editors

G.T. Szeifert, *Budapest*
D. Kondziolka, *Pittsburg, Pa.*
M. Levivier, *Brussels*
L.D. Lunsford, *Pittsburg, Pa.*

131 figures, 66 in color, and 33 tables, 2007

KARGER

Basel · Freiburg · Paris · London · New York ·
Bangalore · Bangkok · Singapore · Tokyo · Sydney

George C. Tsokos
Founder of the Series

György T. Szeifert, MD, PhD
National Institute of Neurosurgery and
Department of Neurological Surgery
Semmelweis University
Budapest, Hungary

Marc Levivier, MD, PhD
Centre Gamma Knife
Hôpital Académique Erasme
Université Libre de Bruxelles
Brussels, Belgium

Douglas Kondziolka, MD, FACS, FRCS(C)
Center for Image-Guided
Neurosurgery
Department of Neurological Surgery
University of Pittsburgh
Pittsburgh, Pa., USA

L. Dade Lunsford, MD, FACS
Center for Image-Guided
Neurosurgery
Department of Neurological Surgery
University of Pittsburgh
Pittsburgh, Pa., USA

Library of Congress Cataloging-in-Publication Data
Radiosurgery and pathological fundamentals / volume editors, G.T. Szeifert
. . . [et al.].
p. ; cm. – (Progress in neurological surgery ; v. 20)
Includes bibliographical references and indexes.
ISBN-13: 978-3-8055-8200-1 (hardcover: alk. paper)
ISBN-10: 3-8055-8200-5 (hardcover: alk. paper)
1. Radiosurgery. 2. Pathology, Surgical. I. Szeifert, G. T. (György T.)
II. Series.
[DNLM: 1. Radiosurgery–methods. 2. Brain–pathology. 3. Brain
Diseases–surgery. W1 PR673 v.20 2007 / WL 368 R1293 2007]
RD594.15.R338 2007
617.4′81059–dc22
2006038289

Bibliographic Indices. This publication is listed in bibliographic services, including Current Contents® and Index Medicus.

Disclaimer. The statements, options and data contained in this publication are solely those of the individual authors and contributors and not of the publisher and the editor(s). The appearance of advertisements in the book is not a warranty, endorsement, or approval of the products or services advertised or of their effectiveness, quality or safety. The publisher and the editor(s) disclaim responsibility for any injury to persons or property resulting from any ideas, methods, instructions or products referred to in the content or advertisements.

Drug Dosage. The authors and the publisher have exerted every effort to ensure that drug selection and dosage set forth in this text are in accord with current recommendations and practice at the time of publication. However, in view of ongoing research, changes in government regulations, and the constant flow of information relating to drug therapy and drug reactions, the reader is urged to check the package insert for each drug for any change in indications and dosage and for added warnings and precautions. This is particularly important when the recommended agent is a new and/or infrequently employed drug.

www.karger.com
Printed in Switzerland on acid-free paper by Reinhardt Druck, Basel
ISSN 0079–6492
ISBN-10: 3–8055–8200–5
ISBN-13: 3–8055–8200–1

Editor

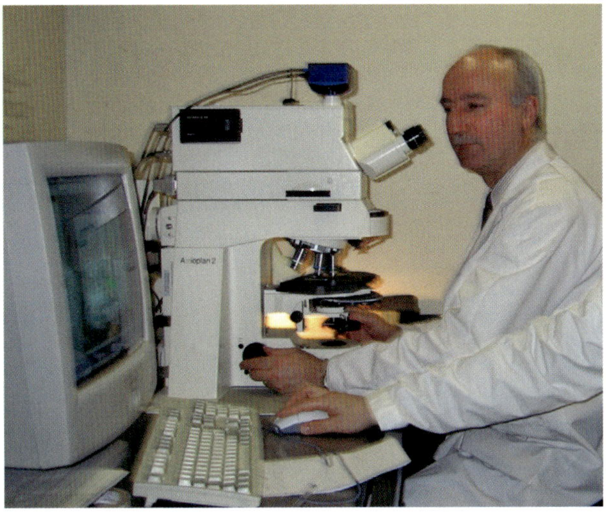

György T. Szeifert, MD, PhD

National Institute of Neurosurgery and Department of Neurological Surgery, Semmelweis University, Budapest, Hungary

Co-Editors

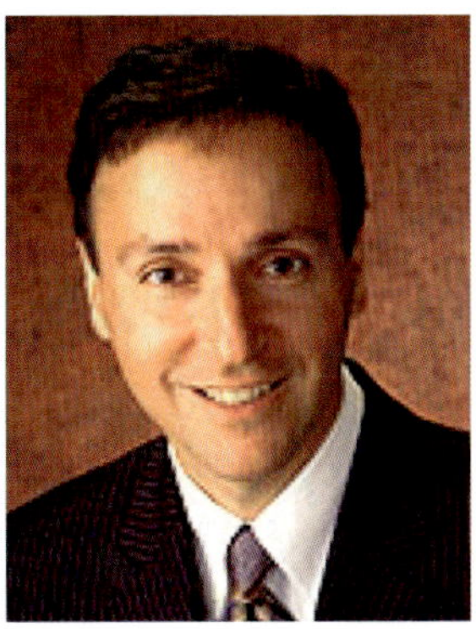

Douglas Kondziolka, MD, FACS, FRCS(C)

Center for Image-Guided Neurosurgery, Department of Neurological Surgery, UPMC Presbyterian Hospital, University of Pittsburgh, Pittsburgh, Pa., USA

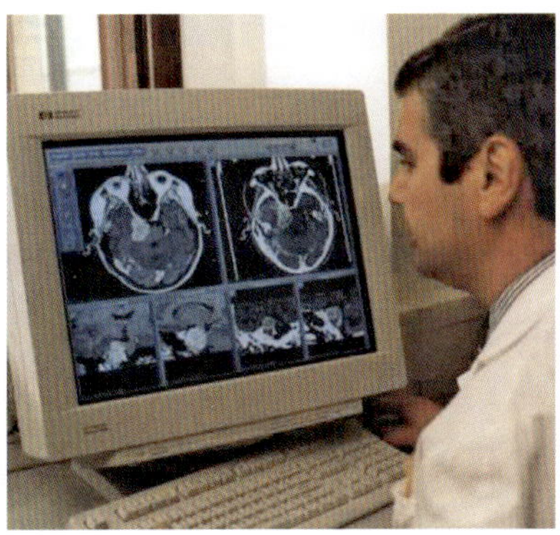

Marc Levivier, MD, PhD

Centre Gamma Knife, Department of Neurosurgery, Hôpital Académique Erasme, Université Libre de Bruxelles, Brussels, Belgium

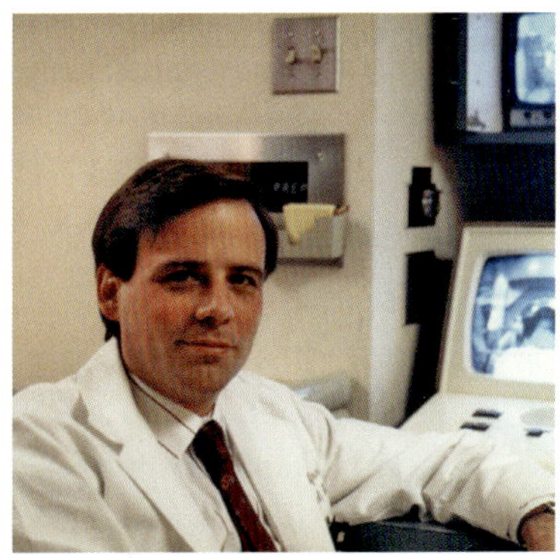

L. Dade Lunsford, MD, FACS

Center for Image-Guided Neurosurgery, Department of Neurological Surgery, UPMC Presbyterian Hospital, University of Pittsburgh, Pittsburgh, Pa., USA

List of Contributors

Erik-Olof Backlund, MD, PhD
Department of Neurosurgery
exp. US plan 17
University Hospital
SE–581 85 Linköping (Sweden)
E-Mail eo.backlund@swipnet.se

Nicholas M. Barbaro, MD
Box 0112, Department of
Neurological Surgery
University of California at
San Francisco
San Francisco, CA 94143 (USA)
E-Mail barbaron@neurosurg.ucsf.edu

Jacques Brotchi, MD, PhD
President of the WFNS
Department of Neurological Surgery
Hôpital Académique Erasme
Université Libre de Bruxelles
Route de Lennik 808
BE–1070 Brussels (Belgium)
E-Mail jb.wfns@ulb.ac.be

Christopher Duma, MD, FACS
Department of Neurosurgery
Hoag Memorial Hospital
Presbyterian,
351 Hospital Drive, #401
Newport Beach, CA 92660 (USA)
E-Mail cduma@mindspring.com

John C. Flickinger, MD, FACR
Center for Image-Guided
Neurosurgery
Department of Neurological Surgery
University of Pittsburgh
UPMC Presbyterian/Suite B-400
200 Lothrop Street
Pittsburgh, PA 15213 (USA)
E-Mail flickingerjc@upmc.edu

Peter Gerszten, MD
Department of Neurological Surgery
University of Pittsburgh Medical
Center
200 Lothrop Street, Suite B-400
Pittsburgh, PA 15213 (USA)
E-Mail gersztenpc@upmc.edu

Jenö Julow, MD, PhD
Department of Neurological Surgery
St. John's Hospital
Diósárok u. 1–3
HU–1125 Budapest (Hungary)
E-Mail h12494jul@helka.iif.hu

Andras A. Kemeny, MD, FRCS
National Centre for Stereotactic Radiosurgery
Department of Neurological Surgery
Royal Hallamshire Hospital
Sheffield S10 2JF (UK)
E-Mail a.kemeny@shef.ac.uk

Tatsuya Kobayashi, MD, PhD
Nagoya Radiosurgery Center
Nagoya Kyoritsu Hospital
1-172 Hokke, Nakagawa
Nagoya, Aichi 454-0933 (Japan)
E-Mail ttkobayashi@kaikou.org.jp

Douglas Kondziolka, MD, FACS, FRCS(C)
Center for Image-Guided Neurosurgery
Department of Neurological Surgery
University of Pittsburgh
UPMC Presbyterian/Suite B-400
200 Lothrop Street
Pittsburgh, PA 15213 (USA)
E-Mail kondziolkads@upmc.edu

John Y.K. Lee, MD
Department of Neurosurgery
University of Pennsylvania
Penn Gamma Knife at Pennsylvania Hospital
330 South 9th Street
Pennsylvania Neurological Institute
4th Floor
Philadelphia, PA 19107 (USA)
E-Mail leejohn@uphs.upenn.edu

Dan Leksell, MD
Karlavägen 63
SE–114 49 Stockholm (Sweden)
E-Mail dan.leksell@elekta.com

Marc Levivier, MD, PhD
Centre Gamma Knife
Hôpital Académique Erasme
Université Libre de Bruxelles
Route de Lennik 808
BE–1070 Brussels (Belgium)
E-Mail Marc.Levivier@ulb.ac.be

Roman Liščák, MD
Stereotactic and Radiation Neurosurgery Department
Hospital Na Homolce, Roentgenova 2
CZ–150 30 Prague 5 (Czech Republic)
E-Mail Roman.Liscak@homolka.cz

L. Dade Lunsford, MD, FACS
Center for Image-Guided Neurosurgery
Department of Neurological Surgery
University of Pittsburgh
UPMC Presbyterian/Suite B-400
200 Lothrop Street
Pittsburgh, PA 15213 (USA)
E-Mail lunsfordld@upmc.edu

Ottó Major, MD, PhD
National Institute of Neurosurgery
Amerikai út 57
HU–1145 Budapest (Hungary)
E-Mail majoott@mailer.oiti.hu

Nicolas Massager, MD
Centre Gamma Knife
Hôpital Académique Erasme
Université Libre de Bruxelles
Route de Lennik 808
BE–1070 Brussels (Belgium)
E-Mail nmassage@ulb.ac.be

Ajay Niranjan, MBBS, MS, MCh
Center for Image-Guided
Neurosurgery
Department of Neurological Surgery
University of Pittsburgh
UPMC Presbyterian/Suite B-400
200 Lothrop Street
Pittsburgh, PA 15213 (USA)
E-Mail niranjana@upmc.edu

István Nyáry, MD, PhD
National Institute of Neurosurgery and
Department of Neurological Surgery,
Semmelweis University
Amerikai út 57
HU–1145 Budapest (Hungary)
E-Mail nyary@oiti.hu

Bruce E. Pollock, MD
Department of Neurological Surgery
Mayo Clinic
200 First Street N.W.
Rochester, MN 55905-0001 (USA)
E-Mail pollock.bruce@mayo.edu

Jean Régis, MD, PhD
Centre Gamma Knife
C.H.U. La Timone
264 rue Saint-Pierre
FR–13385 Marseille Cedex 05
(France)
E-Mail jregis@mail.ap-hm.fr

Jason Sheehan, MD, PhD
Lars Leksell Center for Gamma
Knife Surgery
Box 800-212
University of Virginia Health
Sciences Center
Charlottesville, VA 22908 (USA)
E-Mail jps2f@virginia.edu

Stéphane Simon, MS
Centre Gamma Knife
Hôpital Académique Erasme
Université Libre de Bruxelles
Route de Lennik 808
BE–1070 Brussels (Belgium)
E-Mail gamma.knife@ulb.ac.be

György T. Szeifert, MD, PhD
National Institute of Neurosurgery and
Department of Neurological Surgery
Semmelweis University
Amerikai út 57
HU–1145 Budapest (Hungary)
E-Mail gyorgyszeifert@yahoo.com

David Wikler, MS
Centre Gamma Knife
Hôpital Académique Erasme
Université Libre de Bruxelles
Route de Lennik 808
BE–1070 Brussels (Belgium)
E-Mail David.Wikler@ulb.ac.be

Masaaki Yamamoto, MD
Katsuta Hospital, 5125-2 Nakane
Hitachi'naka, Ibaraki 312-0011
(Japan)
E-Mail BCD06275@nifty.com

Contents

In Memoriam Prof. Lars Leksell (1907–1986)

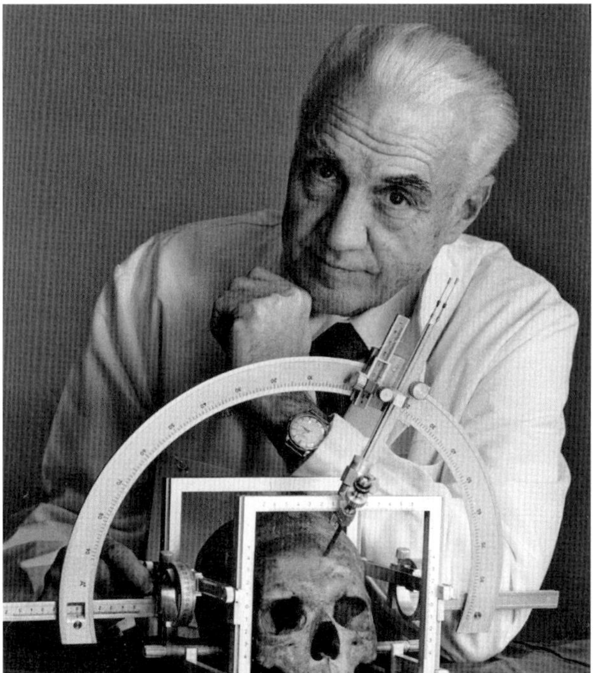

'I was born under the sign of Sagittarius and I liked the motto: to ride, to shoot with the bow, and to tell the truth.'

Acknowledgement

Dr Szeifert and this project were partly supported by a Congress of Neurological Surgeons/Elekta Clinical Fellowship in Radiosurgery, and by the Hungarian Ministry of Health and Welfare (ETT: grant 12980-9/2003-1018EKU; 395/KO/03). [TONE].

Foreword

Within the past 3 decades, and more precisely within the last 5 years, radiosurgery has become a fundamental arm in neurosurgery.

Starting with arteriovenous malformations, it is currently a basic treatment for grade I and II vestibular schwannomas, cavernous sinus meningiomas, recurrent pituitary tumors, metastases, and recently also for trigeminal neuralgia, temporal lobe epilepsy and other functional neurosurgery indications. A new door has recently been opened for spinal tumors.

But, in spite of a very wide clinical experience, one should recognize the lack of fundamental researches, the need for a better understanding of radiobiology and for more pathological studies. That is one of the major contributions of the monograph edited by G.T. Szeifert, D. Kondziolka, M. Levivier and L.D. Lunsford entitled *Radiosurgery and Pathological Fundamentals*.

A better understanding of radiobiological processes will enhance the quality of radiosurgery, focus the indications together with new applications.

The sterile fight between conventional microneurosurgery and radiosurgery is behind us. Today, it is clear that both modalities are complementary. But when there is a choice, the best should be offered to the patient, taking into consideration medical treatment, risk of therapy with an ultimate goal – quality of life.

Jacques Brotchi
President of the WFNS

Preface

It's been a great pleasure working with Professors Szeifert, Kondziolka and Levivier in the preparation and review of the current Volume 20 of *Progress in Neurological Surgery.* Stereotactic radiosurgery has turned out to be not just a small blip on the great ocean of brain surgery, but in fact a veritable ocean liner. It has had amazing staying power related to its original goal; a minimally invasive low risk strategy designed as an alternative or primary management for difficult tumors, vascular malformations, movement disorders, pain problems, and epilepsy. It has spawned a remarkable re-evaluation of radiobiology, and has emphasized that when done with precision, small volumes of tissue can be inactivated or eradicated using closed skull radiosurgery. What has been missing to a large extent has been a long-term analysis of the mechanisms of the pathologic substrate, as well as better understanding of adverse radiation effects. This is in part related to the successful outcomes that most patients obtain after radiosurgery, which limits the amount of eventual histopathological data. I believe that this volume helps address that question.

Professor Szeifert, perhaps the only neurosurgeon who trained as a neuropathologist (in addition to being a concert organist) is an individual uniquely equipped to be able to lead the team of authors who assembled this monograph. Many of the chapters provide new insights into the field of radiosurgery. Pay special attention to the introductory chapter of my own personal mentor, Professor Erik Olof Backlund. He gives a unique historical summary of the early days of radiosurgery under the guidance of the great Swedish innovative neurosurgeon, Lars Leksell. The timing of this book is also a fitting memorial to the vision and creativity of Professor Leksell who was born in 1907. On the

100th Anniversary of his birth, many surgeons who are first-, second- or third-generation disciples of Leksell assisted in this volume. Lars Leksell envisioned this concept and defined the term stereotactic radiosurgery in 1951. In this half a century, and especially in the last 25 years, the knowledge base of the field of stereotactic radiosurgery has dramatically increased. The procedure has tremendous staying power. At many neurosurgical centers of excellence across the world, it accounts for 10% or more of all intracranial brain surgery being done.

L. Dade Lunsford, MD

Szeifert GT, Kondziolka D, Levivier M, Lunsford LD (eds): Radiosurgery and Pathological Fundamentals. Prog Neurol Surg. Basel, Karger, 2007, vol 20, pp XXI–XXVIII

Gamma Knife – The Early Story: Memoirs of a Privileged Man

Erik-Olof Backlund

Department of Neurosurgery, University Hospital, Linköping, Sweden

In the fall of 1960, a few months after my beginning as a resident of the Department of Neurosurgery at the Karolinska Institute in Stockholm, Lars Leksell came to this Department as the new Professor and Chairman, succeeding Herbert Olivecrona, the founder of Swedish neurosurgery. I became immediately acquainted with Leksell's on-going and indeed very exciting experiments together with the radiobiologist Börje Larsson in Uppsala, on trying to develop 'stereotactic radiosurgery', aimed at lesioning in the central brain in functional operations such as thalamotomy and capsulotomy. Clinical experiments using a proton beam were initiated at the Gustav Werner Institute in Uppsala, and a few patients had been treated [1]. Experiences from these led Leksell to design a multi-source 'beam knife', which became ready for use in 1967 [2] as the first 'Gamma Knife' (GK). It was financed by nongovernmental funding and installed at the private hospital Sophiahemmet in Stockholm as a clinical research unit to be run by the staff at the Department of Neurosurgery of the Karolinska Institute/Hospital.

The basic concept of the GK was that extremely well-collimated beams from a large number of Cobalt-60 sources, distributed around a half-spherical collimator helmet, would allow a circumscribed focus of beams to be produced in the central part of the patient's skull. The direction of beams and the placement of this focus should be guaranteed by stereotactic measures. Although the primary aim with the GK was to offer 'nonsurgical' lesioning in the central gray for functional surgery, it seemed obvious that it would also offer precision irradiation of small intracranial tumors, e.g. those of the pituitary. This latter concept, using proton beams, had already been exploited at a few other centers in other countries [3–5].

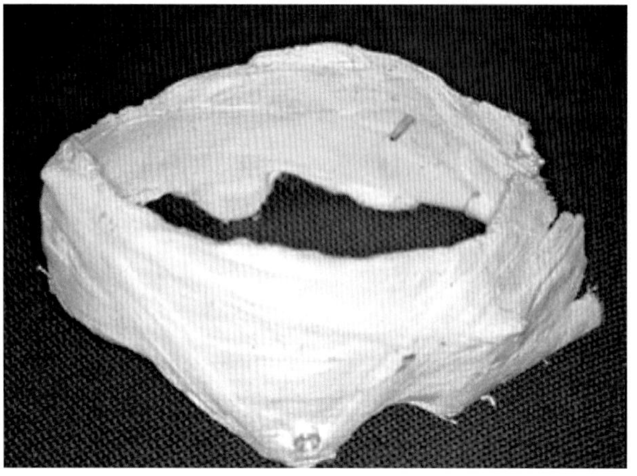

Fig. 1. The plaster of Paris cap used for the first GK patient in 1967 (now on display at Dade Lunsford's OR in Pittsburgh, Pa., USA).

The arrival of the GK did matter a lot to me personally, just leaving behind the final phase of my specialization, to be intimately acquainted with the principle of 'bloodless surgery'. For example it would enable me to be instrumental in starting new and tentative projects within my own fields of interest, precision irradiation of pituitary tumors in particular. First of all, I eagerly wanted to include the longed for GK alternative in my protocol for stereotactic craniopharyngioma treatment. Moreover, I had plans to try a noninvasive/outpatient technique for destruction of the normal pituitary in cases of advanced mammary carcinoma, a current therapeutic principle during the 1960s.

This might explain why I, together with Leksell himself and Börje Larsson in October 1967 came to constitute the first GK operation team in history. The case was one of a series of craniopharyngiomas, later constituting the case material of my own PhD thesis. The patient was a young man with a craniopharyngioma where the cystic part had been treated previously by intracavitary irradiation, using Yttrium-90 colloid [6]. The solid tumor remnant was of appropriate size for one single lesion using the smallest (5 × 3 mm) collimator alternative, and 20 Gy were given to the center of the tumor. A plaster of Paris cap (fig. 1), secured to the patient's skull by three aluminum screws was used as a mechanical interface, allowing the head to be attached to the axis trunnions of the GK in agreement with precalculated stereotactic coordinates. Unexpectedly the patient died from an acute shunt obstruction 4 months later, allowing us to study the radiation effect at autopsy. A small crescent of surviving tumor tissue was found, surrounding a central tumor necrosis [7]. This first case was fol-

Table 1. GK I: the first ten operations

Patient	Diagnosis	Irradiation date	Max. dose, Gy
FE	Craniopharyngioma	October 1967	20
ÖD	Pituitary adenoma	January 27, 1968	28
EN	Intractable cancer pain	February 22, 1968	~150
JO	Intractable cancer pain	February 23, 1968	~150
WA	Intractable cancer pain	March 27, 1968	~150
JO2	Intractable cancer pain	April 24, 1968	~150
BE	Craniopharyngioma	May 21, 1968	50
BL	Intractable cancer pain	May 29, 1968	~200
EL	Intractable cancer pain	June 29, 1968	~200

lowed by a pituitary adenoma patient (see below), a few patients with intractable cancer pain for 'gamma-thalamotomy' [8], and another craniopharyngioma patient (summarized data in table 1).

The second case in table 1 (ÖD) was a man who had a 'chromophobe adenoma' removed transfrontally by me in 1967. Postoperative irradiation was part of the routine for these tumors at that time. Having the sophisticated GK single-dose technique at our disposal, our oncology colleagues agreed to use that alternative for the irradiation. An arbitrary dose of 28 Gy was given to the center of the sella, the dose level chosen with the regard to the assumed radiation tolerance of the optic pathways. The optic chiasm was assessed to have received less than 5–6 Gy. During a 2-year follow-up, there was radiological evidence of a slight shrinkage of the irradiated volume.

These pilot cases stimulated the GK staff to design virtual research protocols for further systematic studies, and principal investigatorships were defined for each project. For example under my mentorship, the two senior residents Tiit Rähn and Georg Norén were given personal tasks with pituitary and acoustic tumors, respectively. Over the coming years, these two young colleagues presented reports on patients with Cushing's disease and vestibular schwannomas treated with the GK, which must be considered seminal, each in its field, for the further progress of radiosurgery [9, 10]. Ladislau Steiner, already in charge of the routine vascular surgery, received the paramount responsibility for the most exciting GK project, the irradiation of intracranial arteriovenous malformations (AVMs). We were all spellbound over the results in the latter, where already in the first tentative cases a marvelous disappearance of the malformation could be seen (fig. 2).

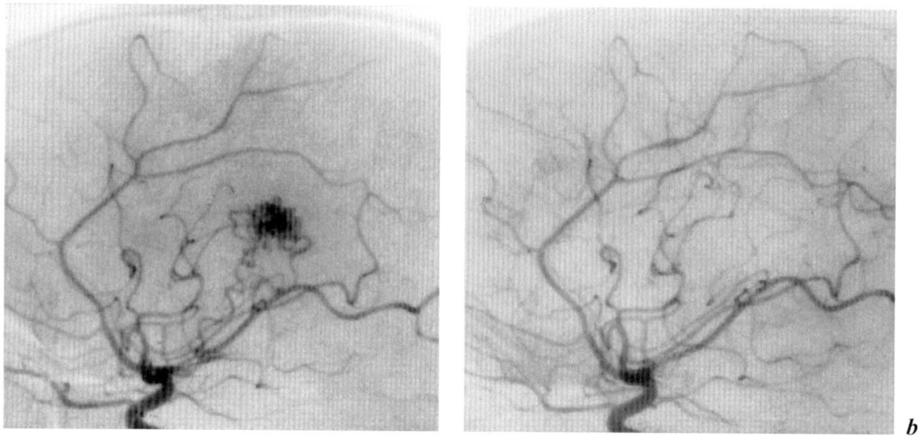

Fig. 2. Radiological findings in one of the first AVM patients. Carotid angiography before (***a***) and 2 years after GK irradiation (***b***).

Table 2. Original papers from the GK I group, 1968–1980

Year	Author(s)	Topic
1968	Leksell [8]	Gammathalamotomy
1969	Backlund [7]	Craniopharyngioma
1971	Leksell [11]	Acoustic tumor
1971	Leksell [12]	Trigeminal neuralgia
1972	Steiner et al. [13]	AVM
1972	Backlund et al. [14]	Pituitary ablation
1974	Backlund et al. [15]	Pineal tumors
1978	Thorén et al. [9]	Cushing's disease
1979	Leksell and Backlund [16]	Gammacapsulotomy

Professor Leksell himself was strongly involved in the treatment of patients with intractable cancer pain, not least to try to develop peroperative pain tests for assessing the expected radiolesions in the nonspecific pain pathways in centrum medianum. Personally, I also foresaw a project on pineal tumors, together with Tiit Rähn, enabling us to avoid, by stereotactic biopsy, the common diagnostic 'guessing' in these lesions, after which GK lesioning should be made in suitable, i.e. circumscribed and nonmalignant tumors.

The gradual emergence of tentative scientific reports during the first decade is summarized in table 2.

Snapshots

The famous pituitary surgeon Jules Hardy had just postulated that the most common location for ACTH adenomas in Cushing' syndrome is in the most anterior part of the anterior pituitary lobe. Thus Tiit and I decided, as a first step in a new case, to irradiate this part only, and wait for any hormonal response. To our satisfaction, this seemed to be correct. As many as 48% of those treated with this very limited field only went into remission, and could escape adrenalectomy. Those who did not respond had a second (or third, or even fourth) GK course, for the remaining gland. The overall results from this step-by-step irradiation protocol were very rewarding [9].

Snapshot: Tiit patiently contemplating at the light box, meticulously examining serial X-rays and tomographies of Cushing patients, looking for irregularities of the sellar floor, possibly disclosing the extension and location of the ACTH adenoma. Together with previous pneumoencephalographic findings, any such sellar pathology guided the dose planning. The CT technique was still in the future.

In the AVM patients, there was empirical evidence that the 'shunting compartment' of the malformation might be the critical volume for irradiation. Thus, scrutinizing analysis of the angiograms was crucial. But out of the AVM patients admitted, who should be irradiated, and who should not? Of those irradiated, why did some respond well and in a reasonable time, and some not?

Snapshot: Ladislau contemplating for hours in his office, at his light box, discussing preoperatively various collimator alternatives and field configurations with the radiophysicist, and subtle if any changes in early postirradiation angiograms with the neuroradiologist.

Lars Leksell himself actualized important ethical issues. One example: in contrast to the 'reasonable' doses given in tumors and AVMs, for capsulotomy very high doses were deemed necessary, performed as they should be in presumably 'radioresistant' normal brain tissue. For doses around 150 or 200 Gy, an irradiation time of many hours would then be necessary. It was tempting to divide such a tedious procedure into two parts, with a night in between, thus the first part could serve the purpose of a sham operation. Would that be ethically tolerable?

Snapshot: Lars telling me that after serious consideration he did not find such a two-step operation violating ethical standards, as the intermission (1) would be nothing but extremely relaxing for the patient, and moreover (2) would do no harm whatsoever.

Georg had a less enviable situation in his task to 'hit' properly the smaller acoustic tumors selected for the GK. For the dose planning, he had to get the tumor visualized on the stereotactic X-ray, notably without the possibility to include, in the GK procedure, pneumoencephalography, the common and the only road to radiological diagnosis at that time.

Snapshot: The radiologist and Georg climbing around in the X-ray lab, intermittently and quickly turning the patient to head positions optimal for a small amount of positive contrast (intrathecal metrizamide) to be captured on the film.

The main aim of a tentative study in 8 patients with advanced mammary carcinoma was to explore the possibility of halting the disease by 'gamma-hypophysectomy'. My preliminary impression was that we failed as the pituitary hormonal levels were found essentially unchanged after the GK irradiation, and moreover the cancer continued to ruin the patient's life.

Snapshot: Tiit stubbornly emphasizing – in retrospect and after regretting publication of a preliminary report [14] – that we might not have failed completely, as all the 'gamma-hypophysectomy' patients were pain free after the GK treatment. We might have been, without fully appreciating it, on the tracks of the up to that time unknown pituitary-related endorphin system.

Methodological Progress

In a historical account like this, it would be unfair not to mention how many of us involved had to solve purely practical/technical problems of joint responsibility related to the irradiation procedure proper. We had the machine, in splendid sophistication, but regarding its practical use, a number of details were less than obvious. A few examples are given here.

(1) The Attachment

The dimensions of the collimator helmets of the GK were set from the radiophysical requirements. In principle and ideally, the patient's head should be placed as close as possible to the radiation sources (i.e. the inner aperture of each of the 198 collimators) to avoid any surplus scattered radiation contributing to an unwanted integral dose. To satisfy this, the space within the collimator helmet had been made very narrow, not allowing any stereotactic frame to be used for the alignment of the patient to the GK. Leksell had foreseen a routine where less space-occupying, individually modeled and disposable fixtures should solve the problem of mechanically securing the patient. As mentioned above, the first patient had a plaster of Paris cap made around his head, secured to the skull by metal screws. Leksell later substituted the plaster of Paris by Thermoplast (fig. 3). Both myself and my younger associates found the 'cap' technique less

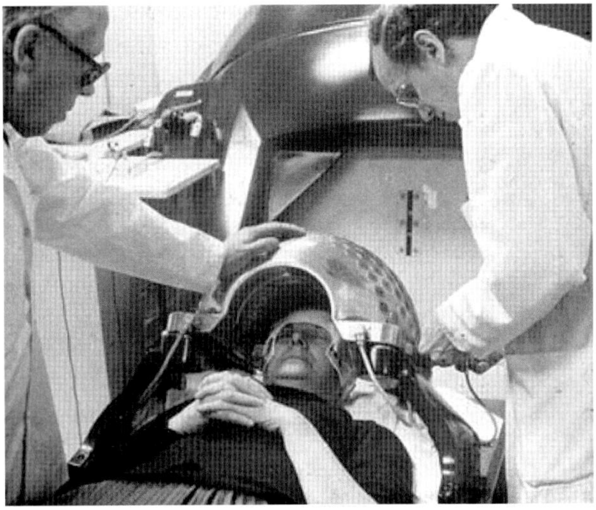

Fig. 3. Capsulotomy patient in position in GK I, just before attachment to the trunnion axes. The lateral stereotactic coordinate is set on the left axis (by the author, right). In this case, an Orthoplast cap was used. (Research engineer Bengt Jernberg to the left.)

convenient for the surgeon and indeed unpleasant for the patient. Thus some standardized aluminum interphases, a kind of 'pseudo-frames', were designed. An important additional reason to give up the 'cap' technique (allowing nothing but a one-isocenter irradiation) was that we wanted eagerly to introduce a multi-target (field cluster) technique for the larger tumors. The 'pseudo-frames' worked very well for this purpose, and it was not until the Elekta company introduced the so-called G-frame (for GK II), that the attachment technique was standardized. One of the 'pseudo-frames' is shown in figure 4. An example of a cluster irradiation using this frame is shown in figure 5.

(2) Individual Adjustments of Radiation Parameters

For the planning of each individual treatment, it was crucial to know the dimensions and form of the radiation field, as well as the irradiation time necessary for a certain radiation dose. We then profited from the thorough 3-dimensional calculations made during the GK construction work, and used a few standardized, 'average' dose diagram templates to superimpose directly upon the diagnostic X-rays. This was a tolerable compromise when it came to single-isocenter irradiations and the small apertures. But as soon as we introduced double- (or multi-) target irradiations, the individual, composite isodose

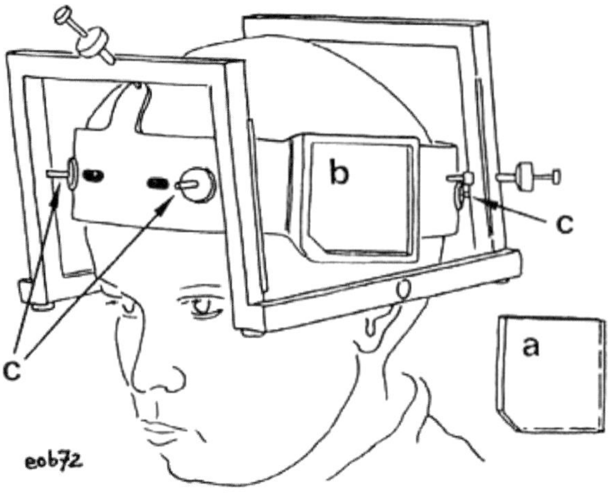

Fig. 4. The standard Leksell stereotactic frame attached outside a 'pseudo-frame', designed for cluster irradiations. Guided by the former, a pattern of drill holes (for the axis trunnions) representing the configuration of the dose diagram was made in plexiglass sheets ***(a)*** fitting into a 'box' on the 'pseudo-frame' (***b***), during the irradiation.

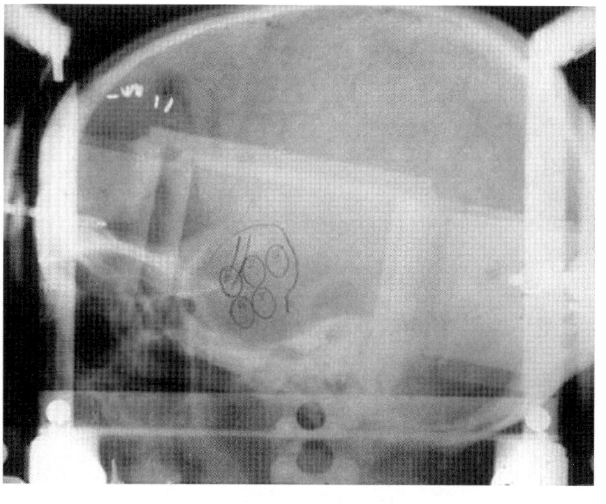

Fig. 5. Cluster irradiation of a giant recurrent pituitary adenoma (in October 1969), using the 'pseudo-frame' shown in figure 4. The 3 × 5 collimator alternative is used in five isocenters.

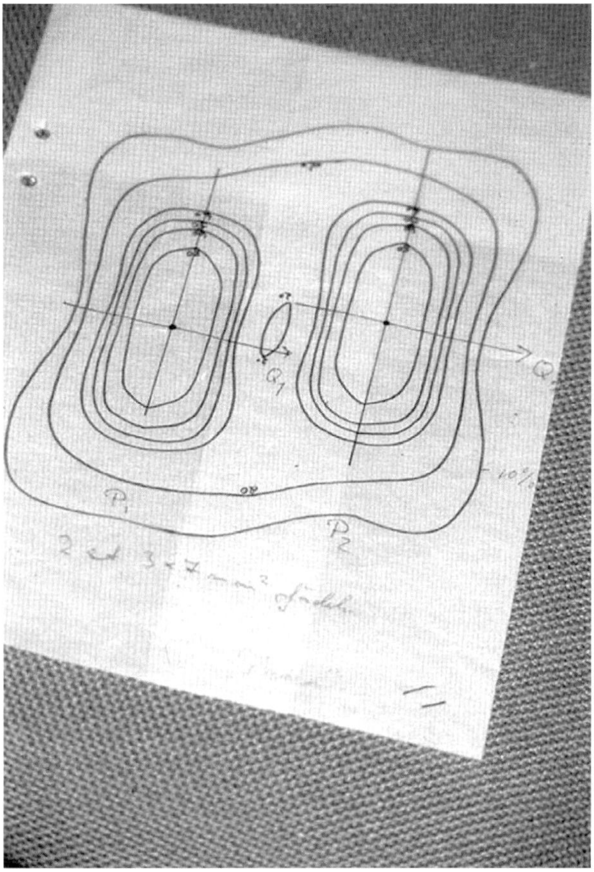

Fig. 6. Hand-drawn dose diagram (up-scaled to 10:1) of a double-isocenter target for the 3 × 7 mm collimator alternative (of GK I).

diagrams had to be 'hand-calculated' and hand-drawn, by the radiophysicist as computed dose planning was still far ahead (fig. 6).

(3) Treatment Nomogram

As the radiation source was Cobalt-60, with a defined decay over time, the operation planning had to take the actual irradiation date into consideration. Although most of the irradiation targets were rather centrally located in the head, the degree of 'eccentricity' of the focus (i.e. the average distance from skin to target) moreover influenced the dose rate (and thus the irradiation/'exposure'

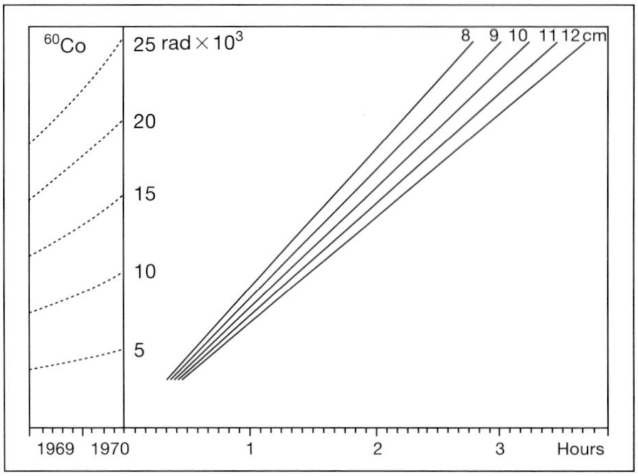

Fig. 7. By plotting (1) the figures for the patient's 'head radius' (i.e. the average distance from skin to target, in cm), (2) the desired target dose and (3) the irradiation date, the irradiation/exposure time (in h) was easily obtained from this 'adjustment nomogram'.

time) in the individual case. To facilitate such individual adjustments without separate calculations, I designed a smart 'nomogram' (fig. 7).

(4) GK – The Second Generation

Lars Leksell's original and basic idea with the GK was to obtain a new kind of surgical tool for 'cutting' in the brain, for tractotomy, thalamotomy, etc. However, the first years with a number of tentative cluster irradiations in the first GK clearly showed the need for a modified, second-generation machine, allowing (more) spherical radiation fields to be produced, using cylindrical collimators. This work for a GK II started immediately. I suggested that two (or three) collimator alternatives should be made, each with the cross-section of the individual cylindrical beam in the target area to be 4, 8 and 14 mm. The latter two alternatives were chosen for the GK II, taken into use in 1974. It was installed at the Karolinska Hospital in Stockholm (fig. 8), where a dedicated radiosurgical OR was built. One year later, when professor Leksell retired, I was appointed to a formal position as Chief of the Stereotactic Service at the Karolinska Hospital, including the GK.

Concluding Reflections

This very comprehensive account, a few personal impressions a bit out of an official record, mirrors a short, intense and indeed exciting decade of

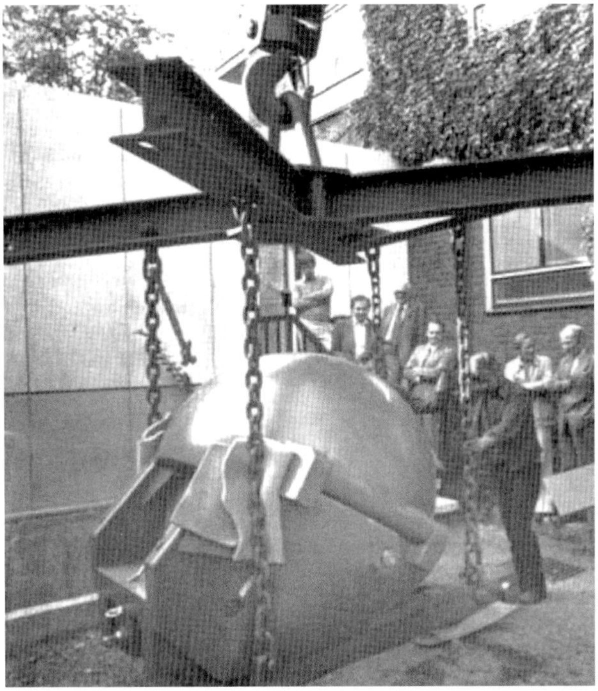

Fig. 8. Arrival of GK II to the Karolinska in 1974. The spectators in the background are (from left) Drs Norén, Rähn, Leksell, Melander (oncologist), Backlund and Sarby (physicist).

neurosurgical history, initiated by one of the most innovative minds of the neurosurgical community, Lars Leksell. In his absolutely indefatigable creativity, he led his team with steady but generous hands; thus every individual around the first GK was given his particular role and a certain freedom, fostering both self-esteem and responsibility. And we learned, like maybe few other clinicians, to appreciate the indispensable intimate collaboration with people off the clinical floor, radiobiologists, physicists, technicians. We shared each other's ideas and suggestions in a mode probably not so often seen among tight groups of people in the van.

Notably, moreover, we spontaneously never saw this new field of work as a branch of any 'radiation therapy'. Indeed, it was natural to look upon it as a branch of surgery, radiosurgery. I have previously published a thorough discussion on the arguments for that [17].

Finally, it must not be forgotten that we saw but few, if any, appreciating glances from the neurosurgical community in the world around, notably not even in Sweden; 'no one is a prophet in his native city'. Particularly our work was far from recognized as a step forward by influential microsurgeons, who had difficulties to see the potentiality in this new therapeutic concept. To some, the provocative principle of 'not removing a tumor but inactivating or obliterating it' primarily with the aim of minimizing the risk for the patient was even awfully insulting.

Being the first of Lars Leksell's pupils to be involved in the GK project, and presumably being the one most intimately engaged in it during the first few years, indeed I consider myself most privileged, and I have collected these small memoirs with pride but also in great gratitude.

References

1 Larsson B, Leksell L, Rexed B: The use of high-energy protons for cerebral surgery in man. Acta Chir Scand 1963;125:1–7.

2 Leksell L: Stereotaxis and radiosurgery. An operative system. Springfield, Charles C Thomas, 1971.

3 Linfoot JA, Lawrence JH, Born JL, Tobias CA: The alpha particle of proton in surgery of the pituitary gland for Cushing's disease. N Engl J Med 1963;269:597–601.

4 Kjellberg RN: Stereotactic Bragg peak proton radiosurgery method; in Szikla G (ed): Stereotactic Cerebral Irradiation. Amsterdam, Elsevier, 1979, pp 93–100.

5 Minakova EI, Krymskii VA, Luchi EI, Serbinenko FA, Liass FM: [Proton therapy in clinical neurosurgery] (In Russian). Med Radiol (Mosk) 1987;32:36–42.

6 Backlund EO, Johansson L, Sarby B: Studies on craniopharyngiomas II. Treatment by sterotaxis and radiosurgery. Acta Chir Scand 1972;138:749–759.

7 Backlund EO: Stereotaxic treatment of craniopharyngiomas; in Hamberger CA, Wersäll J (eds): Nobel Symposium 10: Disorders of the Skull Base Region. Stockholm, Almquist & Wiksell, 1969, pp 237–244.

8 Leksell L: Cerebral radiosurgery I. Gammathalamotomy in two cases of intractable pain. Acta Chir Scand 1968;134:585–595.

9 Thorén M, Rähn T, Hall K, Backlund EO: Treatment of pituitary dependent Cushing's syndrome with closed stereotactic radiosurgery by means of Co-60 gamma radiation. Acta Endocrinol (Copenh) 1978;88:7–17.

10 Norén G, Arndt J, Hindmarsch T: Stereotactic radiosurgery in acoustic neurinoma: Further experiences. Neurosurgery 1983;13:12–22.

11 Leksell L: A note on the treatment of acoustic tumors. Acta Chir Scand 1971;137:763–765.

12 Leksell L: Stereotaxic radiosurgery in trigeminal neuralgia. Acta Chir Scand 1971;137:311–314.

13 Steiner L, Leksell L, Greitz T, Backlund EO: Stereotaxic radiosurgery for cerebral arteriovenous malformations. Report of a case. Acta Chir Scand 1972;138:459–464.

14 Backlund EO, Rähn T, Sarby B, de Schryver A, Wennerstrand J: Closed stereotaxic hypophysectomy by means of Co-60 gamma radiation. Acta Radiol (Ther Phys Biol) 1974;11:545–555.

15 Backlund EO, Rähn T, Sarby B: Treatment of pinealomas by stereotaxic radiation surgery. Acta Radiol (Ther Phys Biol) 1974;13:368–376.

16 Leksell L, Backlund EO: Stereotaxic gammacapsulotomy; in Hitchcock ER, Ballantine HT, Meyerson BA (eds): Modern Concepts in Psychiatric Surgery. Elsevier/North-Holland Biomedical Press, 1979, pp 213–216.

17 Backlund EO: The history and development of radiosurgery; in Lunsford LD (ed): Stereotactic Radiosurgery Update. Amsterdam, Elsevier Science, 1992, pp 3–9.

Erik-Olof Backlund, MD, PhD
Department of Neurosurgery, exp. US plan 17, University Hospital
SE–581 85 Linköping (Sweden)
Tel. +46 13 143386, E-Mail eo.backlund@swipnet.se

Szeifert GT, Kondziolka D, Levivier M, Lunsford LD (eds): Radiosurgery and Pathological Fundamentals. Prog Neurol Surg. Basel, Karger, 2007, vol 20, pp 1–15

1. Introduction: The Contribution of Pathology to Radiosurgery

György T. Szeifert[a], Douglas Kondziolka[b], L. Dade Lunsford[b], István Nyáry[a], Zoltán Hanzély[a], Isabelle Salmon[c], Marc Levivier[c]

[a]National Institute of Neurosurgery and Department of Neurological Surgery, Semmelweis University, Budapest, Hungary; [b]Center for Image-Guided Neurosurgery, Presbyterian University Hospital, Pittsburgh, Pa., USA; [c]Centre Gamma Knife, Hôpital Académique Erasme, Université Libre de Bruxelles, Brussels, Belgium

Abstract

The term radiosurgery signifies any kind of application of ionizing radiation energy, in experimental biology or clinical medicine, aiming at the precise and complete destruction of chosen target structures containing healthy and/or pathological cells, without significant concomitant or late radiation damage to adjacent tissues. The goal of this study is to explore the short- and long-term pathophysiological effects of high-dose focused irradiation on neural tissue and its pathologies with histological, electron-microscopical tissue culture and biological-biochemical methods. Radiosurgical pathology focuses its scope and microscope on tissue, cellular, genetic and molecular changes in the human organism and experimental animals, or in cell lines and other in vitro experiments, generated by the ionizing radiation delivered from radiosurgical devices.

'Fons floiritionis medicinae modernae in anatomia pathologica quaerendus est'

Ignatius Philippus Semmelweis, 1844 [1]

Radiosurgery, invented by Prof. Lars Leksell [2, 3], has become a successful treatment modality in the neurosurgical realm during the past 4 decades. Since December, 1967, when the first patient suffering from a craniopharyngioma was treated at the Sophiahemmet Hospital in Stockholm, Sweden, with the prototype Gamma Knife, more than 400,000 cases have already been operated on worldwide with the Gamma Knife. In addition to this, many patients were treated with other radiosurgical methods like linear accelerators or charged particle devices. Although the treatment indications and the number of treated patients has been increasing continuously, we know relatively little about the pathological background of radiosurgery explaining radiobiology and pathophysiological mechanisms leading to therapeutic or undesired side effects. The future of radiosurgery beyond technical advancements will be built on better understanding of the biological basis of radiation, which will enable treatment of new disorders [4]. Considering, that huge clinical experience has already been accumulated in radiosurgery during the past 4 decades, it would be timely to process out systematically pathological fundamentals of the effect of single high-dose irradiation, to understand better radiobiology for radiosurgically treatable diseases. Medicine has been built from experience. As it had happened in the ancient times, clinical studies progressed much more ahead than the exploration of pathological radiobiological mechanisms of radiosurgical disorders. The father of pathological anatomy, Giovanni Battista Morgagni (1682–1771), had started his regular autopsy studies because he was not happy with the unexplainable physical signs and symptoms, and wanted to reveal the overlying pathophysiological process leading to disturbance of the human organism. Although anatomical lessons had been performed before Morgagni as well, the systematic comparison of clinical symptoms and signs with anatomic findings and logical correlation between the two graduated him as a dedicated master of clinical pathology [5].

The term radiosurgery signifies any kind of application of ionizing radiation energy, in experimental biology or clinical medicine, aiming at the precise and complete destruction of chosen target structures containing healthy and/or pathological cells, without significant concomitant or late radiation damage to adjacent tissues [6]. Therefore, the goal of radiosurgical pathology should be to study the short- and long-term effects of high-dose focused radiation on neural tissue and its pathologies with histological, electron-microscopical tissue culture and biological-biochemical methods. Radiosurgical pathology focuses its scope and microscope on tissue, cellular, genetic and molecular changes in the human body and experimental animals, or in cell lines and other in vitro experiments, generated by the ionizing radiation delivered from radiosurgical devices.

Historical Antecedents

The genesis, structure and function of the human organism and the central nervous system has attracted the fantasy and interest of many artists or scientists since centuries, especially during the Renaissance (fig. 1), including even the most unsurpassable individual masters with the highest intellectual talent

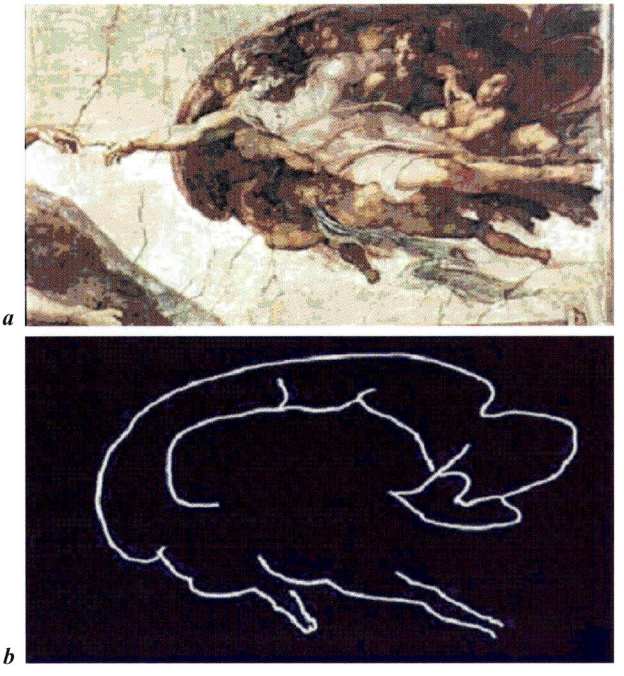

Fig. 1. ***a*** One of Michelangelo's most fascinating gigantic frescos, 'Creation of Adam' (painted between 1508–1512), on the ceiling of the Sistine Chapel in the Vatican (courtesy of Prof. Roberto Toni and Editrice Kurtis). ***b*** The background and contour of the image is reminiscent of a midline sagittal section of the brain for some scientists [50, 51].

like Michelangelo Buonarroti (1475–1564). The first remarkable human anatomical image collection was created by the prominent humanist, artist and scholar Leonardo da Vinci (1452–1519) as early as the 15th century (fig. 2a–c). However, from the medical point of view systematic anatomical lessons were performed by Andreas Vesalius (1514–1564) one century later. His experience was based totally on human autopsy studies and collected it in the book *De humani corporis fabrica libri septem* published in 1543 (fig. 3). In this way the anatomical teachings of Galenos, which came mainly from animal investigations, were developed. Another century ahead, and Giovanni Battista Morgagni (1682–1771), professor of medicine in Padova, Italy, started to collate on a regular basis clinical symptoms and signs with anatomical alterations in the human body. He explained different disorders as consequences of morphological disturbances in the structure of organs therefore we can regard him as the founder of clinical pathology (fig. 4). His fundamental work *De sedibus et*

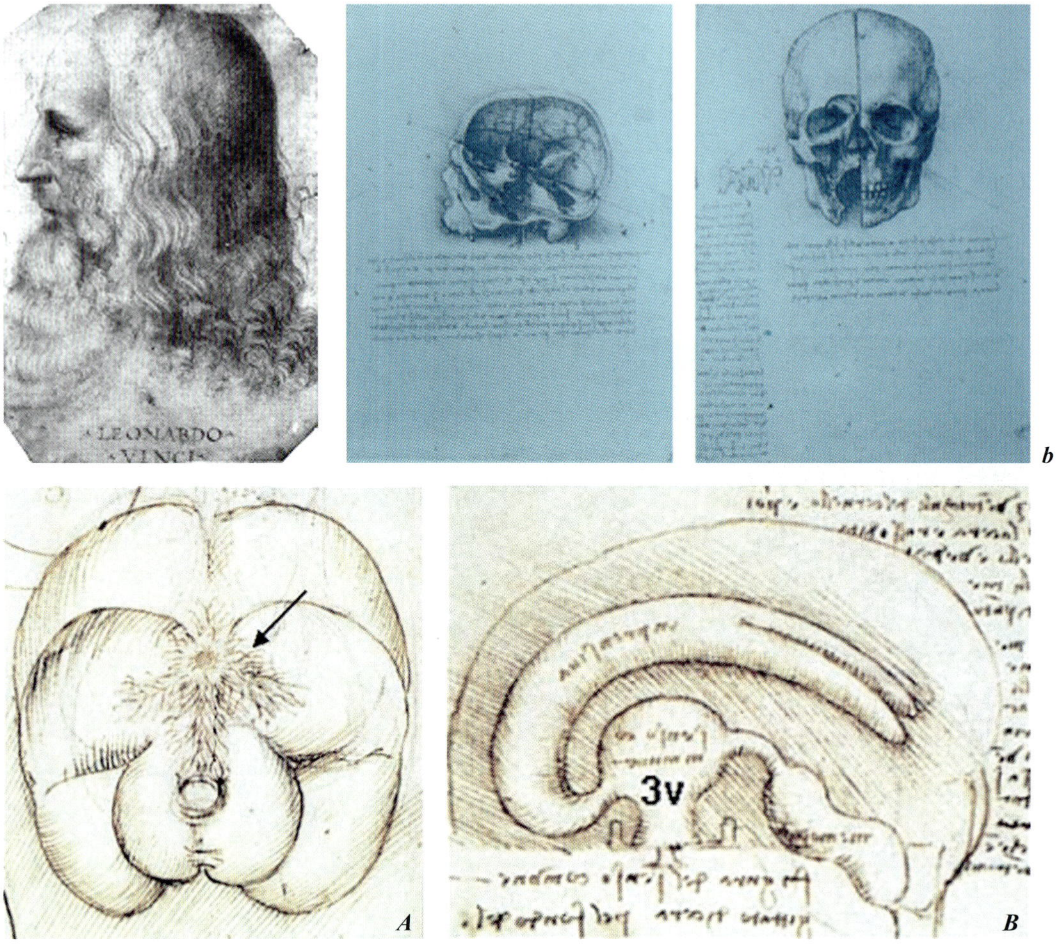

Fig. 2. ***a*** A portrait of Leonardo da Vinci (1452–1519). ***b*** Skull delineation. ***c*** The basal surface of the brain (**A**) with the rete mirabilis around the pituitary stalk (arrow), and a 3D reconstruction of cerebral ventricles (**B**) from da Vinci's anatomical image collection (1508–1509; 'Codici di Anatomia').

causis morborum per anatomen indagatis libri quinque was published in 1761. Antonie van Leeuwenhoek (1632–1723) did a meaningful contribution by the use of microscope for scientific investigations. The pioneer of microscopic anatomy was Marcello Malpighi (1628–1694) with regular microscopical examinations of various organs. Different tissue elements of the organism were discovered by Marie Françoise Xavier Bichat (1771–1802). He suggested that

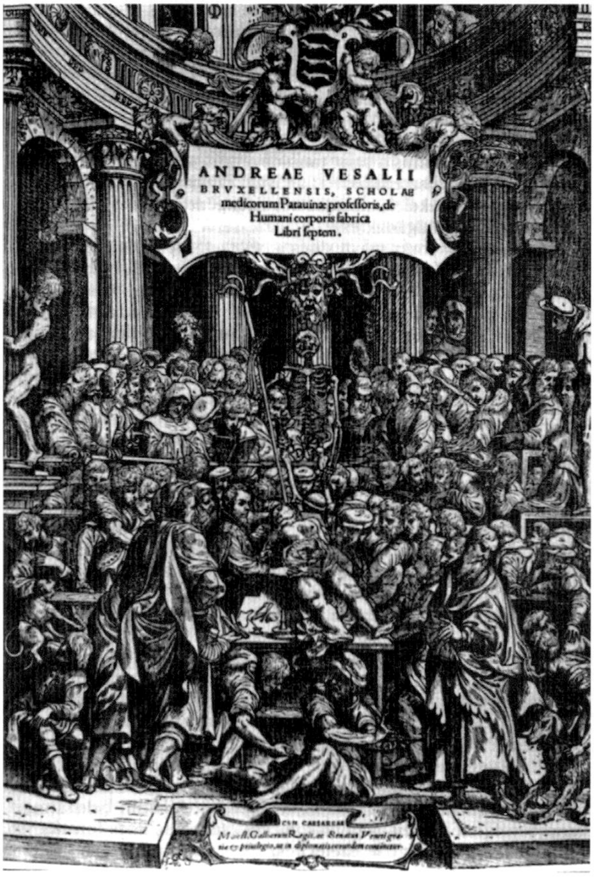

Fig. 3. The front page of Vesalius' anatomical book (1543).

diseases propagate along tissues and established modern histology. An outstanding observation in morphological research came from Mathias Jakob Schleiden (1804–1881) and Theodor Schwann (1810–1882). They realized that the cell is the basic unit of every living organism in 1838. Since then, the humoral pathophysiological theory was changed for the cellular approach. Earliest Japanese anatomical studies were found in the books of Zoshi (1754) and Kaitai Shinsho (1774). Two centuries later, in 1958, the basic histopathological lesion in radiosurgery was published by Larsson et al. in *Nature* [7]. In that landmark paper, they stated that in animal experiments 'with high-energy protons a sharply delimited lesion can be made at any desired site in the central nervous system'.

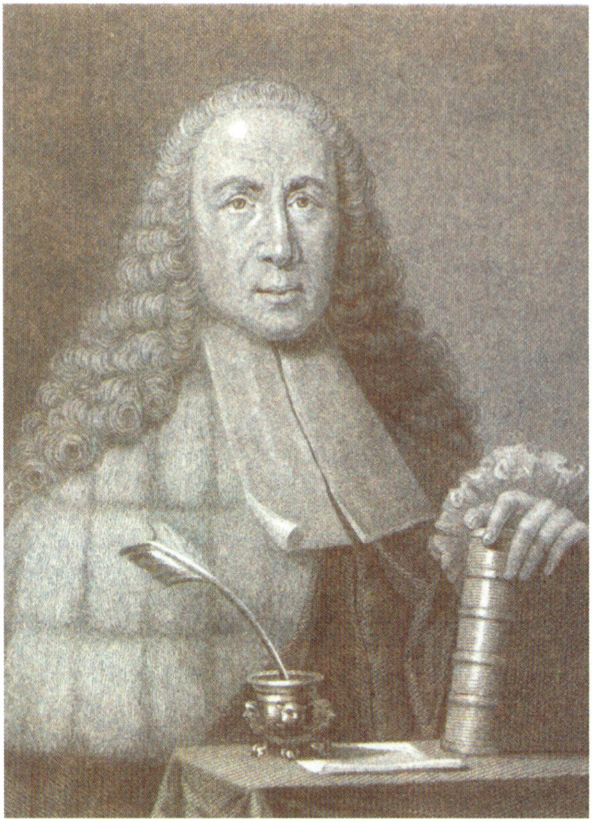

Fig. 4. Giovanni Battista Morgagni, the father of pathology (1682–1771).

Pathological Fundamentals

The basic histopathological radiolesion produced by high-energy ionizing radiation in neural tissue is a coagulation necrosis (fig. 5). This can be found within the target volume, its size does not change in time, and the boundary between the necrosis and the surrounding structures is distinct, according to the sharp radiation fall-off [7–11]. Lesions appeared in the spinal cord following irradiation with doses of 400 and 200 Gy on the 3rd and 9th day, respectively. They were sharply defined and had about the same width as the beam. In the cerebral hemispheres, the earliest lesions were observed 14 days after irradiation with 200 Gy, and the changes between 2 and 8 weeks were similar. Macroscopically, corresponding to the path of the beam, a groove appeared on the upper surface, and a sharply defined narrow band of discoloration was seen

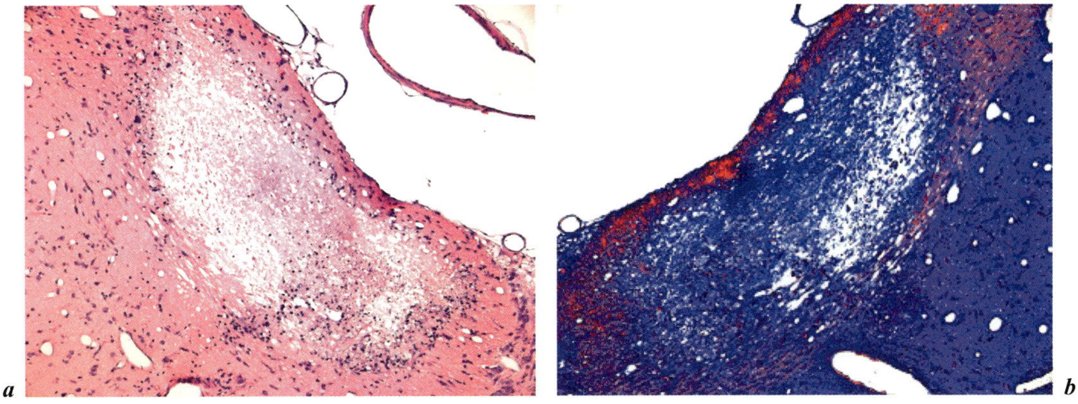

Fig. 5. Sharply demarcated gamma-radiolesion (i.e. coagulation necrosis) towards surrounding brain tissue in rat brain 6 months after 160-Gy irradiation. ***a*** HE. ×100. ***b*** Masson's trichrom for fibrin stain, ×100.

beneath the hemispheres. Histologically, within the lesions necrosis of nerve cells, myelin sheaths and axons occurred. Small perivenous hemorrhages were present at the margin of the lesions, and occasionally in the center of the damaged tissue, particularly in the gray matter. Collections of leukocytes were seen in the necrotic zone and around it proliferation of astrocytes. These were the early experimental pathological changes following high-dose irradiation. This phase of postirradiation changes was also mentioned as the necrotic stage in the literature [11].

The next period of postradiosurgery changes is the stage of resorbtion. This stage is characterized by resorbtion of cellular debris and beginning glial scar formation. Here, phagocytic cells are actively eliminating necrotic debris from the central part of the lesion, being maximal at the end of the necrotic stage this activity gradually decreases. It is generally presented by astrocyte proliferation around the necrotic area and occasional giant cells which sometimes have large lobed nuclei. This marginal zone also discloses a chronic inflammatory reaction with congested vessels and formation of new capillaries, often with endothelial thickening, and round cell proliferation. These changes were observed in goat experiments between 18 and 28 months following high-dose irradiation.

The late stage was characterized histologically by prominent glial scar formation surrounding a cavity. Around this scar, there were myelinated fibers and nerve cells with an astrocytic reaction sometimes containing calcium concrements. There was no inflammatory reaction, no giant cells, no proliferation of vessels, teleangiectasis or hemorrhage. These observations were made 39–48 months after experimental radiosurgery.

In summary, experimental histopathological investigations had given a qualitative picture on morphological changes of radiolesions in the brain after single high-dose irradiation which expressed time and dose dependence. After a standard 200-Gy irradiation, the period which followed the acute degenerative phase was divided into three stages:

1 *Necrotic stage*: acute degenerative changes, necrosis and inflammatory reaction occur approximately after the 2nd week following irradiation.
2 *Stage of resorption*: elimination of necrotic debris several months following irradiation.
3 *Late stage*: replacement of necrotic debris by scar tissue years after focused irradiation.

In human brain, the morphology of radiolesions is quite similar. The temporal development of radiation-induced changes is divided into three phases in the human oncology practice [12]. The immediate response occurs milliseconds to hours after initiation of exposure, usually less than 24 h. Pathologically and clinically, the lesions are acute. The early reaction develops days to weeks after initial exposure. Often 24 h to 2 months. Morphologically and clinically, the lesions may be acute or subacute. The delayed response evolves months to years after exposure. Often 2 months to many years. Morphologically and clinically, the lesions may be acute, subacute, or chronic.

Pathologically, the acute type lesions are characterized mainly by necrotic changes and polymorphonuclear leukocyte infiltration (fig. 6a). The subacute type tissue reaction consists of mostly macrophages with phagocytotic activity removing necrotic debris accompanied by small vessel proliferation (fig. 6b). In chronic type tissue responses, the most prominent cellular elements are lymphocytes (fig. 6c), later replaced by hypocellular scar tissue undergoing hyaline degeneration or even calcification in end-stage lesions (fig. 6d).

The first available pathological report about the morphology of a human radiolesion observed in a patient operated on with 200-Gy proton beam radiosurgery for intractable pain because of metastasizing carcinoma was published by Larsson et al. [9] in 1963. At autopsy, the radiolesion macroscopically demonstrated a well-demarcated necrotic area surrounded by a zone of slight cellular reaction 2 months after radiosurgery. The necrosis measured about 2–4 mm along the three major axes. Microscopically, there was a complete destruction of axons, myelin and glial cells. In the marginal zone of the lesion, nuclear debris and macrophages had collected. The latter were filled with particles of broken down myelin. Small hemorrhages were seen near vessels with necrotic walls in the central part of the lesion. Such hemorrhages were also observed at the periphery, associated with vessels of small caliber and collageneous walls, containing red

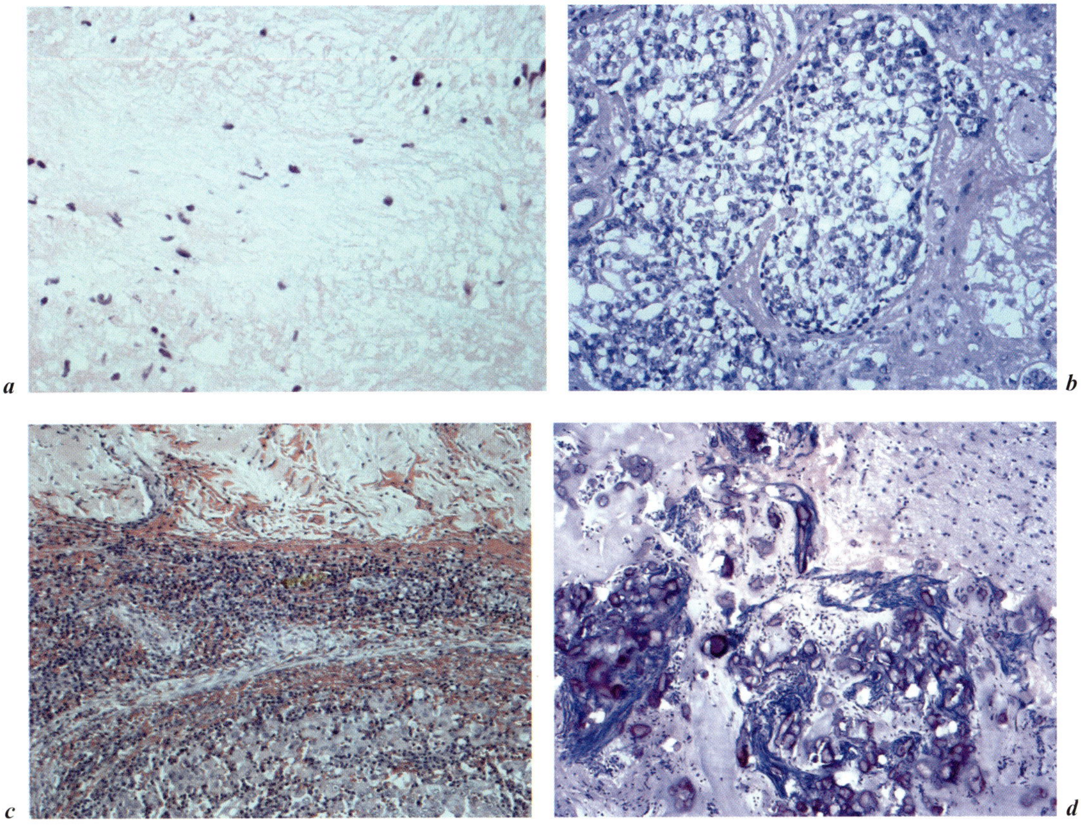

Fig. 6. Tissue responses following radiosurgery. ***a*** Acute type tissue response with necrotic changes and scattered pycnotic, apoptotic cells from a vestibular schwannoma 2.5 months following radiosurgery. HE. ×300. ***b*** Subacute type tissue reaction consisting of mostly macrophages in a GBM 3.5 months after radiosurgery. HE. ×200. ***c*** Chronic type infiltration with prominent lymphocytic component in a metastatic melanoma 12 months following radiosurgery. HE. ×100. ***d*** End-stage lesion consisting of hypocellular scar tissue with hyaline degeneration and dystrophic calcification, sharply demarcated towards brain tissue in a breast CC metastasis 15 months after radiosurgery. HE. ×200.

blood corpuscles. Congestion of vessels occurred in a zone adjacent to the necrotic region. There was no widespread macrophage infiltration of the tissue surrounding the necrotic zone, and no marked proliferation of astrocytes. The axons appeared normal in juxtaposition to the zone of the cellular reaction.

Considering that the synchrocyclotron producing high-energy proton beams had been too complicated for general neurosurgical application, the Gamma Knife was designed specifically for brain radiosurgical purposes and incorporated in the stereotactic system by Leksell in 1967 [2]. The gamma radiolesions investigated in two autopsy cases (with 3 lesions) treated with 20- and 25-Gy gamma thalamotomy for intractable cancer pain expressed similar morphological characteristics like the proton radiolesion. Macroscopically, there were well-defined lesions in the targeted areas. Histological examinations revealed sharply demarcated areas from the surrounding brain tissue 10, 14 and 20 weeks after the operation. The lesions consisted mainly of dense necrosis with few distinguishable cellular components. The necrosis was more dense in a narrow zone at the periphery of the lesion. There was a narrow region of astrocytic gliosis, about 0.3 mm thick, surrounding the lesion. Outside this gliosis, the brain parenchyma had a normal appearance. The blood vessels in the center of the lesions were thrombotic and had necrotic walls, while at the periphery of the lesions the vessel walls were somewhat fibrotic but their lumen remained patent. There was virtually no histological difference among the three gamma lesions. In 1970, a histopathological review was given on 9 patients treated with a dose of 180–250 Gy for intractable pain and in whom autopsy was performed 3 weeks to 7.5 months after irradiation [10]. The histopathological changes were fairly uniform in all cases in spite of the difference in the age of the lesions. They were well demarcated from the undamaged surrounding tissues. The lesions were necrotic and in them thrombosed vessels with necrotic walls could be identified, sometimes surrounded by small hemorrhages. In lesions older than 3 weeks, the necrosis was also infiltrated by macrophages and some round cells. Immediately around the necrotic tissue was a spongy zone, 0.3–0.5 mm wide, which presented a moderate increase in the number of vessels, which were often congested and had a thickened intima. Sometimes the vessels were also thrombosed. In this zone, there was also a slight astrocytic proliferation and a moderate infiltration of round cells and macrophages. Perivascular cuffing with round cells or macrophages was also seen. Some of the nerve cells in this perinecrotic zone were shrunken and hyperchromatic. The myelin sheaths and axons were swollen. The tissue around this zone appeared normal. These histological observations were very similar to those produced by single-proton high-dose irradiation; however, the gamma radiolesions were more sharply demarcated and the histological picture was highly uniform. These morphological findings might supply pathological background to the high precision of Gamma Knife radiosurgery.

Steiner et al. [13] have demonstrated that at least 140 Gy was necessary to produce a lesion in the human brain after radiosurgery. With more than 160 Gy the lesions were consistently observed, and the optimal dose appeared to be around 170–180 Gy. Higher doses, up to 250 Gy, did not change the physical characteristics of the lesion, which was due to the sharp dose gradient.

The pathological effect of radiosurgical interventions on the central nervous system tissue can be reflected in degenerative and proliferative changes as well. Endothelial cell injury, apoptosis, coagulation necrosis, fibrinoid and hyaline degeneration are the most frequent degenerative processes. These might be the result of the cytotoxic effect of radiosurgery. They play important role in the destruction of malignant tumors, or normal tissue structures in functional neurosurgery [14–18]. On the other hand, granulation tissue formation, proliferation of fibrocytes, fibroblasts, myofibroblasts, astrocytic elements, capillaries or other vessels, inflammatory cells and production of collagen or glial fibers appear as commonest proliferative responses after radiosurgery. This is the pathological situation mostly in the obliteration process of vascular malformations [19–27]. Radiosurgery seems to cause a proliferative vasculopathy within the blood vessels of AVMs that begins with endothelial cell injury [28, 29]. It appears that the abnormal vessels of neoplasms or vascular malformations have a relative sensitivity to radiosurgery in comparison with normal surrounding or feeding arteries [30]. Kondziolka et al. [31] believe that the radiobiological effect on meningiomas, schwannomas, pituitary tumors, and other benign neoplasms is a combination of both cytotoxic and delayed vascular effects. This theory was supported by further investigations [32].

Quo Vadis?

Is radiosurgical pathology a new subspeciality? Do we need it? We think that we are at the beginning of a long and interesting road. Our purpose is to collect and process systematically potential radiosurgical pathology cases. That is, to follow all those cases where a radiosurgical intervention had been performed as a first step, then the patient underwent open conventional craniotomy-related operation or autopsy for some reason. We have to compare imaging data, treatment parameters, modern functional methods [33–36], follow-up material with surgical pathology or autopsy macroscopical and histological findings (fig. 7). Results of experimental pathology should be included and considered as well [37–48]. In this way, systematic comprehensive comparative investigations could become part of the broader radiobiology concept that would draw our attention and direct our activity towards radiosurgical pathology [49].

Conclusions

'Mortui vivos docent' was the original intention of pathology. Our hope is that radiosurgical pathology will promote better understanding of morphological changes, biological and pathophysiological mechanisms behind therapeutic

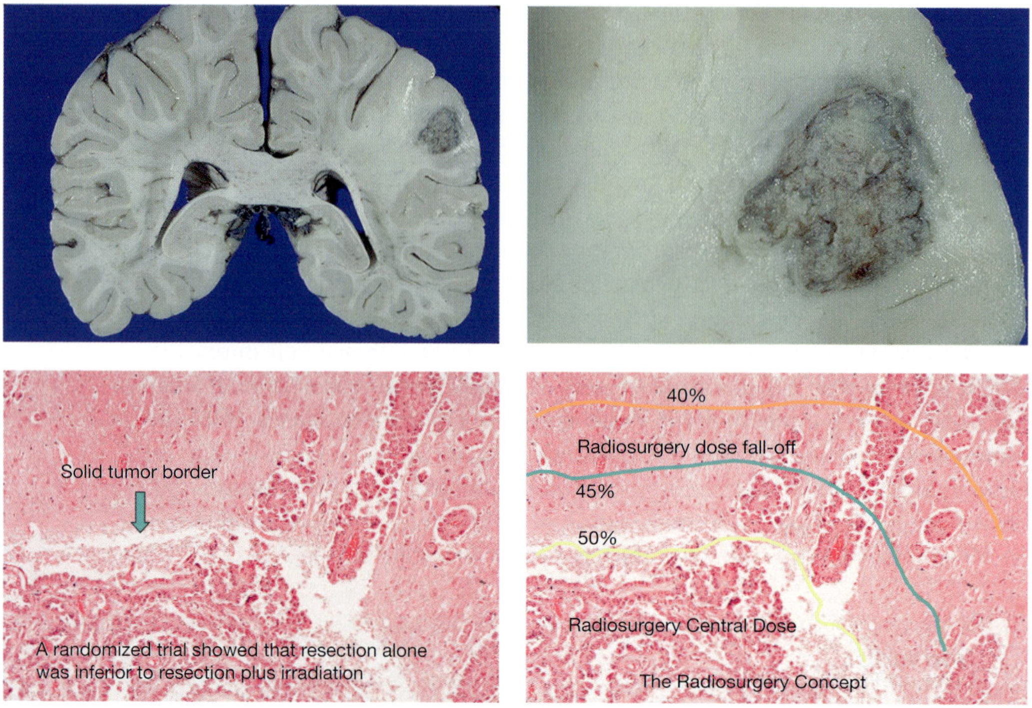

Fig. 7. Comparison of radiosurgical dosimetry parameters with autopsy findings. Histopathological investigation revealed microscopic cancer nests infiltrating brain tissue outside of the 50% treatment isodose line, imperceptible with routine imaging techniques. ***a*** A metastatic lung adenocarcinoma in the left parietal region. ***b*** Higher magnification: macroscopically the lesion seems to be 'soliter' with sharp demarcation. ***c*** Histopathology demonstrates infiltrating microscopic tumor extensions spreading from the main bulk of the neoplasm. HE. ×200. ***d*** Correlation with delivered isodose profile discloses carcinoma cell nests beyond the effective therapeutic dose line. HE. ×200.

radiosurgical interventions. In this way it would serve more sophisticated treatment planning of current and future potential radiosurgical disorders for the benefit of our patients in need.

Acknowledgement

This paper was dedicated in honor of Professor Emeritus *Szabolcs Gomba,* Department of Pathology, University Medical School of Debrecen, Hungary, for his 70th birthday, recognizing his commitment to education and pathology.

References

1 Semmelweis IP: Dissertatio inauguralis sistens tractatum de vita plantarum. Vindobonae, Ueberreuter, 1844, p 31.

2 Leksell L: The stereotaxic method and radiosurgery of the brain. Acta Chir Scand 1951;102: 316–319.

3 Leksell L: Cerebral radiosurgery. I. Gammathalamotomy in two cases of intractable pain. Acta Chir Scand 1968;134:585–595.

4 Kondziolka D, Lunsford LD, Witt TC, Flickinger JC: The future of radiosurgery: radiobiology, technology, and applications. Surg Neurol 2000;54:406–414.

5 Andrioli G, Trincia G: Padua: the Renaissance of Human anatomy and medicine. Neurosurgery 2004;55:746–755.

6 Larsson B: Radiobiological fundamentals in radiosurgery; in Steiner L, Lindquist C, Forster D, Backlund EO (eds): Radiosurgery: Baseline and Trends. New York, Raven Press, 1992.

7 Larsson B, Leksell L, Rexed B, Sourander P, Mair W, Andersson B: The high-energy proton beam as a neurosurgical tool. Nature 1958;182:1222–1223.

8 Leksell L, Larsson B, Andersson B, Rexed B, Sourander P, Mair W: Lesions in the depth of the brain produced by a beam of high energy protons. Acta Radiologica 1960;54:251–264.

9 Larsson B, Leksell L, Rexed B: The use of high energy protons for cerebral surgery in man. Acta Chir Scand 1963;125:1–7.

10 Wennerstrand J, Ungerstedt U: Cerebral radiosurgery. II. An anatomical study of gamma radiolesions. Acta Chir Scand 1970;136:133–137.

11 Andersson B, Larsson B, Leksell L, Mair W, Rexed B, Sourander P, Wennerstrand J: Histopathology of late local radiolesions in the goat brain. Acta Radiologica Therapy Physics Biology 1970;9:385–394.

12 Fajardo L-GLF, Berthrong M, Anderson RE (eds): Radiation Pathology. New York, Oxford University Press, Inc., 2001.

13 Steiner L, Forster D, Leksell L, Meyerson BA, Boëthius J: Gammathalamotomy in intractable pain. Acta Neurochir 1980;52:173–184.

14 Szeifert GT, Salmon I, David P, Devriendt D, De Smedt F, Rorive S, Brotchi J, Levivier M: Tumor control and growth in a patient with two cerebral metastases treated with the Leksell Gamma Knife; in Kondziolka D (ed): Radiosurgery. Basel, Karger, 2002, vol 4, pp 152–161.

15 Szeifert GT, Massager N, Brotchi J, Levivier M: Morphological redifferentiation in a malignant astrocytic tumor after gamma knife radiosurgery. J Neurosurg 2002;97(suppl 5):627–630.

16 Thompson BG, Coffey RJ, Flickinger JC, Lunsford LD: Stereotactic radiosurgery of small intracranial tumors: neuropathological correlation in three patients. Surg Neurol 1990;33:96–104.

17 Hirato M, Hirato J, Zama A, Inoue H, Ohye C, Shibazaki T, Andou Y: Radiobiological effects of Gamma Knife radiosurgery on brain tumors studied in autopsy and surgical specimens. Stereotact Funct Neurosurg 1996;66(suppl 1):4–16.

18 Szeifert GT, Salmon I, Rorive S, Massager N, Devriendt D, Simon S, Brotchi J, Levivier M: Does gamma knife radiosurgery stimulate cellular immune response to metastatic brain tumors? A histopathological and immunohistochemical study. J Neurosurg 2005;102(suppl):180–184.

19 Yamamoto M, Jimbo M, Kobayashi M, Toyoda C, Ide M, Tanaka N, Lindquist C, Steiner L: Long-term results of radiosurgery for arteriovenous malformation: neurodiagnostic imaging and histological studies of angiographically confirmed nidus obliteration. Surg Neurol 1992;37:219–230.

20 Yamamoto M, Jimbo M, Ide M, Kobayashi M, Toyoda C, Lindquist C, Karlson B: Gamma Knife radiosurgery for cerebral arteriovenous malformations: an autopsy report focusing on irradiation-induced changes observed in nidus-unrelated arteries. Surg Neurol 1995;44:421–427.

21 Szeifert GT, Kemeny AA, Major O, Timperley WR, Forster DMC: Histopathological changes in cerebral arteriovenous malformations following stereotactic irradiation with the Gamma Knife; in Kondziolka D (ed): Radiosurgery 1997. Basel, Karger, 1998, vol 2, pp 129–136.

22 Szeifert GT, Kemeny AA, Timperley WR, Forster DMC: The potential role of myofibroblasts in the obliteration of arteriovenous malformations after radiosurgery. Neurosurgery 1997;40: 61–66.

23 Szeifert GT, Vandersmissen B, Taib NOB, Balériaux D, Rodesch G, Salmon I, Brotchi J, Levivier M: Recurrent hemorrhage in a radiosurgically obliterated cerebral arteriovenous malformation; in Kondziolka D (ed): Radiosurgery. Basel, Karger, 2002, vol 4, pp 34–41.
24 Szeifert GT, Salmon I, Balériaux D, Brotchi J, Levivier M: Immunohistochemical analysis of a cerebral arteriovenous malformation obliterated by radiosurgery and presenting with re-bleeding. Case report. Neurol Res 2003;25:718–721.
25 Szeifert GT, Major O, Nyáry I: Pathobiology of human cerebrovascular malformations: basic mechanisms and clinical relevance. Neurosurgery 2005;56:1166.
26 Szeifert GT, Major O, Kemeny AA: Ultrastructural changes in arteriovenous malformations after gamma knife surgery: an electron microscopic study. J Neurosurg 2005;102(suppl):289–292.
27 Nyáry I, Major O, Hanzély Z, Szeifert GT: Histopathological findings in a surgically resected thalamic cavernous hemangioma 1 year after 40-Gy irradiation. J Neurosurg 2005;102 (suppl):56–58.
28 Schneider BF, Eberhard DA, Steiner LE: Histopathology of arteriovenous malformations after Gamma Knife radiosurgery. J Neurosurg 1997;87:352–357.
29 Szeifert GT: Radiosurgery and AVM histopathology. J Neurosurg 1998;88:356–357.
30 Szeifert GT, Major O, Fazekas I, Nagy Z: Effects of radiation on Cerebral vasculature: a review. Neurosurgery 2001;48:452–453.
31 Kondziolka D, Lunsford LD, Flickinger JC: The radiobiology of radiosurgery. Neurosurg Clin N Am 1999;10:157–166.
32 Szeifert GT, Massager N, Devriendt D, David P, De Smedt F, Rorive S, Salmon I, Brotchi J, Levivier M: Observation of intracranial neoplasms treated with gamma knife radiosurgery. J Neurosurg 2002;97(suppl 5):623–626.
33 Levivier M, Wikler D, Goldman S, David P, Metens T, Massager N, Gerosa M, Devriendt D, Desmedt F, Simon S, Van Houtte P, Brotchi J: Integration of the metabolic data of positron emission tomography in the dosimetry planning of radiosurgery with the gamma knife: early experience with brain tumors. J Neurosurg 2000;93(suppl 3):233–238.
34 Levivier M, Wikler D, Goldman S, Massager N, Szeifert GT, David P, Devriendt D, Desmedt F, Simon S, Van Houtte P, Brotchi J: Positron emission tomography-guided radiosurgery: early experience with the integration of metabolic data in the dosimetry planning with the Leksell Gamma Knife; in Kondziolka D (ed): Radiosurgery. Basel, Karger, 2002, vol 4, pp 123–133.
35 Levivier M, Massager N, Wikler D, Lorenzoni J, Ruiz S, Devriendt D, David P, Desmedt F, Simon S, Van Houtte P, Brotchi J, Goldman S: Use of stereotactic PET images in dosimetry planning of radiosurgery for brain tumors: clinical experience and proposed classification. J Nucl Med 2004;45:1146–1154.
36 Pirotte B, Goldman S, Massager N, David P, Wikler D, Lipszyc M, Salmon I, Brotchi J, Levivier M: Combined use of ^{18}F-fluorodeoxyglucose and ^{11}C-methionine in 45 positron emission tomography-guided stereotactic brain biopsies. J Neurosurg 2004;101:476–483.
37 Lunsford LD, Altschuler EM, Flickinger JC, Wu A, Martinez AJ: In vivo biological effects of stereotactic radiosurgery: a primate model. Neurosurgery 1990;27:373–382.
38 Kondziolka D, Lunsford LD, Claassen D, Maitz AH, Flickinger JC: Radiobiology of radiosurgery: Part I – the normal rat brain model. Neurosurgery 1992;31:271–279.
39 Kondziolka D, Lunsford LD, Claassen D, Pandalai S, Maitz AH, Flickinger JC: Radiobiology of radiosurgery: Part II – the rat C6 glioma model. Neurosurgery 1992;31:280–288.
40 Kamiryo T, Kassel NF, Thai QA, Lopes MB, Lee KS, Steiner L: Histological changes in the normal rat brain after gamma irradiation. Acta Neurochir (Wien) 1996;138:451–459.
41 Kamyrio T, Lopes MB, Kassel NF, Steiner L, Lee KS: Radiosurgery-induced microvascular alterations precede necrosis of the brain neuropil. Neurosurgery 2001;49:409–415.
42 Major O, Kemeny AA, Forster DMC, Walton L, Szeifert GT: Time modulation effect of taxol on vasoreactivity of rat middle cerebral artery after single dose gamma irradiation; in Kondziolka D (ed): Radiosurgery 1997. Basel, Karger, 1998, vol 2, pp 183–196.
43 Kondziolka D, Couce M, Niranjan A, Maesawa S, Fellows W: Histology of the 100-Gy thalamotomy in the baboon; in Kondziolka D (ed): Radiosurgery. Basel, Karger, 2002, vol 4, pp 279–284.
44 Liscak R, Vladyka V, Novotny J Jr, Brozek G, Namestkova K, Mares V, Herynek V, Jirak D, Hayek M, Sykova E: Leksell gamma knife lesioning of the rat hippocampus: the relationship between radiation dose and functional and structural damage. J Neurosurg 2002;97(suppl 5):666–673.

45 Major O, Szeifert GT, Radatz MWR, Walton L, Kemeny AA: Experimental stereotactic gamma knife radiosurgery. Vascular contractility studies of the rat middle cerebral artery after chronic survival. Neurol Res 2002;24:191–198.
46 Major O, Szeifert GT, Fazekas I, Vitanovics D, Csonka É, Kocsis B, Bori Z, Kemeny AA, Nagy Z: Effect of a single high-dose gamma irradiation on cultured cells in human cerebral arteriovenous malformation. J Neurosurg 2002;97(suppl 5):459–463.
47 Niranjan A, Gobbel GT, Kondziolka D, Flickinger JC, Lunsford LD: Experimental radiobiological investigations into radiosurgery: present understanding and future directions. Neurosurgery 2004;55:495–505.
48 Szeifert GT, Major O, Nyáry I: Pathobiology of human cerebrovascular malformations: basic mechanisms and clinical relevance. Neurosurgery 2005;56:1166.
49 Szeifert GT, Kondziolka D, Lunsford LD, Hanzély Z, Nyáry I, Salmon I, Levivier M: What can we learn from pathology? From the beginnings towards radiosurgical pathology; in Kondziolka D (ed): Radiosurgery. Basel, Karger, 2004, vol 5, pp 13–21.
50 Meshberger FL: An interpretation of Michelangelo's 'Creation of Adam' based on neuroanatomy. JAMA 1990;10:1837–1841.
51 Toni R, Malaguti A, Benfenati F, Martini L: The human hypothalamus: a morpho-functional perspective. J Endocrinol Invest 2004;27(suppl 6):73–94.

György T. Szeifert, MD, PhD
National Institute of Neurosurgery and Department of Neurological Surgery
Semmelweis University
Amerikai út 57
HU–1145 Budapest (Hungary)
Tel. + 36 1 2512 999, Fax +36 1 2515 678, E-Mail gyorgyszeifert@yahoo.com

Szeifert GT, Kondziolka D, Levivier M, Lunsford LD (eds): Radiosurgery and Pathological Fundamentals. Prog Neurol Surg. Basel, Karger, 2007, vol 20, pp 16–27

2. Radiobiology of Radiosurgery

Douglas Kondziolka[a,b], *Ajay Niranjan*[a], *L. Dade Lunsford*[a,b], *John C. Flickinger*[a,b]

Departments of [a]Neurological Surgery and [b]Radiation Oncology, University of Pittsburgh, and the Center for Image-Guided Neurosurgery, UPMC Presbyterian Pittsburgh, Pennsylvania, Pa., USA

Abstract

The effects of radiosurgery on brain tumor tissue remain to be defined. Effects are dose, volume, time, and tumor histology dependent. In this report, we discuss data from resected specimens after radiosurgery, and work to develop a classification method for radiosurgery effects.

Radiosurgery is the precise destruction of a chosen target containing healthy and/or pathological cells, without significant concomitant or late radiation damage to adjacent tissues [28]. Leksell's initial radiosurgery concept was for the management of functional neurologic disorders but the number of clinical indications has increased greatly. The current radiosurgery concept is that damage to tissue within the target volume (either normal or lesional) is the desired effect. In radiosurgery, the physician does not attempt to spare some tissues and treat others, but to achieve a total destructive effect within the targeted volume. Conformal irradiation using image guidance serves to spare regional structures.

van der Kogel [45] wrote that effects of radiosurgery, in radiobiological concepts, were no different from the effects of fractionated irradiations. The difference between radiosurgery and radiotherapy generally is the size of the treatment volume, and the dose delivered during that single session. While volume is important, it is the surgeons ability to deliver precise and accurate radiation to a defined target during one procedure that provides the powerful radiobiologic effect. This effect often is not identified after standard dose fractionated radiotherapy either to target or to surrounding brain. Accurate targeting opens the door for the powerful radiobiologic effect of radiosurgery.

Since fractionated radiation therapy treats a relatively large tissue volume that incorporates both lesion and normal parenchyma, the physician must exploit some therapeutic ratio that injures tumor cells but maintains normal brain integrity. Consequently, the delivered dose is often relatively low. Many tumors are considered somewhat radioresistant (meningiomas, schwannomas, melanomas, sarcomas) to these doses. Precise and accurate radiation delivery in radiosurgery means that lesions which do not contain normal tissue can be irradiated at a high dose provided that only a fraction of the dose is received by the surrounding brain [27]. The technology used must provide a steep fall-off in radiation delivery. These powerful doses transcend the modern concept of 'radiation resistance'. Meningiomas, schwannomas, melanomas, and sarcomas respond favorably and consistently to radiosurgery [43].

Hall and Brenner [13] agreed with the use of radiosurgery for benign brain lesions such as arteriovenous malformations (AVMs) and benign tumors but questioned its role for the management of malignant tumors. They derived data to argue that the treatment of malignant tumors with a single radiation fraction would result in a suboptimal therapeutic ratio between tumor control and the late response. An improved ratio would be expected from fractionation [13]. Their argument was based on the concept that hypoxic cells could reestablish their oxygenated state and become more sensitive to irradiation when treated with multiple fractions. Since AVMs and benign tumors are late-responding tissues, nothing was felt to be gained by fractionation. The performance of stereotactic fractionated radiotherapy for acoustic tumors may lessen the radiobiological effect on cranial nerves [27] (perhaps to overcome dose planning and delivery issues posed by some radiosurgery systems), but the early published data do not support any improvement in nerve preservation. Fractionation is unlikely to increase the therapeutic schwannoma response.

We advocate radiosurgery as a boost to fractionated radiotherapy in the management of malignant gliomas and not as the sole radiation approach. On the other hand, fractionated radiation may not improve the results of treatment for brain metastases. These benefits may be dose-related. Since whole brain irradiation is limited by brain tolerance, a powerful effect on the small tumor and surrounding brain may not be possible without a high rate of tissue injury. When radiosurgery is used as the sole treatment for a solitary metastasis, the problems of whole brain tolerance are eliminated and the physician can focus on the delivery of a high dose to the tumor itself. Such an approach provides excellent local control (approximately 90% for most tumors) with concomitant longer survival [9]. The benefits of whole brain radiotherapy for potential remote disease remain to be defined.

Larson et al. [27] placed the different targets for radiosurgery into four categories. Category 1 included a late-responding target embedded within late-responding normal tissue (e.g. AVM). Radiosurgery was believed an appropriate biologic strategy with no advantage to fractionation. In category 2, a late-responding target was surrounded by late-responding normal tissue (i.e. meningioma or other tumor that does not invade normal brain parenchyma). Again this category was believed to be appropriate for radiosurgery. Category 3 included early-responding targets embedded within late-responding normal tissue (i.e. astrocytoma). In this tumor, both normal glial cells and neoplastic cells exist within the target volume. One might anticipate a poor therapeutic ratio with radiosurgery although our early reports on pilocytic astrocytoma have shown a favorable response with radiosurgery. For the most part, such tumors are of small volume and mainly in children where both the physician and family would like to avoid large field irradiation in the developing brain. Category 4 included early-responding tissue surrounded by late-responding normal tissue (i.e. brain metastases). In this lesion, the target volume contains mainly malignant cells. Radiosurgery would be expected to kill oxygenated cells but might do less damage to hypoxic cells. As noted above, clinical reports do not support this concept since tumor control rates are high and morbidity rates low. Larson et al. [27] state that most fractionated regimens have not provided the radiobiologic effect that is administered during radiosurgery.

The Effect of Dose Rate

Reducing the dose rate of irradiation has an effect similar to fractionation. Over time, cells can repair sublethal radiation-induced damage [15]. The rate of repair (expressed as the half-time for disappearance of repairable injury) is approximately 1.5 h in the central nervous system [45]. An obvious effect of dose rate that pertains to radiosurgery systems is the decay in cobalt activity found with the Gamma Knife. Since the half-life of cobalt is approximately 5 years, a dose rate effect can be postulated. In our clinical experience however, we have not been able to define an effect of dose rate within our own patient series. Larson hypothesized that the concept of microfractionation might be important in reducing morbidity simply by delaying treatment times between radiosurgery isocenters at different stereotactic coordinates (within the same overall procedure) [26]. A study by Shaw et al. [38] showed poorer tumor control rates with linear accelerator-based radiosurgery than with Gamma Knife radiosurgery. One explanation for this result might be that the much lower dose rate of linear accelerator irradiation led to a reduced tumor biologic effect. Despite the potential importance of dose rate, no study has shown conclusively the effect of this factor. An analysis of postradiosurgery imaging changes in 307 AVM patients managed at our center did not find any correlation with the dose rate at the periphery of the AVM nidus targeted [11]. The lack of correlation in this study indicates only that the dose rate effect appears to be small within the range seen for the clinical use of the Gamma Knife.

Experimental Laboratory Comparisons between Radiosurgery and Fractionation

A number of experimental models have studied the effects of radiosurgery [32]. The magnitude of radiosurgical effects remain poorly understood, especially when described in terms of conventional radiation therapy doses. Although it is difficult to select a dose for each approach or tumor type that might be radiobiologically equivalent, use of information provided by Larson et al. [27] would be one starting point. In their report, for early-responding tissue such as a malignant neoplasm ($\alpha/\beta = 10$), a radiosurgery dose of 20 Gy was hypothesized to equal a fractionated dose of 50 Gy. We were interested in comparing single to multiple fraction irradiation in an animal model. Calculated α/β ratios for different malignant glioma cell lines showed a mean value of 10.4 [14, 30, 41, 48]. Thus, we realized that an α/β ratio of 10 was an assumption, and may not exactly reflect the tumor studied. Using this model, 35 Gy radiosurgery (to the 50% isodose) would be biologically equivalent to 85 Gy in 10 fractions [24].

The increased use of stereotactic radiosurgery and stereotactic fractionated irradiation as an addition or alternative to conventional therapy for malignant brain tumors mandates investigation into the relative effects of these approaches [27, 34, 37]. We hypothesized that radiosurgery alone or in combination with whole brain irradiation, would increase animal survival rates in comparison to no treatment or whole brain irradiation alone [3, 39, 46], and that a histologic correlate could be defined with the survival response. Such a comparison is clinically relevant since there is an increasing use of stereotactic radiation therapy approaches for brain tumors (as an alternative to radiosurgery), despite limited knowledge regarding the number of fractions or dose necessary that might compare with radiosurgery. Rats were randomized to control ($n = 54$) or treatment groups after implantation of C6 glioma cells into the right frontal brain region [22, 35].

When compared to the control group ($n = 54$, median survival = 22 days), prolonged survival was identified after radiosurgery ($p < 10^{-4}$), radiosurgery plus radiation therapy ($p < 10^{-4}$), whole brain radiation therapy alone ($p = 0.0002$), hemibrain radiation therapy to 85 Gy ($p < 10^{-4}$), and 35-Gy hemibrain single fraction irradiation ($p = 0.005$) [24]. There was no difference between the 'biologically equivalent' groups of radiosurgery and 10-fraction radiotherapy ($p = 0.45$), nor between radiosurgery and single-fraction non-stereotactic irradiation at the same 35-Gy margin dose ($p = 0.8$). Compared to the control group (mean, 6.8 mm), the mean tumor diameter was reduced in all treatment groups except whole brain radiation therapy alone. However, at the higher fractionated dose of 85 Gy, a significant reduction in tumor size was found (mean $= 5.4 \pm 1.6$ mm; $p = 0.004$), which was similar to the radiosurgery arm.

Radiosurgery ($p = 0.006$) and radiosurgery plus radiation therapy ($p = 0.009$) showed reduced tumor cell density when compared with control, a finding not observed after any fractionated regimen. Increased intratumoral edema was identified after radiosurgery ($p = 0.03$) and combined treatment ($p = 0.05$), but not after fractionated radiation therapy or 35-Gy single fraction hemibrain irradiation. In this animal model, the addition of radiosurgery significantly increased tumor cytotoxicity, potentially at the expense of radiation effects to regional brain. The histologic responses after radiosurgery were generally greater than those achieved with biologically equivalent doses of fractionated radiation therapy [24]. These effects may represent apoptosis, necrosis, or both. In experimental tumor models, we have identified apoptosis beginning in the early hours after radiosurgery [47]. It would be logical to expect a greater decrease in tumor size or even less tumor cellularity after combined radiosurgery/radiotherapy than in the other groups since more radiation was administered. However, in the 'biologically equivalent' groups of 35-Gy radiosurgery and 10-fraction 85-Gy radiotherapy, and even when compared to the single-fraction 35-Gy arm, radiosurgery led to greater cytotoxic effects as noted by a greater reduction in cellular density. This was most likely due to the variation in the distribution of dose delivered across the tumor in radiosurgery (35 Gy at the margin, increasing to 70 Gy at the center), versus a much more uniform dose delivered across the tumor in the other regimens.

This finding suggests that dose heterogeneity within solid neoplasms may be of benefit. Such higher central doses, as well as a delayed vascular response from vessels irradiated at the tumor periphery, are likely responsible for the marked loss of central contrast enhancement often found after human acoustic tumor radiosurgery [10, 34].

The Issue of Dose Homogeneity

There are only limited studies that attempt to address the effect of dose inhomogeneity on complications. Dose inhomogeneity within a small radiosurgery treatment volume that matches the target volume should have little or no effect on the risk of complications. There is also support for the conclusion that dose inhomogeneity can increase the risks of complications for large target volumes treated with radiosurgery treatment volumes that are less than perfect matches for the target. The seemingly conflicting findings of the Harvard JCRT series [31] and the University of Pittsburgh data on the relationship of dose inhomogeneity to complications seem to be explained by differences in the goodness of fit for the radiosurgery treatment plans. Dose inhomogeneity did not seem to be a problem with conformal multiple-isocenter Gamma Knife treatment plans, while less elaborate two-isocenter LINAC radiosurgery plans with possible high-dose overlap regions extending into normal tissue, were associated with a higher risk of complications. If radiosurgery volumes do not match well the treatment volume, then plans should be homogeneous to reduce complication risks. Our knowledge of complication risks from radiosurgery does not allow us to know to what extent different degrees of imperfection in matching a treatment volume to a target can be compensated for by plans with greater dose homogeneity.

Because charged particle beams (proton beams) can create custom-shaped treatment volumes just as easily at the 90 or 95% isodose level as with lower isodoses like 50%, there is a natural tendency for investigators treating with this equipment to believe that dose homogeneity is important for avoiding complications. Gamma Knife users have historically favored irradiating with 50% isodose volumes (the isodose percentage is always relative to the maximum dose in Gamma Knife prescriptions). The greater ease of producing custom-tailored multiple isocenter treatment plans with this isodose level compared to using more homogeneous plans makes it natural for Gamma Knife users to favor this or similar isodoses.

Benign Tumor Radiosurgery

Benign tumor radiosurgery has grown to become one of the most frequent indications. Since the majority of these patients remain alive and few have had their tumors removed, little postradiosurgery tissue has been available for histologic study. We believe that the radiobiologic effect on meningiomas, schwannomas, pituitary tumors, and other benign neoplasms is a combination of both cytotoxic and delayed vascular effects. Animal models such as the athymic mouse subrenal capsule xenograft technique have proved suitable to study radiosurgery effects.

For human vestibular schwannomas grafted into the subrenal capsule of nude mice [29], the model permitted accurate quantitation of small changes in tumor size and vascularity. The same model was used for the evaluation of human meningioma tumors. After both vestibular schwannoma and meningioma radiosurgery, we found significant reductions in tumor volume observed after 40 Gy (within 2 weeks) and after 1 month in the 20 Gy group [29]. Similarly, tumor surface vascularity was reduced in the 20 Gy and 40 Gy groups (but not in the 10 Gy group) after 3 months of follow-up. The model proved to be an excellent technique to study the in vivo radiobiology of benign tumors after radiosurgery. In this early analysis, we believed that tumor size reduction was due to neoplastic cell death [20]. Current studies are being performed to evaluate growth factor production after meningioma or vestibular schwannoma radiosurgery using this xenograft model.

Some investigators have reported that apoptosis may play a significant role in the early effects of radiosurgery for benign and malignant tumors. Since cell death may be either apoptotic or necrotic, and the temporal nature of these events different, it is important to understand how and when radiosurgery exerts an effect [47]. We found a doubling of the number of apoptotic cells after radiosurgery when compared to controls, within the first 48 h after irradiation. Apoptosis is characterized by cell shrinkage and pyknosis without an overt inflammatory reaction. One characteristic early stage of apoptosis is deoxyribonucleic acid (DNA) cleavage. Although apoptosis may involve cell membrane or organelle effects (that later translate into DNA damage), many investigators believe that the first effect is nuclear. Tsuzuki et al. [44] theorized that the response of tumors to low-dose Gamma Knife radiosurgery may be due to apoptosis since these doses would be less likely to cause vascular effects or inflammation. They evaluated expression of proliferating-cell nuclear antigen (PCNA) in tumors before low-dose Gamma Knife radiosurgery. Interestingly, they found that all cases of malignant lymphoma showed strong positive staining for PCNA, and rapid reduction of tumor volumes after Gamma Knife radiosurgery (sometimes with tumor margin doses as low as 8 Gy). They suspected that these cells received DNA damage and then rapidly entered the cell cycle leading to apoptotic death. In contrast, most benign tumors showed negative staining for PCNA and little radiographic response to low-dose radiosurgery [44].

Vascular Effects

Radiosurgery at doses used to manage tumors or vascular malformations appears to inflict little injury on normal brain vessels. Even the higher doses used in functional radiosurgery do not appear to cause vascular injury with proper targeting. Available information from AVM radiosurgery or meningioma radiosurgery has shown that normal vessels rarely decrease in size or occlude after radiosurgery [48]. Since angiograms show only blood vessels greater than 1 mm in diameter, no comment can be made regarding the response of smaller diameter vessels using this imaging technique. Nevertheless, in our benign tumor experience, no occurrence of perforator occlusion leading to an infarct has been identified. It appears that the abnormal vessels of neoplasms or vascular malformations have a relative sensitivity to radiosurgery in comparison to normal surrounding vessels.

Radiosurgery appears to cause a proliferative vasculopathy within the blood vessels of an AVM that begins with endothelial cell injury [36]. Blood vessels become hyalinized, thickened, and eventual luminal closure occurs. Granulation tissue may surround the AVM. This process takes many months and probably begins with an acute inflammatory reaction to radiosurgery. When this response becomes chronic, fibroblasts replace much of the mass of the AVM. Szeifert et al. [42] showed that myofibroblasts could be identified within the AVM and may provide some element of contractility to the obliteration process. Schneider et al. [36] reported a recent review of the histopathology of AVM radiosurgery from nine specimens up to 60 months after irradiation. In most patients where histology has been obtained, only subtotal obliteration had been found (hence the need for AVM removal). We anticipate that a similar response would occur in AVMs that proceed to complete obliteration. Analysis of the complications of AVM radiosurgery [11] shows that effects in surrounding brain most likely occur from a combination of hemodynamic changes as well as parenchymal irradiation. Flickinger's group found that the volume surrounding the malformation that received 12 Gy was predictive of a symptomatic imaging change following irradiation. It may be that this volume has an increased sensitivity to radiation, perhaps from regional ischemia surrounding the malformation.

Functional Radiosurgery

Simple animal models using rat, rabbit, goat, and baboon provided the basis for functional radiosurgery. Experiments in the 1960s showed that high radiosurgical doses (above 150 Gy) delivered to small volumes (3 × 5 mm diameter) caused consistent tissue necrosis that occurred within 1 month and did not change significantly over time [1, 19, 28]. Similar findings were identified in the rat brain where doses of 150 or 200 Gy led to tissue necrosis by 3 weeks [21]. In 1980, Steiner et al. [40] reported an autopsy series of Gamma Knife thalamotomy in the management of cancer pain and recommended that a dose of 150 Gy was necessary for the reproducible creation of a brain lesion. Subsequent rat experiments showed that a dose of 100 Gy caused necrosis in most (but not all) animals within 5 months and that even a dose of 50 Gy could cause complete volume necrosis in some baboons when an 8-mm collimator was used [21]. Thus, the lesion is both dose, volume, and time dependent. Reproducible radiosurgery lesions in humans were created using the 4-mm collimator of the Gamma Knife with a dose of 120–200 Gy. When volume was increased, such as when two 4-mm isocenters were used, the response became less predictable and larger lesions were sometimes created [18]. As a result, consistent lesion generation is best achieved when a single 4-mm isocenter is used (or at least the smallest volume necessary for the desired clinical result). For human thalamotomy, we have used doses of 130–140 Gy. Histologically, the radiosurgery lesion consists of coagulative necrosis within the target volume, a thin gliotic rim, and rapid normalization of parenchyma within 1–2 mm [21]. Although imaging studies may show long TR signal changes in white matter tracts surrounding the lesion, these are usually asymptomatic. Lower radiosurgery doses (i.e. 80 Gy) used for trigeminal neuralgia radiosurgery cause enhancement of the nerve and incomplete axonal degeneration [20]. We evaluated these effects in a baboon model, 6 months after 80- or 100-Gy radiosurgery.

Potential Pharmacologic Radioprotection for Radiosurgery

Future improvements in the results of stereotactic radiosurgery will be related to better patient selection, dose planning, radiosensitization of the target [8], and possibly protection of the brain surrounding the target. Prior investigations into radiation protection have examined myelin and lipid effects, as well as vascular effects [33]. We previously investigated the potential radioprotectant effects of high-dose pentobarbital; however, we detected no specific benefit in our radiosurgical model [23]. Bernstein et al. [4] reported that the 21-aminosteroid U-74389G reduced brachytherapy-induced brain injury in a rat model and Buatti et al. [7] reported that U-74389G provided radiation protection in a model where cats received either 21-aminosteroid or corticosteroid. 21-aminosteroids may provide protection against brain radiation injury by inhibition of lipid peroxidation and a selective action on vascular endothelium [2, 5, 6, 12]. We hypothesized that the 21-aminosteroid U-74389G would reduce radiosurgery-related brain injury without attenuating the target volume response. Kallfass et al. [17], using a celiac artery irradiation model, demonstrated inflammatory vascular effects within 24 h. As a membrane stabilizer, 21-aminosteroids block the release of free arachidonic acid from injured cell membranes [12]. The pharmacologic prevention of this early response might prevent a reactive cascade that would otherwise end in a chronic radiation vasculopathy.

Hornsey et al. [16] studied the effects of vasoactive drugs such as dipyramidole and desferrioxamine, and found reduction of spinal cord radiation damage. They postulated that the beneficial effect was due to improved spinal cord blood flow. Whether an agent selective to blood vessels could improve regional blood flow or provide regional vascular stability with limitation of regional edema remains to be identified. Braughler et al. [6] reported that the effects of

21-aminosteroid were 100 times more potent than desferrioxamine. In a separate study using cultured bovine endothelial cells, Audus et al. [2] showed that 21-aminosteroids associate with the hydrophobic segments of endothelial cell membranes, and thus can exert their action on the local cerebrovasculature. Oxygen radical-initiated peroxidation of vascular membranes is catalyzed by free iron release from hemoglobin, ferritin, and transferrin. If not prevented, lipid peroxidation progresses over the surface of the cell membrane to cause disruption of phospholipid-dependent enzymes, ionic gradients, and later membrane lysis. Repair of these effects will be manifest as a radiation-induced vasculopathy. U-74389G as a lipid antioxidant and free-radical scavenger was found in our study to limit radiation-induced vessel changes and prevent regional edema [25].

The 21-aminosteroid U-74389G provided protection after a single intravenous 15-mg/kg dose against 100-Gy radiation-induced vasculopathy and edema [25]. High-dose 21-aminosteroids appeared to have optimal properties for radiosurgery: surrounding brain protection without reducing the therapeutic effect desired within the target volume. We found a dose-response relationship for prevention of vascular effects, and that this likely translated into prevention from the development of regional cerebral edema. Our next experiment showed that this drug did not appear to protect a malignant glioma treated radiosurgically in the rat brain. Animals that received 21-aminosteroid before radiosurgery survived longer than either control animals or rats that had radiosurgery alone. Unfortunately, no clinical trials have yet evaluated pharmacologic radioprotection for use in stereotactic radiosurgery.

References

1 Andersson B, Larsson B, Leksell L, et al: Histopathology of late local radiolesions in the goat brain. Acta Radiol Ther Phys Biol 1970;9:385–394.

2 Audus KL, Guillot FL, Braughler JM: Evidence for 21-aminosteroid association with the hydrophobic domains of brain microvessel endothelial cells. Free Radic Biol Med 1991;11: 361–371.

3 Barker M, Deen DF, Baker DG: BCNU and X-ray therapy of intracerebral 9L rat tumors. Int J Radiat Oncol Biol Phys 1979;5:1581–1583.

4 Bernstein M, Ginsberg H, Glen J: Protection of iodine-125 brachytherapy brain injury in the rat with the 21-aminosteroid U-74389G. Neurosurgery 1992;31:923–928.

5 Braughler JM: Lipid peroxidation-induced inhibition of gamma-aminobutyric acid uptake in rat brain synaptosomes: protection by glucocorticoids. J Neurochem 1985;44:1282–1288.

6 Braughler JM, Pregenzer JF, Chase RL, Duncan LA, Jacobsen EJ, McCall JM: Novel 21-aminosteroids as potent inhibitors of iron-dependent lipid peroxidation. J Biol Chem 1987;262: 10438–10440.

7 Buatti JM, Friedman WA, Theele DP, Bova FJ, Mendenhall WM: The lazaroid U74389G protects normal brain from stereotactic radiosurgery-induced radiation injury. Int J Radiat Oncol Biol Phys 1996;34:591–597.

8 Cohen JD, Robins HI, Javid MJ: Radiosensitization of C6 glioma by thymidine and 41.8°C hyperthermia. J Neurosurg 1990;72:782–785.
9 Flickinger J, Kondziolka D, Lunsford LD, et al: A multi-institutional experience with stereotactic radiosurgery for solitary brain metastases. Int J Radiat Oncol Biol Phys 1994;28:797–802.
10 Flickinger JC, Kondziolka D, Pollock B, et al: Evolution of technique for vestibular schwannoma radiosurgery and effect on outcome. Int J Radiat Oncol Biol Phys 1996;36:275–280.
11 Flickinger JC, Kondziolka D, Pollock B, et al: Complications from arteriovenous malformation radiosurgery: multivariate analysis and modeling. Int J Radiat Oncol Biol Phys 1997;38:485–490.
12 Hall ED, Travis MA: Inhibition of arachidonic acid-induced vasogenic brain edema by the non-glucocorticoid 21-aminosteroid U-74006F. Brain Res 1988;451:350–352.
13 Hall EJ, Brenner DJ: The radiobiology of radiosurgery: rationale for different treatment regimes for AVMs and malignancies. Int J Radiat Oncol Biol Phys 1993;25:381–385.
14 Henderson SD, Kimler BF, Morantz RA: Radiation therapy of 9L rat brain tumors. Int J Radiat Oncol Biol Phys 1981;7:497–502.
15 Hornsey S, Morris CC, Myers R: The relationship between fractionation and total dose for X-ray induced brain damage. Int J Radiat Oncol Biol Phys 1981;7:393–396.
16 Hornsey S, Myers S, Jenkinson T: The reduction of radiation damage to the spinal cord by post-irradiation administration of vasoactive drugs. Int J Radiat Oncol Biol Phys 1990;18:1437–1442.
17 Kallfass E, Kramling HJ, Schultz-Hector S: Early inflammatory reaction of the rabbit coeliac artery wall after combined intraoperative and external irradiation. Radiother Oncol 1996;39: 167–178.
18 Kihlstrom L, Guo W, Lindquist C, et al: Radiobiology of radiosurgery for refractory anxiety disorders. Neurosurgery 1995;36:294–302.
19 Kihlstrom L, Hindmarsh T, Lax I, et al: Radiosurgical lesions in the normal human brain 17 years after gamma knife capsulotomy. Neurosurgery 1997;41:396–402.
20 Kondziolka D, Lacomis D, Niranjan A, Maesawa S, Mori Y, Fellows W, Lunsford LD: Histologic effects of trigeminal nerve radiosurgery in a primate model: implications for trigeminal neuralgia radiosurgery. Neurosurgery 2000;46:971–977.
21 Kondziolka D, Lunsford LD, Claassen D, et al: Radiobiology of radiosurgery: Part 1. The normal rat brain model. Neurosurgery 1992;31:271–279.
22 Kondziolka D, Lunsford LD, Claassen D, et al: Radiobiology of radiosurgery: Part II. The rat C6 glioma model. Neurosurgery 1992;31:280–288.
23 Kondziolka D, Somaza S, Flickinger JC, et al: Cerebral radioprotective effects of high-dose pentobarbital evaluated in an animal radiosurgery model. Neurol Res 1994;16:456–459.
24 Kondziolka D, Somaza S, Comey C, Lunsford LD, Claassen D, Pandalai S, Maitz A, Flickinger JC: Radiosurgery and fractionated radiation therapy: comparison of different techniques in an in vivo rat glioma model. J Neurosurg 1996;84:1033–1038.
25 Kondziolka D, Somaza S, Martinez AJ, et al: Radioprotective effects of the 21-aminosteroid U-74389G for stereotactic radiosurgery. Neurosurgery 1997;41:203–208.
26 Larson DA: Radiosurgery and fractionation. Radiosurgery 1996;1:261–267.
27 Larson DA, Flickinger JC, Loeffler JS: The radiobiology of radiosurgery. Int J Radiat Oncol Biol Phys 1993;25:557–561.
28 Larsson B, Leksell L, Rexed B, et al: The high-energy proton beam as a neurosurgical tool. Nature 1958;182:1222–1223.
29 Linskey ME, Martinez AJ, Kondziolka D, et al: The radiobiology of human acoustic schwannoma xenografts after stereotactic radiosurgery evaluated in the subrenal capsule of athymic mice. J Neurosurg 1993;78:645–653.
30 Malaise EP, Fertil B, Chavaudra N, et al: Distribution of radiation sensitivities for human tumor cells of specific histological types: comparison of in vitro to in vivo data. Int J Radiat Oncol Biol Phys 1986;12:617–624.
31 Nedzi L, Kooy H, Alexander E, et al: Variables associated with the development of complications from radiosurgery of intracranial tumors. Int J Radiat Biol Phys 1991;21:591–599.
32 Niranjan A, Gobbel G, Kondziolka D, Flickinger JC, Lunsford LD: Experimental radiobiological investigations into radiosurgery: present understanding and future directions. Neurosurgery 2004;55: 495–505.

33 Olson JJ, Friedman R, Orr K, Delaney T, Oldfield EH: Cerebral radioprotection by pentobarbital: dose response characteristics and association with GABA agonist activity. J Neurosurg 1990;72:749–758.

34 Pollock BE, Lunsford LD, Kondziolka D, et al: Outcome analysis of acoustic neuroma management: a comparison of microsurgery and stereotactic radiosurgery. Neurosurgery 1995;36: 215–229.

35 San-Galli F, Vrignaud P, Robert J, et al: Assessment of the experimental model of transplanted C6 glioblastoma in Wistar rats. J Neurooncol 1989;7:299–304.

36 Schneider BF, Eberhard DA, Steiner LE: Histopathology of arteriovenous malformations after gamma knife radiosurgery. J Neurosurg 1997;87:352–357.

37 Schwachenwald R, Engebraten O, Valen H, et al: A technique for studying single-dose radiation effects on glioma invasiveness in tissue culture – a pilot study; in Steiner L (ed): Radiosurgery: Baseline and Trends. New York, Raven Press, 1992, pp 101–109.

38 Shaw E, Scott C, Souhami L, et al: Radiosurgery for the treatment of previously irradiated recurrent primary brain tumors and brain metastases: initial report of radiation therapy oncology group protocol 90–05. Int J Radiat Oncol Biol Phys 1996;34:647–654.

39 Steinbok P, Mahaley MS, U R, et al: Treatment of autochthonous rat brain tumors with fractionated radiotherapy: the effects of graded radiation doses and of combined therapy with BCNU or steroids. J Neurosurg 1980;53:68–72.

40 Steiner LE, Forster D, Leksell L, et al: Gammathalamotomy in intractable pain. Acta Neurochir 1990;52:173–184.

41 Stuschke M, Budach V, Sack H: Radioresponsiveness of human glioma, sarcoma, and breast cancer spheroids depends on tumor differentiation. Int J Radiat Oncol Biol Phys 1993;27:627–636.

42 Szeifert G, Kemeny AA, Timperley W, et al: The potential role of myofibroblasts in the obliteration of arteriovenous malformations after radiosurgery. Neurosurgery 1997;40:61–66.

43 Thompson BG, Coffey RJ, Flickinger J, et al: Stereotactic radiosurgery of small intracranial tumors: neuropathological correlation in three patients. Surg Neurol 1990;33:96–104.

44 Tsuzuki T, Tsunoda S, Sakaki T, et al: Tumor cell proliferation and apoptosis associated with the Gamma knife effect. Stereotact Funct Neurosurg 1996;66(suppl 1):39–48.

45 van der Kogel A: Central nervous system radiation injury in animal models; in Gutin P, Leibel S, Sheline G (eds): Radiation Injury to the Nervous System. New York, Raven Press, 1991, pp 91–111.

46 Wheeler KT, Kaufman K: Influence of fractionation schedules on the response of a rat brain tumor to therapy with BCNU and radiation. Int J Radiat Oncol Biol Phys 1980;6:845–849.

47 Witham T, Kondziolka D, Niranjan A, Fellows W, Chambers W: The characterization of tumor apoptosis after experimental radiosurgery. Stereotactic Funct Neurosurg (in press).

48 Yamamoto M, Jimbo M, Kobayashi M, et al: Long-term results of radiosurgery for arteriovenous malformation: neurodiagnostic imaging and histological studies of angiographically confirmed nidus obliteration. Surg Neurol 1992;37:219–230.

Douglas Kondziolka, MD, MSc, FRCS(C)
Professor of Neurological Surgery and Radiation Oncology
Suite B-400,UPMC Presbyterian 1
200 Lothrop Street
Pittsburgh, PA 15213–2582 (USA)
Tel. +1 412 647 6782, Fax +1 412 647 0989, E-Mail Kondziolkads@upmc.edu

Szeifert GT, Kondziolka D, Levivier M, Lunsford LD (eds): Radiosurgery and Pathological Fundamentals. Prog Neurol Surg. Basel, Karger, 2007, vol 20, pp 28–42

3. Dose Selection in Stereotactic Radiosurgery

John C. Flickinger[a,b], *Douglas Kondziolka*[a,b], *Ajay Niranjan*[b], *L. Dade Lunsford*[a–c]

Departments of [a]Radiation Oncology, [b]Neurological Surgery, and [c]Radiology, University of Pittsburgh School of Medicine, Pittsburgh, Pa., USA

Abstract

Selecting optimal doses for radiosurgery requires a thorough consideration of existing dose-response data for radiation injury of brain and surrounding structures and of the dose-response for the desired endpoint (tumor control, obliteration of a vascular malformation, relief of trigeminal neuralgia, etc.). This paper reviews the radiobiological and physics principles that should be considered in dose selection as well as information from retrospective and prospective clinical investigations of radiosurgery.

Basic Principles

Selecting a prescription dose is the final step in radiosurgery treatment planning. In the process of dose selection, physicians should take into account all of the information known about both the expected level of treatment success (tumor control, obliteration of arteriovenous malformations, AVMs, etc.) and complication risks at various doses in order to select a dose that is optimum for the individual patient. The paired sigmoid dose-response curves in figure 1 illustrate the balance between increasing the desired response and increasing complications with higher radiation treatment doses. The separation between these curves is commonly referred to as the therapeutic window. Accurately predicting complication risks for individual patients is a complex undertaking that depends on the radiosurgery treatment volume, the target location, and the nature of the target [1–4]. Dose-response data for desired endpoints from radiosurgery (tumor control, AVM obliteration, etc.) are sparse and difficult to

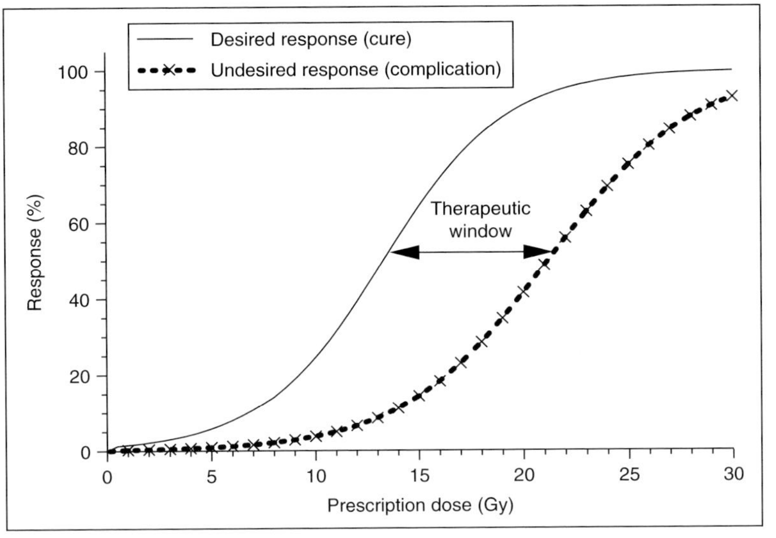

Fig. 1. Theoretical paired sigmoid dose-response curves for desired response (tumor control or cure) versus complications.

interpret for most indications, with perhaps the exception of AVM obliteration and trigeminal neuralgia treatment [5, 6]. This paper will review the principles governing dose selection as well as evolving outcome data that should be considered in dose prescription for radiosurgery.

The creation of a radiosurgical treatment plan is a multiple step process. After first defining the target volume on stereotactic images, we next tailor a radiosurgery treatment volume to closely match it, and then finally we must decide what radiation dose will be prescribed. We follow radiobiological principles to understand and interpret the limited outcome data from past radiosurgery experience to select the optimal dose for individual patients.

Treatment Planning and 'Minimum' Tumor Dose

Radiation oncologists have been accustomed to treating tumors with conventional fractionated radiotherapy, using 10- to 30-mm normal tissue margins around tumors for the planning treatment volume (PTV). A radiation treatment plan to cover the PTV is then generated and the radiation oncologist selects the highest treatment isodose (usually 90–99% with respect to the maximum dose) that completely encloses the tumor plus the margin (PTV) for the 'minimum tumor dose' prescription. If the margin is large enough to ensure that the tumor remains within the treatment volume for every fraction, the 'minimum tumor dose' prescribed represents the true minimum dose that the tumor receives.

The rigid stereotactic fixation used with radiosurgery allows the use of a treatment volume that matches the target volume without any additional margin. Physicians usually choose an isodose for the dose prescription that matches the tumor volume closely, but does not necessarily enclose 100% of the tumor. In a typical radiosurgery treatment plan, the treatment or prescription isodose (often referred to as a 'minimum tumor dose') encloses 90–99% of the tumor or target volume. When dose-volume histograms are analyzed, the true 'minimum tumor dose' is often 67–80% of the prescription dose. Often with this type of plan, the portion receiving less than 90% of the prescription dose is ≤0.5% the tumor. It is unclear how much tumor control probability is affected when a tiny fraction of a tumor receives a lower dose than the rest of the tumor. In the past, most Gamma Knife radiosurgery was done without drawing tumor contours, and therefore without dose-volume histograms. Unfortunately, interpreting dose-volume histogram data is difficult because any uncertainties in drawing the tumor volume will cause substantial variation in the part of the dose-volume histogram less than the prescription dose (including the true 'minimum tumor dose').

Dose-Volume Effects for Complications

One of the most important concepts behind radiosurgery is that the ability of normal tissue to tolerate radiation highly depends on the tissue volume irradiated, particularly at small volumes. Because stereotactic fixation eliminates the need for treating the target with an additional margin, radiosurgery allows dramatically smaller treatment volume to be safely irradiated to high doses when the target volumes are small. The variation in radiation tolerance across the range of treatment volumes used in radiosurgery is tremendous compared with the variation seen over the range of volumes treated in conventional fractionated radiotherapy. As shown in figure 2, reducing the treatment volume with improved treatment planning shifts the complication dose-response curve to the right, thereby increasing the therapeutic window.

Early Dose-Volume Guidelines for Brain Tolerance

Although Leksell published the concept of high-dose small-volume stereotactic brain irradiation and coined the term 'radiosurgery' as far back as 1951 [6], there was only sparse data from laboratory and clinical investigation to define dose-volume effects when photon radiosurgery began in the United States in the 1980s. Kjellberg and his colleagues plotted 1 and 99% dose-volume isoeffect lines for brain necrosis on log-log axes using data from animal experiments and limited human clinical experience with photon and proton beams to guide his subsequent dose prescriptions for proton beam radiosurgery [7].

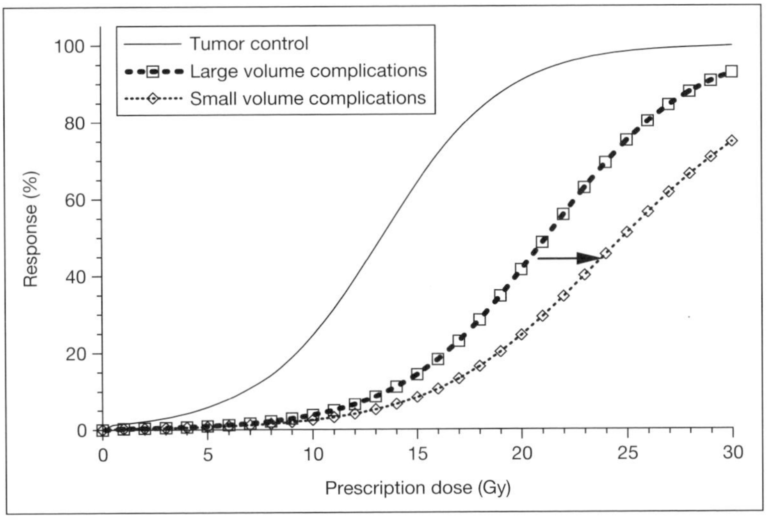

Fig. 2. The complication dose-response curve was shifted to the right by reducing the treatment volume. This increased the separation between complications and tumor control (the therapeutic window).

Leksell's group in Stockholm changed their dose prescriptions for the Gamma Knife over the years as they accumulated clinical and laboratory experience. By the mid-1980s, they felt that marginal doses of 25 Gy appeared optimal for treating AVMs, acoustic neuromas and meningiomas.

In 1987, the new Pittsburgh Gamma Unit was one of the earliest equipped with 18-mm diameter collimators (in addition to the 4-, 8-, and 14-mm collimators with prior models). Larger collimators and better treatment planning software made it easier to treat larger volumes than Stockholm had treated in the past. The Harvard Joint Center started treating patients a year earlier with Linac radiosurgery using Kjellberg's 1% dose-volume (or more precisely dose-diameter) isoeffect guideline for brain necrosis to prescribe marginal doses usually to the 80% isodose treatment volume [8]. Although we considered following Kjellberg's 1% isoeffect guideline, we questioned whether isoeffect lines for relatively homogenous, single-isocenter, proton beam irradiation with different-sized circular collimators would serve as reasonable guidelines for multiple isocenter photon radiosurgery with differing degrees of dose inhomogeneity. In addition, there was no way to estimate the contribution of whole-brain irradiation to brain tolerance for subsequent radiosurgery of brain metastasis patients. The integrated logistic formula was developed to estimate brain necrosis risk from radiosurgery dose-volume histograms [9]. The formula

Table 1. A comparison of dose-volume prescription guidelines from Kjellberg's 1% radionecrosis isoeffect line, 3% necrosis risk predictions from the integrated logistic formula (ILF), and the RTOG phase I maximum tolerated doses for <20% grade 3–5 toxicity sequelae within 3 months[a] [8, 9, 14]

Diameter, mm	Volume, cm^3	1% isoeffect, Gy	3% ILF, Gy	RTOG, Gy
12.5	1.02	27.5	34.0	24[a]
15.0	1.77	25.0	29.0	24[a]
17.5	2.81	22.5	23.0	24[a]
20.0	4.19	20.0	18.0	24[a]
22.5	5.96	18.7	16.5	18
25.0	8.18	17.5	14.5	18
27.5	10.9	16.5	13.5	18
30.0	14.1	15.0	13.0	18
32.5	18.0	14.0	12.5	15

[a]Maximum tolerated dose was not reached for tumors <2 cm in diameter.

parameters were fitted to the scant clinical and laboratory data available at the time, with the intent of refitting them to new data as they became available.

We hoped to limit brain necrosis risk from radiosurgery to 3% or less by following the 3% isoeffect curve for brain necrosis predicted by the integrated logistic formula. Subsequent reviews of the clinical experience with Gamma Knife radiosurgery at the University of Pittsburgh following this guideline documented that the risk of long-term sequelae of radiosurgery (radiation necrosis) to be in the 3–5% range, as expected. The 3% isoeffect curve for brain necrosis predicted with the integrated logistic formula called for almost the same doses as Kjellberg's 1% isoeffect line for similar volumes. Both of these dose-volume guidelines were widely used to guide radiosurgery dose prescriptions. Table 1 compares these two guidelines for spherical targets of different diameter. Both the integrated logistic formula and Kjellberg's 1% isoeffect line were intended to predict only parenchymal brain necrosis. They were not expected to be able to predict injury to cranial nerves, which were known to be more sensitive to injury from conventional radiotherapy than other brain structures.

Brain Tolerance Studies from AVM Radiosurgery

Recent detailed analyses of clinical experience with AVM radiosurgery have provided reliable predictions of brain tolerance to help guide radiosurgery dose prescription. Volume and location effects can be examined in detail in these studies since AVM come in all different sizes and locations. Most importantly,

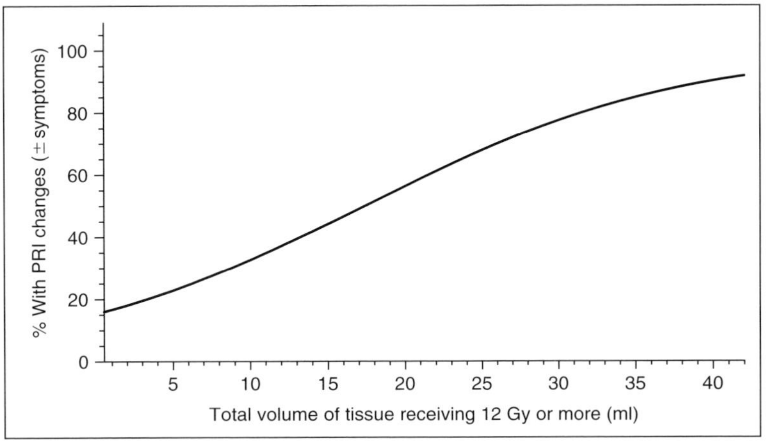

Fig. 3. Risk prediction curves that correlate the probability of developing any (symptomatic or asymptomatic) PRI changes for AVM patients (n = 307) undergoing radiosurgery with the volume of all tissue receiving 12 Gy or more (correlation: $p > 0.0001$).

follow-up data of AVM radiosurgery patients are more reliable and easier to obtain than for radiosurgery of malignant tumors.

We evaluated 307 AVM patients who received Gamma Knife radiosurgery at the University of Pittsburgh between 1987 and 1993 [3]. All patients had regular clinical or imaging follow-up for a minimum of 2 years (range: 24–96 months, median = 44 months). The rate of developing any postradiosurgery imaging (PRI) changes 2 (and 7) years after radiosurgery was 30.5%; while 10.5% of patients (included in that 30.5% total) developed symptomatic changes. Symptomatic PRI changes resolved in 53% of patients within 3 years of onset, a significantly lower resolution rate ($p = 0.0274$) than the 95% resolution rate for 20% of patients who developed asymptomatic PRI changes. The actuarial rate for developing persistent symptomatic PRI changes (radiation necrosis) was 5.05% at 7 years.

Multivariate analysis of various treatment parameters identified a significant correlation of any PRI change only with the total volume of AVM plus surrounding tissue receiving a radiation dose greater than 12 Gy, termed the 12-Gy volume. None of the other factors tested including target dose inhomogeneity, dose rate, number of isocenters, maximum or minimum AVM nidus dose, or treatment volume were independently correlated with PRI changes in any significant way. The 12-Gy volume reflects both the treatment volume and the minimum dose to the AVM nidus used in the radiosurgical treatment but is better correlated with the risk of radiation sequelae than either one of those factors individually. The risk of developing PRI changes for AVM patients is shown in figure 3.

Location Effects and AVM Radiosurgery Tolerance

The chance of causing symptomatic radiation injury to the brain from radiosurgery is effected dramatically by location. Since there are not dramatic differences in cell composition of the brain parenchyma from one region to another, differing locations of the brain should not have significantly different risks of temporary or permanent parenchymal injury from radiosurgery detectable on imaging studies or histological sections at autopsy. We found this to be true in studying the effect of location on PRI changes detectable by magnetic resonance imaging (MRI) scans [4]. The function of some regions of the brain is much more important in the functions of daily life than others (so called 'eloquent' versus 'silent' regions). Accordingly, the chance that a postradiosurgery injury reaction is symptomatic varies dramatically with location.

We modeled location effects using data from 85 AVM patients who developed symptomatic complications following Gamma Knife radiosurgery, and 337 control patients with no complications were evaluated as part of another multi-institutional study [4]. After excluding patients with easily resolvable sequelae (headaches and seizures) out of the 85 patients with complications in this series, 38 patients were classified as having permanent symptomatic sequelae (necrosis), the endpoint for this study. AVM marginal doses varied from 10 to 35 Gy and treatment volumes from 0.26 to 47.9 cm^3. Median follow-up for patients without complications was 45 months (range: 24–92).

We constructed a multivariate model of the effects of AVM location and the volume of tissue receiving 12 Gy or more (12-Gy volume) for the risk of developing permanent postradiosurgery sequelae. To rate the risk of complications for each location, we developed a 'significant postradiosurgery injury expression' or 'SPIE' score. The variation in risk with location and 12-Gy volume is shown in figure 4. Table 2 lists the risks of permanent symptomatic sequelae for AVMs measuring 1, 2, 3, and 4 cm in average diameter by location from radiosurgery to doses following the 3% integrated logistic formula guidelines. It must be remembered that this model was constructed with a limited amount of data (38 complications) and a large number of variables (10 different locations), so the risk predictions for some locations (such as very small brainstem locations) may be unreliable. As can be seen in table 2, the expected complication risks are extremely high for 4-cm diameter AVMs in all nonfrontal locations. For this reason, we recommend a volume-staged approach in patients with large AVMs (15 cm^3 or more in volume). With volume staging, the AVM is treated in two or three 7- to 15-cm^3 volume portions, preferably with a 5- to 6-month rest in between portions to allow normal tissue radiation injury repair.

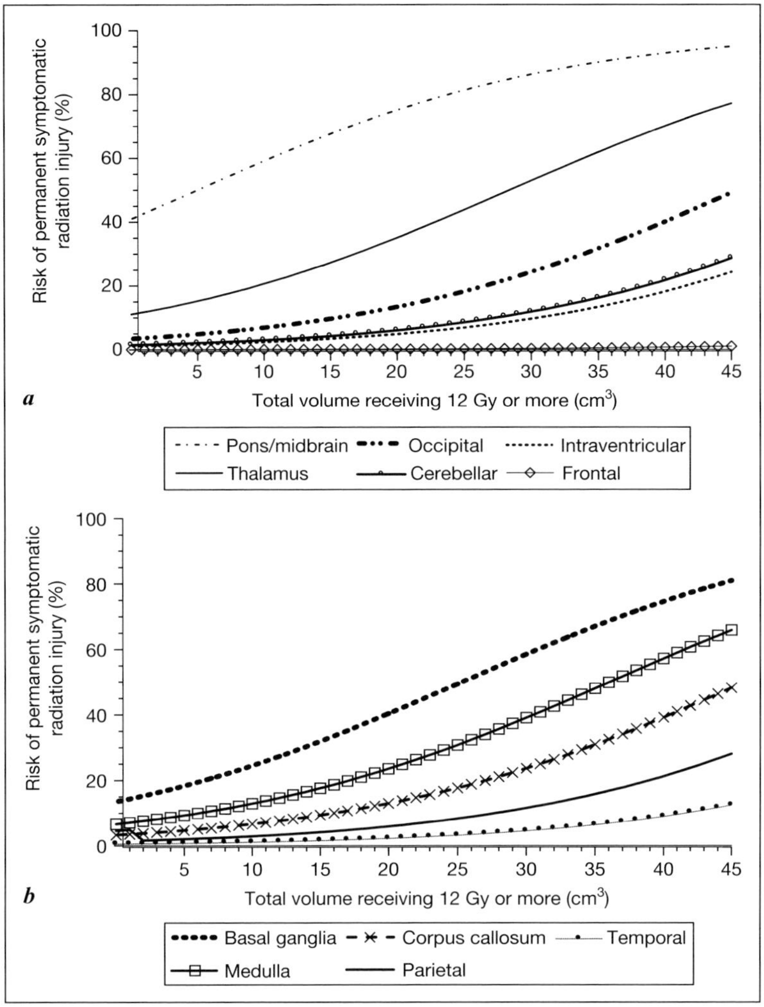

Fig. 4. Risk prediction curves for AVM patients that correlate the12-Gy volume with risks for developing symptomatic postradiosurgery sequelae separately according to location.

Cranial Nerve Tolerance to Radiosurgery

It has long been known that several of the cranial nerves, and specifically the optic chiasm/nerves, are more susceptible to injury from fractionated radiotherapy than the rest of the brain [10–12]. There appear to be differences in radiation sensitivity among the different cranial nerves. Special sensory nerves (optic and auditory) are the most sensitive, followed by somatic sensory nerves,

Table 2. Estimated % risk of permanent symptomatic postradiosurgery sequelae (radiation necrosis) for AVMs measuring 1, 2, 3, and 4 cm in average diameter by different location

Location	Percent risk			
	1-cm AVMs	2-cm AVMs	3-cm AVMs	4-cm AVMs
Pons/midbrain	44.02	55.89	66.19	96.46
Basal ganglia	15.01	22.15	30.54	85.95
Thalamus	12.36	18.51	25.98	83.00
Medulla	7.43	11.46	16.66	73.55
Occipital	3.87	6.09	9.11	58.23
Corpus callosum	3.73	5.88	8.8	57.32
Parietal	2.61	2.55	3.88	35.99
Cerebellar	1.65	2.62	4.00	36.68
Intraventricular	1.32	2.11	3.22	31.63
Temporal	0.59	0.94	1.45	16.95
Frontal	0.04	0.07	0.11	1.48

Marginal doses were chosen according to 3% guidelines from the integrated logistic formula [9].

and then motor nerves as the least sensitive [12]. Cranial neuropathy risk depends upon dose and the length of the nerve irradiated [12]. We recommend limiting the maximum dose to the optic nerve to 8 Gy for radiosurgery [10]. Because the consequences of injury to other cranial nerves are not as severe as blindness, it is reasonable to treat them with higher doses and to accept greater risks of injury to improve chances for tumor control or vascular obliteration.

After analyzing optic nerve complications, a combined Harvard/Pittsburgh study of radiosurgery complications recommended 8 Gy as the safe dose limit for the optic nerves/chiasm [10]. The lowest optic chiasm dose at which radiation-induced optic neuropathy developed in that study was 9.7 Gy. The same study had difficulty correlating injury to the cranial nerves 3–6 with anything except that it did not occur with maximum doses <15 Gy. The chief limitation of this study was the lack of high-resolution images in the early radiosurgery experience (using CT planning) to precisely define the entire length of the optic nerves/chiasm to define the true maximum dose and perform a dose-volume histogram analysis.

Stafford et al. [11] reviewed the Mayo Clinic experience with using a dose limit for the optic nerves/chiasm higher than 8 Gy. In their series, 4/215 patients developed optic neuropathy after Gamma Knife radiosurgery to median dose to the optic nerves/chiasm of 10 Gy. Limitations of that study are the lack of a dose-volume histogram analysis and some mixture in the analysis of patients treated by single-session radiosurgery, patients treated after recent or remote fractionated radiotherapy (XRT) and patients who underwent radiosurgery more than once. Only one case developed after radiosurgery alone. That patient received a maximum optic nerve chiasm dose of 12.8 Gy. It appears from the article that 28 patients received a comparable dose, which means the risk at 12–13 Gy should be approximately 1/28. Three cases with a history of prior XRT developed optic neuropathy following doses of 58.8 Gy XRT with 7 Gy from SRS, 45 Gy XRT with 9 Gy from SRS, and 50.4 Gy XRT followed by 9 Gy from SRS 1 and 12 Gy from SRS 2. It therefore appears that 12 Gy should be a reasonable limit for a 3% risk of optic neuropathy.

Based on these studies, what dose limit should be chosen for the optic nerve chiasm? That depends somewhat on the risk level that is appropriate for the patient. A 3% risk limit of 12 Gy or perhaps even higher would be appropriate for treating a previously unirradiated malignant tumor with a steep dose-response near the prescription dose. On the other hand, a 3% risk is inappropriate for a benign tumor such as a nonfunctional pituitary adenoma or meningioma that could be treated with fractionated radiotherapy with lower risk and where surgery or repeat radiation treatment can be effective options for salvage treatment of radiosurgery failures. In those cases, sticking with the 8-Gy limit for the optic system to keep the optic neuropathy risk to <1/1,000 is more appropriate and should allow tumors to be safely retreated with radiosurgery or fractionated radiotherapy in the future, if necessary. The optic nerve/chiasm limit for radiosurgery after full-dose radiotherapy should be 6–7 Gy depending on the total dose of prior XRT and how long ago it was given (>6 months ago versus recent). It is unclear whether in the future these maximum dose limits will prove too conservative for limiting maximum optic doses from dose-volume histograms (which tend to be higher) or whether a certain dose-volume limit will prove a better guideline.

Dose-response curves for cranial nerves 5, 7 and 8 that depend on the length of the nerve irradiated have been published [12]. With modern acoustic neuroma radiosurgery to 12–13 Gy, the risks of any drop in Gardner-Robertson hearing level, loss of all testable hearing (deafness), facial numbness/abnormal sensation, or facial weakness are approximately 25–30, 8, 3, and 0.2%, respectively [13].

The RTOG Phase I Maximum Tolerated Doses

Table 1 lists the RTOG dose-volume prescription guidelines. Shaw et al. [14] reported the results of the RTOG Phase I–II dose escalation study of radiosurgery in 102 analyzable patients with recurrent brain metastases or primary brain tumors. For tumors <20 mm, minimum tumor dose levels (D_{min}) of 18, 21,

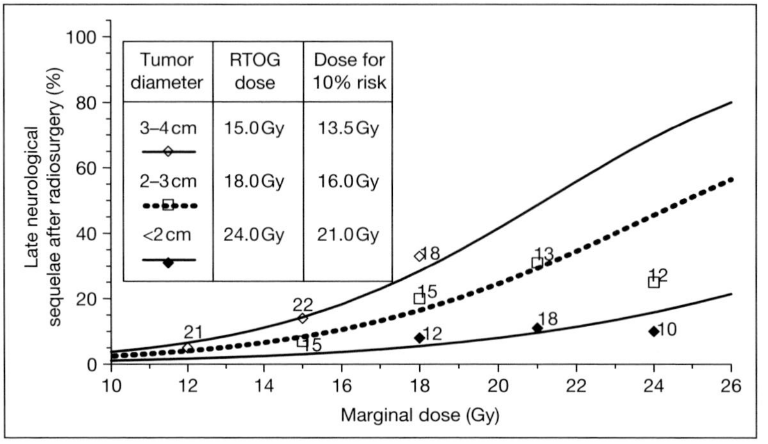

Fig. 5. Data from the RTOG radiosurgery dose-escalation study for recurrent metastatic or primary brain tumors [14] fit to logistic dose-response curves.

24 Gy were tested with 0/40 patients developing a CNS toxicity grade of ≥3. For tumors 21–30 mm in diameter, marginal doses of 15, 18 and 21 Gy were tested. Two out of 42 of these patients developed grade 3 CNS toxicity at dose levels of 15 and 21 Gy. For 31- to 40-mm tumors, dose levels of 12, 15, and 18 Gy were tested. After a dose level of 12 Gy, 1/21 developed grade 5 toxicity (death). At 15 Gy, 0/22 patients had grade 3 or greater toxicity, but at 18 Gy, 4/18 patients developed significant toxicity (2 with grade 3 and 2 with grade 4). The maximum tolerated dose for 3- to 4-cm diameter tumors was judged to be 15 Gy. Dose-response curves constructed from this data are shown in figure 5.

Target or Tumor Dose-Response Curves

Introductory radiotherapy texts often show steep sigmoid dose-response curves for tumor control derived from uniform laboratory models such as cell cultures. This leads to the expectation that minor changes in a radiotherapy prescription dose will always dramatically effect tumor control. With radiosurgery as in fractionated radiotherapy, it is hard to identify any clear change in the control of most benign and many malignant tumors within the range of doses commonly used. In several thorough analyses, we have not as yet been able to find any correlation between control of acoustic neuromas and meningioma and marginal dose prescribed within the range of 12–20 Gy [13, 15]. Because of this, we recommend prescription doses of 12–13 Gy for benign tumors like meningiomas and acoustic neuromas, assuming that the treatment volume

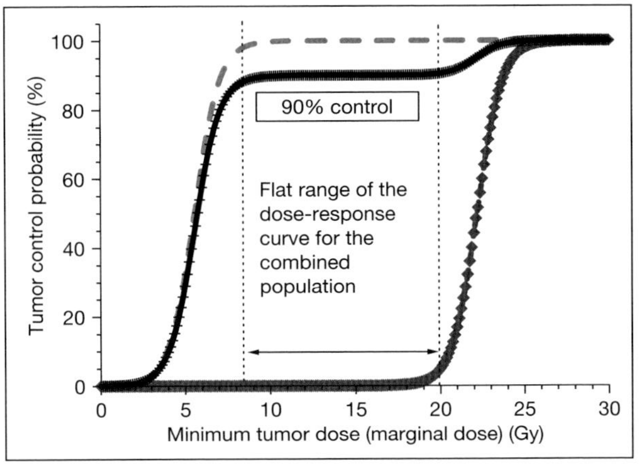

Fig. 6. Composite dose-response curves (solid line) for a heterogeneous population of tumors. The population is composed of 90% of patients with a relatively radiosensitive tumor subtype (the dashed dose-response curve) and 10% with a relatively radioresistant tumor subtype (the dotted dose-response curve with diamond shapes). This results in 90% tumor control from 8 to 20 Gy.

covers more than 90% of the gross tumor volume and the true minimum tumor dose from the dose-volume histogram is greater than 8 Gy. The only exception for this is in radiosurgery of functional pituitary tumors where our policy is to prescribe marginal doses up to 25–30 Gy if possible but limited to lower doses as needed to keep the maximum dose to the optic nerve/chiasm to ≤8 Gy.

Tumor heterogeneity may explain why many tumor dose-response curves are flat within the therapeutic dose range. Figure 6 shows a composite dose-response curve constructed from one tumor subpopulation where the tumors are easily controlled at doses below the usual therapeutic range and a second subpopulation where higher doses are needed. The dose-response curves for each subpopulation are relatively steep, but the composite curve is relatively flat within the therapeutic range.

Functional Radiosurgery

Functional lesion generation is a concept with a long history in neurosurgery. Different functional neurosurgical interventions have been dramatically successful in managing severe chronic pain, disabling tremor, other parkinsonian symptoms, uncontrolled epilepsy, and rare cases of severe, refractory obsessive-compulsive disorder.

Radiosurgery and the other surgical procedures for trigeminal neuralgia (aside from deep brain stimulation) are designed to injure the nerve to interrupt pain transmission. Four-millimeter collimator is used to irradiate the proximal trigeminal nerve at the root entry zone [6]. We found that maximum radiosurgical doses of 70 or 80 Gy provide significant benefit over lower doses (60–65 Gy) for trigeminal neuralgia [6]. To date, sensory loss has been observed after radiosurgery in only 6–8% of patients. Approximately 55% of patients became pain free and another 30% obtained significant pain reduction. We are presently conducting a clinical trial to compare maximum doses of 80 vs. 90 Gy for treatment of typical trigeminal neuralgia.

Despite the dependence on anatomic targeting alone, recent small series report encouraging results for radiosurgical thalamotomy or pallidotomy [16, 17]. It may be useful in patients with coagulopathy or in specific disorders where physiologic data are not believed to be helpful (i.e. cingulotomy, capsulotomy, medial thalamotomy). The optimal dose for lesion generation has not been precisely defined. Steiner et al. [16] reported that radiosurgery doses of ≥180 Gy were needed to reliably create a thalamotomy within the relatively short lifespan of patients with intractable pain from metastatic disease. It is now clear that lower maximum doses of 130–140 Gy with 4-mm diameter collimators are adequate for the creation of necrotic lesions in patients with longer expected survival. Future improvements in imaging, i.e. functional MRI and magnetoencephalography, may further expand the role of functional radiosurgery.

Arteriovenous Malformations

We studied AVM obliteration after Gamma Knife radiosurgery in the University of Pittsburgh experience with 351 patients with 3–11 years of follow-up imaging [5]. The median marginal dose was 20 Gy (range: 12–30) and median treatment volume was 5.7 cm^3 (range: 0.26–24). We developed a mathematical dose-response model for overall obliteration not dependent on any assessment of in-field versus out-of field nidus persistence. Figure 7 shows the AVM obliteration dose-response curve from this data using a maximum obliteration rate model we developed. This model has a maximum overall obliteration rate of 88% with only limited improvement in the obliteration rate above 23 Gy (where 86% obliteration is expected). The maximum obliteration rate model for patients with prior embolization was similar, except that it uses a maximum obliteration rate of 71.7% due to an increased risk of marginal miss (from recanalization of previously embolized nidus, etc.). Two alternate models based on in-field obliteration assessments had maximum obliteration occurring at either 21.75 or 24.75 Gy for all patients (with or without prior embolization). These last two models reflected the fact that a significantly higher proportion (126/135 or 93.3%) of AVM receiving marginal doses of 20–24 Gy (mean dose 20.7 Gy) achieved in-field obliteration compared to the proportion (85/100) obliterated in-field after a marginal dose of exactly 25 Gy ($p = 0.034$, χ^2 test; $p = 0.049$, two-sided Fisher's exact test). From

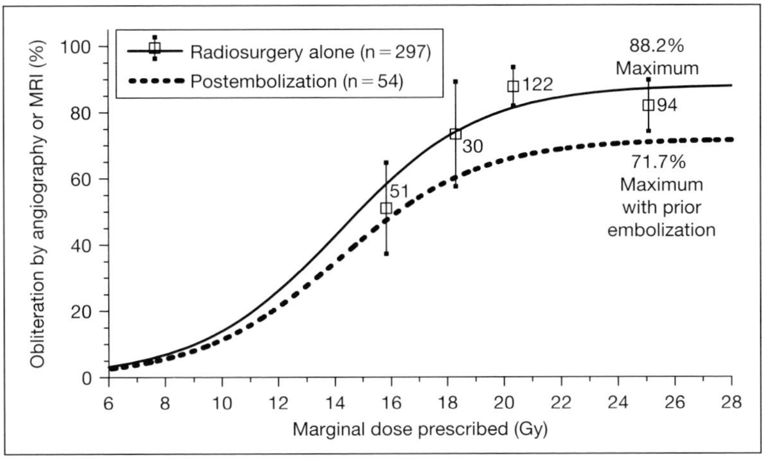

Fig. 7. Dose-response curve for in-field obliteration of AVM nidus according to minimum or marginal dose prescribed. The numbers show the number of patients within each adjacent dose interval. The position of each dose interval reflects the percentage of patients in the group with complete obliteration.

this analysis of the dose-response for AVM obliteration, we feel that there is little gained in treating AVMs with marginal dose above 23 Gy. Likewise, it seems unwise to treat AVMs with doses <15 Gy because of the low obliteration rates.

Malignant Tumors

Our prescription policy with malignant tumors (brain metastasis or glioblastoma) originally was to follow the guidelines of the integrated logistic formula for limiting complication risk to approximately 3% [9]. After the maximum tolerated doses were defined from the RTOG dose-escalation study, we switched to using those doses for most recurrent tumors [14]. Based on the Brown University report that there was no added benefit to increasing dose above 20 Gy, we use that dose for primary or metastatic brain tumors <2 cm in diameter [18]. We also use an interpolated dose of 16 Gy for tumors that are 2.8–3.2 cm in average diameter.

References

1 Flickinger JC, Lunsford LD, Kondziolka D: Radiosurgical dosimetry: Principles and clinical implications; in DeSalles AF, Goetsch S (eds): Stereotactic Surgery and Radiosurgery. Madison, Medical Physics Publishing, 1993, pp 293–306.

2 Flickinger JC, Lunsford LD, Kondziolka D, Maitz AM, Epstein A, Simons S, Wu A: Radiosurgery and brain tolerance: an analysis of neurodiagnostic imaging changes following gamma knife radiosurgery for arteriovenous malformations. Int J Radiat Oncol Biol Phys 1992;23:19–25.

3 Flickinger JC, Kondziolka D, Pollock BE, Maitz AH, Lunsford LD: Complications from arteriovenous malformation radiosurgery: multivariate analysis and risk modeling. Int J Radiat Oncol Biol Phys 1997;38:485–490.
4 Flickinger JC, Lunsford LD, Kondziolka D: Development of a model to predict permanent symptomatic post-radiosurgery injury for arteriovenous malformation patients. Int J Radiat Onc Biol Phys 2000;46:1143–1148.
5 Flickinger JF, Kondziolka D, Maitz AH, Lunsford LD: An analysis of the dose-response for arteriovenous malformation radiosurgery and other factors affecting obliteration. Radiother Oncol 2002;63:347–354.
6 Kondziolka D, Lunsford LD, Flickinger JC, Young RF, Vermeulen S, Duma CM, Jacques DB, Rand RW, Regis J, Peragut JC, Epstein M, Lindquiest C: Stereotactic radiosurgery for trigeminal neuralgia: a multi-institution study using the gamma unit. J Neurosurg 1996;84:940–945.
7 Leksell L: The stereotaxic method and radiosurgery of the brain. Acta Chir Scand 1951;102: 316–319.
8 Kjellberg RN, Hanamura T, Davis KR, Lyons S, Butler W, Adams R: Bragg-peak proton-beam therapy for arteriovenous malformations of the brain. N Engl J Med 1983;309:269.
9 Flickinger JC: An integrated logistic formula for prediction of complications from radiosurgery. Int J Radiat Oncol Biol Phys 1989;17:879–885.
10 Tishler RB, Loeffler JS, Lunsford LD, Duma C, Alexander E III, Kooy HM, Flickinger JC: Tolerance of cranial nerves of the cavernous sinus to radiosurgery. Int J Radiat Oncol Biol Phys 1993;27:215–221.
11 Stafford SL, Pollock BE, Leavitt JA, et al: A study on the radiation tolerance of the optic nerves and chiasm after stereotactic radiosurgery. Int J Radiat Oncol Biol Phys 2003;55:1177–1181.
12 Flickinger JC, Kondziolka D, Lunsford LD: Dose and diameter relationships for facial, trigeminal, and acoustic neuropathies following acoustic neuroma radiosurgery. Radiother Oncol 1996;41: 215–219.
13 Flickinger JC, Kondziolka D, Niranjan A, Maitz A, Voynov G, Lunsford LD: Acoustic neuroma radiosurgery with marginal tumor doses of 12 to 13 Gy. Int J Radiat Oncol Biol Phys 2004;60: 225–230.
14 Shaw E, Scott C, Souhami L, et al: Single dose radiosurgical treatment of recurrent previously irradiated primary brain tumors and brain metastases: final report of RTOG protocol 90–05. Int J Radiat Oncol Biol Phys 2000;47:291–298.
15 Flickinger JC, Kondziolka D, Maitz AH, Lunsford LD: Gamma knife radiosurgery of imagining-diagnosed intracranial meningioma. Int J Radiation Oncology Bio Phys 2003;56:801–806.
16 Steiner L, Forster D, Leksell L, Meyerson BA, Boethius J: Gammathalamotomy in intractable pain. Acta Neurochir (Wien) 1980;52:173–184.
17 Niranjan A, Jawahar A, Kondziolka D, Lunsford LD: A comparison of surgical approaches for the management of tremor: radiofrequency thalamotomy, gamma knife thalamotomy and thalamic stimulation. Stereotact Funct Neurosurg 1999;72:178–184.
18 Shehata MK, Young B, Reid B, et al: Stereotatic radiosurgery of 468 brain metastases < or = 2 cm: implications for SRS dose and whole brain radiation therapy. Int J Radiat Oncol Biol Phys 2004;59:87–93.

John C. Flickinger, MD
Joint Radiation Oncology Center
200 Lothrop Street
Pittsburgh, PA 15213 (USA)
Fax +1 412 647 6029, E-Mail flickingerjc@upmc.edu

Szeifert GT, Kondziolka D, Levivier M, Lunsford LD (eds): Radiosurgery and Pathological Fundamentals. Prog Neurol Surg. Basel, Karger, 2007, vol 20, pp 43–49

4. Medical Physics Principles of Radiosurgery

Stéphane Simon[a,b], *Françoise Desmedt*[a,b], *Bruno Vanderlinden*[a,b], *Thierry Gevaert*[a,b], *Christophe Vandekerkhove*[b], *Anne-Sophie Grell*[b], *Marc Levivier*[a,c]

[a]Gamma Knife Center of the Université Libre de Bruxelles, [b]Department of Radiophysics, Jules Bordet Institute, [c]Department of Neurosurgery, Erasme Hospital, Brussels, Belgium

Abstract

Beside basic physical notions such as ionizing radiation, beam production and beam characteristics, this chapter will focus on two major principles that should always be considered in a radiosurgery procedure: conformity and selectivity. Those parameters are influenced by different physical beam properties, by the type of beam delivery device and by the way the dose is delivered. Conformity and selectivity should be evaluated for each treatment with the help of some specific indices, i.e. target volume ratio and normal volume ratio based on the dose-volume histograms.

Only a few months after W. Roengten's fortuitous X-ray discovery in November 1895, the first tangible physiological effect of ionizing radiation was reported in a letter written by a physicist from the Vanderbilt University in Nashville and sent to the editor of *Science*. Interestingly, it was related to a boy who was accidentally shot, received a bullet in his head and had to be operated under X-ray guidance. Although the patient did not show any sign of pain, itching or inflammation of his skin after the surgery, the hair of the large area that was close to the X-ray tube fell out suddenly 3 weeks after the exposure. Fortunately, his hair loss was only temporary and his new hair grew again normally after a few weeks [1, 2].

As a result of intensive and careless X-ray use without any kind of protection, mainly by physicians and physicists, many more accidents followed, were reported and progressively the potential cytotoxic effect of ionizing radiation was highlighted. Since then, ionizing radiation has been used as a therapeutic agent for numerous types of tumors and for benign pathologies.

Ionizing Radiation

Our world is permanently exposed to numerous types of radiation. Radiation in general can be defined as an energy that is emitted from a source and travels through a medium or through space. Heat waves, sound waves and light are some common types of radiation. The light, in particular, is part of the electromagnetic radiation spectrum, like microwaves, UV, radar waves, X-rays and gamma rays. These electromagnetic radiations can be described as the propagation of oscillating electric and magnetic fields perpendicular to each other at the speed of light (roughly 0.3 Gm/s in vacuum). The only difference between all these radiations is the amount of energy they carry. According to Planck-Einstein Law, the energy of such a radiation is given by $E(J) = h \cdot \nu$, where h is the Planck's constant ($6.62\ 10^{-34}\ J \cdot s$) and ν (s^{-1}) is the frequency at which the electromagnetic fields are oscillating. For example, the energy that light carries varies from 1.8 eV (red light) to 3.1 eV (violet light).

An ionizing radiation is defined as any radiation that has enough energy to remove an electron from an atom and thus creates a positive ion. In other words, an ionization is only possible if the radiation energy is bigger than the binding energy of the electron. This binding energy depends on both the chemical nature of the atom (namely the number of protons Z) and on the quantum shell on which the electron is located. The most inner shell (K shell) is associated with the biggest binding energy, this energy is ranging from 13.6 eV (H) to 4 KeV (Ca) in classical atoms found in tissues. In the most outer shell, where the electrons are less tightly bound to their atoms, the typical binding energy value is between 1 and 10 eV. Although a 10-eV radiation could be considered as ionizing, clinical electromagnetic radiosurgery radiation must show enough penetration, and therefore the energy used should be preferably bigger than 1 MeV. If the energy is a major factor for beam attenuation and depth dose deposition, it does not play any part in the distinction between gamma rays and X-rays. Their difference comes in fact from their production origins; gamma rays are coming from a nucleus in an excited state that gets rid of its excess energy by emitting electromagnetic radiation. X-rays have a double electronic origin, either they are produced when high-energy electrons interact with nucleus giving braking radiation (also called Bremsstrahlung), or when a shell vacancy in an ionized atom is filled by an outer shell electron or by a free electron giving characteristic X-rays. Whereas braking radiation shows a continuous energy spectrum from 0 to a maximum energy, gamma rays and characteristic X-rays have discrete energy values [3].

Beside the electromagnetic radiation, particle radiation can be also used in radiosurgery. In that process, materiel particles with very high kinetic energy are produced and will deposit their energy along their track through matter. The easiest particle to accelerate is the electron, but although it is commonly used in therapeutic beams in classical radiotherapy, electron beams are not useful in radiosurgery because they scatter too much and therefore would give significant dose outside the target volume. More useful are heavier high-energy particle beams (protons, neutrons, helium ions, carbon ions, neon ions); the protons and heavy ion beams show a drastic improvement in dose distribution compared to electromagnetic radiation; neutrons and heavy ion beams show different radiobiological properties than electromagnetic radiation [4]. However, the installations that are required to produce such beams are expensive and, as a consequence, the number of accessible facilities is limited.

Clinical Beams for Radiosurgery

Most of the clinical beams used in radiosurgery are produced either by a Cobalt (Co)-60 source or by linear accelerators.

Co-60 is a man-made radioisotope, produced by neutron activation of the naturally occurring stable Co-59. Submitted to a very high neutron flux in a nuclear reactor, Co-59 atom nuclei progressively capture a neutron and transform themselves into Co-60 atoms. This radioisotope emits a β-radiation and transforms itself into a Ni-60 atom, whose nucleus is still in an excited state. The return to the stable state is done with the liberation of two gamma rays in cascade of 1.17 and 1.33 MeV, respectively. The half-life of the Co-60 is 5.26 years and this allows a clinical use of the sources between 5 and 10 years. Because of the high doses generally given in radiosurgery, the activity required to perform the treatment in a reasonable time is in the range of 50–220 TBq (1 TBq = 10^{12} decays per second). Relatively high specific activity of Co-60 makes possible the realization of extremely high radioactive small volume sources, which is a major advantage regarding the definition of the irradiation beam.

Co-60 is the source that is currently used in Leksell Gamma Knives (201 sources of 1.11 TBq), in rotating gamma systems (30 sources of 7.4 TBq), in multiple source isocentric Cobalt units (7 sources of 37 TBq) [5].

The major advantages of Co-60 gamma rays are their reliability and output stability (once corrected for radioactive decay) which makes the quality control much easier. The disadvantages are the continuous presence of radiation, the need to change the source each 5–10 years and the obligation to manage the old source according to the local regulation for nuclear waste.

As opposed to Co-60, the linear accelerator and other similar electrical devices only produce radiation when it is needed. The principle of a linear accelerator is to accelerate electrons until they have a kinetic energy between 3–25 MeV. This acceleration is done using high-frequency electromagnetic waves that travel and combine themselves in a copper wave guide in such a way that a traveling electric field component parallel to the wave guide is created. An electron gun, connected to the wave guide, injects an electron bunch into it, and these electrons are accelerated by the traveling electric field. To convert electron kinetic energy into X-ray braking radiation, accelerated electrons are headed toward a high Z target (usually in tungsten) on the smallest possible spot. This small spot is the source from which X-rays are emitted in every space direction. The beam is then shaped according to clinical needs with different kinds of collimators.

Radiosurgery Principles

When a high precision is required to perform a target irradiation, it is recommended to deliver the treatment in stereotactic conditions. This supposes that each target point (voxel) coordinate is perfectly identified in space during treatment and imaging procedures. One common way to achieve this knowledge for a brain target is to fasten a frame rigidly on the patient's skull with pins. The frame will provide a fixed reference coordinate system applicable for any point in the brain, a fixation mean for the different target localizers (CT, MRI, angiography, PET) equipped with their specific fiducial markers and an accurate immobilized positioning during treatment and imaging procedures.

Noninvasive frame techniques are also possible provided that the patient setup is accurately checked before each treatment beam, for example by means of digital radiographs. These digital radiographs are compared with reference digitally reconstructed radiographs that are created from a CT scan. This check can be done once before the treatment if the patient is perfectly immobilized, or in life, during the treatment, with a potential on-time corrected tracking beam for possible frameless techniques.

Regardless of the stereotactic technique, the treatment is defined as radiosurgery if the total dose is delivered in a single session and as stereotactic radiotherapy when the total dose is given in multiple sessions.

In radiosurgery, it is generally not recommended to add a safety margin outside the tumor in order to define the target volume of a well-delineated lesion. This is due to the fact that a high-accuracy setup position is achieved and the fact that nearby healthy tissues should be protected as much as possible. The isodose line on which the dose is prescribed (also called the prescription isodose) should therefore match as much as possible the shape of the lesion. This matching philosophy, also known as conformity, is the first important principle in radiosurgery. Conformity can be obtained by different means depending on the technology that is used. In single isocenter treatments with a moving gantry, the conformity is improved by shaping the beam section according to the target projection with a micromultileaf collimator. This technique is called Dynamic Arc and has several advantages such as simplicity, short treatment time, smaller leakage dose to the patient, but has also the disadvantage of not being always able to build a horseshoe-shaped isodose. If such a lesion is to be treated with great conformity, the solution is either to use an intensity-modulated radiotherapy technique (nonuniform fluency-generated beams) or to perform the treatment with numerous little beams, each of them covering only a part of the target volume. Typically, this latter approach is realized with Gamma Knife, with linacs that use the multiple static noncoplanar converging arc technique (gantry moving during treatment with a beam shaped by an additional circular collimator) and with cyberknives. Isodose shaping is optimized by changing the number and position of isocenters or beams, the beam diameter and the beam weight.

Apart from the dynamic arc technique, the dose inside the target volume will not be very homogeneous. Whether or not a homogeneous dose distribution within the target must be achieved is still a debated clinical issue.

The second principle of radiosurgery is selectivity. Selectivity is achieved when there is a rapid dose fall-off outside the target area. This fall-off is influenced by the beam penumbra, beam size, mechanical stability and the number of radiation fields. The beam penumbra is usually defined for external radiation fields; it is the distance between two particular isodose lines (often 80 and 20, 100% being the dose in the center of the beam) in a plane perpendicular to the beam axis. The shorter the penumbra, the more specific could be the beam. The penumbra is shortened when the source size is small, when the collimation system is far away from the source, thick enough to avoid significant leakage radiation and focused to the beam. Unavoidable scattered radiation will, on the contrary, tend to increase the penumbra, and the scatter contribution will increase with bigger beam size and with larger depth in the patient. Furthermore, electrons set in motion in the target edge area will spread the dose outside because of their nonnegligible lateral range. This last phenomenon is influenced by the beam energy and is more pronounced for a high-energy photon beam.

The mechanical stability is also an important parameter because any unwanted deviation of the isocenter during treatment will irremediably blur the dose distribution and make the selectivity worse. Very stringent quality controls, for example the Lutz-Winston test [6–8], must therefore be performed prior to treatment for moving devices such as linear accelerators.

A multi-isocentric treatment with numerous small diameter beams is generally more specific than a one isocenter treatment with large fields because the overlap, outside the target, between larger fields is more likely to happen.

Dose-Volume Histograms and Indices

It might be a good practice to assess each radiosurgery treatment in terms of conformity and selectivity. The best way to achieve this assessment is to analyze the dose-volume histograms (DVHs). These calculations are usually provided on the treatment planning systems. The DVH is the relationship between the volume of a structure and the dose this volume is at least receiving. In other words, for a particular isodose line, the DVH gives you the structure volume (or percentage volume) that is located inside the selected isodose [9]. On DVH, the minimum dose of a structure is the largest dose for which there is still a 100% volume coverage, and the maximum dose is the smallest dose for which there is a 0% volume coverage. The difference between the two values is of course the dose range within the structure. If the difference is small, the dose is rather homogenous.

For rather inhomogeneous dose distribution treatments, such as those performed with Gamma Knife, the dose is usually prescribed on an isodose that is in real good conformity with the target volume. Users generally plan the treatment in order to have the 50% (of the maximum dose within the target) isodose line covering 100% of the target volume. Whether a 100% coverage of the target by the prescription isodose is a mandatory criterion to met is still to be assessed, especially for benign tumors for which a 95% volume coverage might be sufficient. In more homogenous dose distribution treatments, the dose is usually prescribed at the 70–80% isodose which has to cover all or almost all the target volume.

The usual way to assess the conformity is to calculate the ratio between the prescription isodose volume and the target volume called the target volume ratio (some use the inverse ratio). This ratio should be as close as possible to 1. If the ratio is much bigger than 1, it means poor conformity. However, a ratio close to 1 is not sufficient by itself to insure a good conformity because it does not tell anything about the intersection of the two volumes. A new index has been created to integrate both concepts – it is the ratio of the prescription isodose volume divided by the target volume and by the fraction of target volume coverage [10]. Doing this, the ratio value is increased when the target is not completely covered by the prescription isodose. One must bear in mind while doing these calculations that absolute volume and its location are clinically more important than the relative ratio value. Furthermore, for very tiny lesions, it is almost impossible to get the ratio close to 1 due to the minimum beam section available.

Similar calculations can be done for the selectivity parameter based on the normal brain DVH. Different ratios could be determined, defined as normal volume ratio (NVR) and equal to the volume included in an isodose value receiving a dose equal to 80, 50, 20 and 5% of the prescription dose divided by the volume of the prescription isodose. The set of values target volume ratio, NVR^{80}, NVR^{50}, NVR^{20}, NVR^{5} would make the comparison between two different dose plans easier and would be a helpful tool to document the conformity and selectivity of a radiosurgery procedure.

References

1. Koll FS: The effects of X-rays on the hair. Elect Eng 1897;23:267.
2. Eisenberg RL: Radiation Injury and Protection; in Radiology. St. Louis, Mosby Year Book, 1992, pp 156–182.
3. Khan FM: The Physics of Radiation Therapy. Philadelphia, Lippincott, Williams & Willkins, 2003.
4. Hall EJ: The particles compared. Int J Radiat Oncol Biol Phys 1982;8:2137–2140.
5. Podgorsak EB, Podgorsak MB: Stereotactic irradiation; in Van Dyk J (ed): The Modern Technology of Radiation Oncology. Madison, Medical Physics Publishing, 1999, pp 589–639.
6. Lutz W, Winston KR, Maleki N: A system for stereotactic radiosurgery with a linear accelerator. Int J Radiat Oncol Biol Phys 1988;14:373.
7. Tsai JS, Buck BA, et al: Quality assurance in stereotactic radiosurgery using a standard linear accelerator. Int J Radiat Oncol Biol Phys 1991;21:737–748.
8. American Association of Physicists in Medicine: Report 54. New York, American Institute of Physics, 1995.
9. Foote KD, et al: Radiosurgical software and dose planning; in Germano IM (ed): LINAC and Gamma Knife Radiosurgery. Park Ridge, AANS, 1999, pp 31–55.
10. Paddick I: A simple scoring ratio to index the conformity of radiosurgical treatment plans. Technical note. J Neurosurg 2000;93(suppl 3):219–222.

S. Simon
Radiophysics Department, Institut Jules Bordet
121, Boulevard de Waterloo
BE–1000 Brussels (Belgium)
Tel. +32 2 541 39 94, Fax +32 2 538 75 42, E-Mail stephane.simon@bordet.be

Szeifert GT, Kondziolka D, Levivier M, Lunsford LD (eds): Radiosurgery and Pathological Fundamentals. Prog Neurol Surg. Basel, Karger, 2007, vol 20, pp 50–67

5. Radiosurgery Techniques and Current Devices

Ajay Niranjan, A.H. Maitz, Andrew Lunsford, Peter C. Gerszten, John C. Flickinger, Douglas Kondziolka, L. Dade Lunsford

Department of Neurological Surgery, University of Pittsburgh, and Center for Image-Guided Neurosurgery, University of Pittsburgh Medical Center, Pittsburgh, Pa., USA

Abstract

Radiosurgery is a minimally invasive technique designed to elicit a specific radiobiologic response at the target tissue using focused ionizing radiation delivered in single procedure. Radiosurgery was originally devised to treat intracranial lesions by delivering a high dose of radiation precisely at the intracranial target using stereotactic guidance. The term was coined and the field defined by Lars Leksell, a visionary leader of neurosurgery at the Karolinska Institute in Stockholm. Refinements in stereotactic methodologies, major improvements in dose planning software, and advances in neurodiagnostic imaging, all facilitated the increasingly broad application of brain radiosurgical methodologies. New technologies have continued to evolve and are still emerging. A variety of different radiosurgery techniques have been developed during the past 4 decades. Radiosurgery is now being used even for extracranial lesions such as spinal tumors, lung, liver, and prostate pathologies. Numerous studies have examined the benefits and risks of radiosurgery performed with various devices. The long-term results of radiosurgery are now available and have established it as an effective noninvasive management strategy for many brain disorders. Radiosurgery is now considered a mainstream neurosurgical modality for treatment of vascular malformations, tumors, trigeminal neuralgia, movement disorders, and perhaps epilepsy. Its role as a tool for spine and body surgery is also under evaluation.

Historical Review

Gamma Knife Radiosurgery

Prof. Lars Leksell first coupled an orthovoltage X-ray tube with his first-generation guiding device to focus radiation on the gasserian ganglion to treat facial pain. He subsequently investigated crossfired protons as well as X-rays from an early-generation linear accelerator (LINAC) for radiosurgery. In the 1960s, he became dissatisfied with the cumbersome nature of crossfired proton beams and remained thoroughly dissatisfied with the unreliability and wobble of then existing LINACs. Leksell and Larsson finally selected Cobalt-60 as the ideal photon radiation source and developed the Gamma Knife [1, 2]. They placed 179 Co-60 sources in a hemispherical array so that all gamma rays (radiation from the decay of Co-60) focused to a single point thereby creating cumulative radiation volume of variable diameter depending on the beam diameter. The first Gamma Knife was designed to create a discoid-shaped lesion suitable for neurosurgical treatment of movement disorders and intractable pain [3, 4]. Clinical work with the Gamma Knife began in 1967 at the manufacturing site, the Motala AB workshop in Linköping, Sweden. The first patient had a craniopharyngioma. The patient's head was immobilized using a plaster-molded headpiece. In 1975, a series of surgical pioneers in Stockholm began to utilize a reengineered Gamma Knife (spheroidal lesion) for the treatment of intracranial tumors and vascular malformations. Units 3 and 4 were placed in Buenos Aires, Argentina, and Sheffield, UK, in the early 1980s. Lunsford's group introduced the first clinical 201-source Gamma Knife unit to North America (the fifth gamma unit worldwide). Lunsford first performed Gamma Knife radiosurgery in August, 1987 at University of Pittsburgh Medical Center [5]. In the US, based on the available published literature, AVMs and skull base tumors that had failed other treatments were considered the initial indications for radiosurgery. A cautious approach was adopted while waiting for increased scientific documentation. The encouraging results of radiosurgery for benign tumors and vascular malformations led to an exponential rise in radiosurgery cases and sales of radiosurgical units. In recent years, metastatic brain tumors have become the most common indication of radiosurgery. Brain metastases now comprise 30–50% of radiosurgery cases at busy centers.

Charged-Particle Radiosurgery

Initial experiments with protons for irradiation of deep-seated targets were performed in the early 1950s using a synchrocyclotron at the Lawrence Livermore Laboratory, Berkeley, Calif., USA. Larsson's group in Uppsala, Sweden, crossfired a 185-MeV proton beam to make small, circumscribed radiation-induced lesions in experimental animals. The first treatment of an intracranial tumor by irradiation with the Bragg peak radiation was carried out in 1957. Beginning in 1958, proton beam irradiation was used to perform functional surgery in patients with advanced Parkinson's disease. In 1961, Kjellberg began performing stereotactic Bragg-peak radiation in a single session, using the 165-MeV proton beam facility in Cambridge, Mass., USA. Their first AVM irradiation was in 1965. Although originally constructed for basic scientific research, these cyclotron units were subsequently reengineered for human use [6–10]. In the US, only few units are currently operational (Loma Linda University Medical Center, Loma Linda, California and Northeast Proton Therapy Center, Massachusetts General Hospital, Boston).

LINAC Radiosurgery

LINACs were developed simultaneously in the US as well as in Britain in the 1950s and became the preferred devices for conventional fractionated photon radiation. LINACs are devices where electrons are accelerated to nearly the speed of light and directed to a metal plate. The resulting interactions produce X-rays, which are aimed at a biological target. Leksell and coworkers at the Karolinska Institute first explored the concept of radiosurgery using a LINAC. The idea was dropped due to low photon energies and the high mechanical inaccuracies of the early machines.

The pioneering work of many researchers in the 1980s led to the gradual modifications of newly redesigned LINACs for use as radiosurgery system. LINAC technologies were modified by incorporating improved guiding (stereotactic) devices and methods to measure accuracy of dose delivery [11–20]. More than 200 such modified LINAC systems are believed to be operating in hospitals across the US, although the frequency of their use for radiosurgery is unknown.

Current Radiosurgical Techniques

Gamma Knife (Models A, B, C, 4-C, and PFX®)

The Gamma Knife has evolved steadily since 1967 [21, 22]. Three commercially produced models are now used worldwide. In the first models (Model U or A) 201 Cobalt sources were arranged in hemispherical array. These units present challenging Cobalt-60 loading and reloading issues. To eliminate this problem, the unit was redesigned so that sources were arranged in a circular (O-ring) configuration (Model B). Gamma Knife radiosurgery usually involves multiple isocenters of different beam diameters to achieve a treatment plan that conforms to the irregular 3-dimensional volumes of most lesions. The total number of isocenters may vary from one to any number greater than one, depending upon the size, shape, and location. The most frequent range of isocenters varies from 8 to 12 per patient. Each isocenter has a set of three X, Y, Z stereotactic coordinates corresponding to its location in three-dimensional (3D) space with respect to the stereotactic frame. In terms of actual dose delivery, this means several changes in the patient's head position within the helmet. In

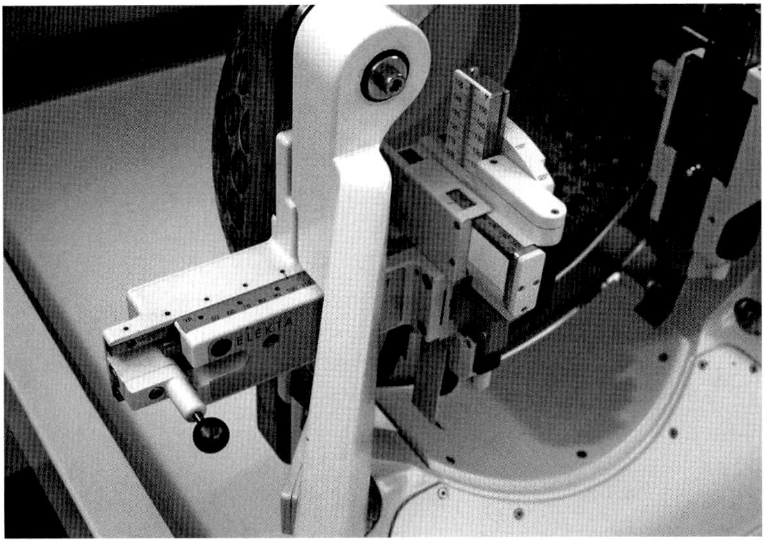

Fig. 1. APS for patient robotic coordinate movement.

1999, the Model C Gamma Knife was introduced. The first Model C in the United States was installed at the University of Pittsburgh Medical Center in March 2000 [23]. This technology combines advances in dose planning with robotic engineering and uses a submillimeter accuracy automated positioning system (APS) in most patients. This obviates the need to manually adjust each set of coordinates in a multiple-isocenter plan. The robotic positioning system (fig. 1) moves the patient's head to the target coordinates defined in the treatment plan. The robot eliminates the time spent removing the patient from the helmet, setting the new coordinates for each isocenter and repositioning the patient in the helmet. This has significantly reduced the total time spent to complete the treatment. Because the treatment time is shortened, a precise 3D plan can be generated using multiple smaller beams. Such an approach results in a steeper dose fall off extending from the target. The other features of the Model C unit include an integral helmet changer, dedicated helmet installation trolleys, and color-coded collimators. In 2005, the fourth generation Leksell Gamma Knife Model 4-C was introduced. The first unit was installed at the University of Pittsburgh in January of 2005 (fig. 2). The Model 4-C is equipped with enhancements designed to improve workflow, increase accuracy and provide integrated imaging capabilities. The integrated imaging, powered by Leksell GammaPlan®, offers ability to fuse images from multiple sources. These images can also be exported on a CD-ROM, so the referring physician can receive pre- or postoperative images for reference and follow-up. The planning

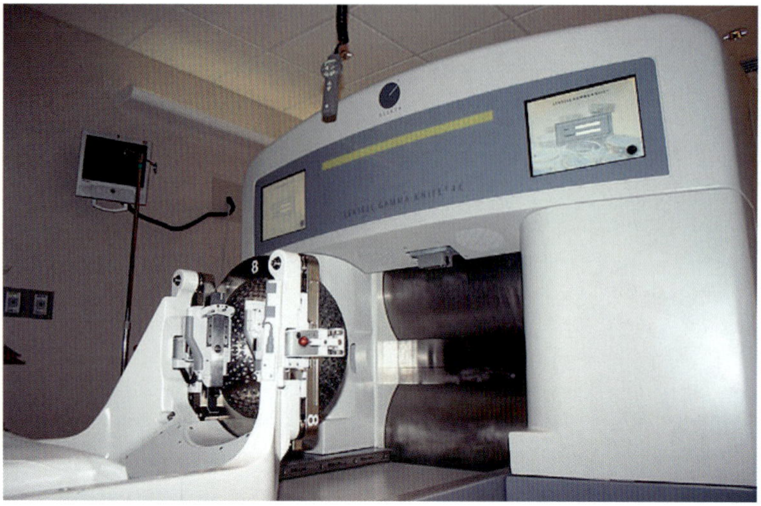

Fig. 2. Model 4-C gamma unit.

information can be viewed on both sides of the treatment couch. The helmet changer and robotic Automatic Positioning System® are faster and reduce total treatment time.

The latest model Leksell Gamma Knife® PERFEXION® was released in 2006. The design of LGK-PFX® allows expanded cranial reach, automatic collimator changes, and automatic beam blocking. LGK-PFX® is equipped with advanced dose planning software that allows composite shots, dynamic shaping, and remote access.

Rotating Gamma System

Recently, a derivative radiosurgery device called the Rotating Gamma System (RGS) has been developed. The RGS (OUR International Inc., Shenzen, China) utilizes 30 Cobalt-60 radiation sources. The radiation sources in the RGS are contained in a revolving hemispherical shell. The secondary collimator is a coaxial hemispheric shell that has six groups of five collimator holes arranged in the same fashion as the radiation sources. By selecting a particular group of collimator holes that can be aligned with the radiation sources, different beam diameters can be achieved. This obviates the need to change helmets manually. The experience with such system is limited. Recently an American-based company American Radiosurgery Inc. of San Diego, Calif, began manufacturing, sales, and marketing of this device.

LINAC-Based Radiosurgery

In LINAC-based radiosurgery, multiple radiation arcs of photons are utilized to crossfire X-rays at a target defined in 3D space. Most of the presently functioning systems use nondynamic techniques in which the patient couch is set at a fixed angle and the head of the LINAC is moved around the patient. The radiation beams enter the skull through these different arcs. In dynamic techniques, both the couch and the arc radiation delivery system move to shape the target volume. The development of dedicated accelerators has improved the accuracy and precision of dose delivery, but at greater cost. Multiple positions are needed for a truly conformal dose distribution. Different techniques and dose planning software have also been developed to enhance conformity of dose planning and delivery using LINAC-based systems. These include beam shaping and intensity modulation radiation therapy. Newer developments include introduction of jaws, noncircular, mini- and microleaf collimators. Single isocenter radiosurgery is now possible with newer LINAC-based systems. The conformal beam can be delivered with the micromultileaf collimation or conformal blocks. Micromultileaf collimation consists of multiple individually motorized tungsten 'leaves' that shape a treatment field. Many LINAC-based systems such as XKnife® (Radionics Inc., Burlington, Mass., USA), Linear Accelerator Scalpel™ (Zmed Inc., Ashland, Mass., USA), Novalis® (BrainLAB, Heimstetten, Germany), the Peacock System® (NOMOS Corp., Sewickley, Pa., USA), and CyberKnife® (Accuray Inc., Sunnyvale, Calif., USA) are commercially available.

The Peacock system (NOMOS Corporation, Sewickley, Pa., USA) uses inverse treatment planning and multileaf wedge-generated intensity modulated beams to increase target conformity using fractionated technology. The CyberKnife, combines X-ray beams, computers, imaging, and robotic technology for target localization and radiation delivery. This system utilizes a 6-MeV LINAC attached to a six-axis robotic manipulator (fig. 3). The robot positions the LINAC at different beam positions always aiming the center of the radiation beam at the target. A stereotactic frame is not used for targeting. Before the radiation is delivered from any position, the patient's movements are tracked using an integrated X-ray image processing system, which consists of two orthogonal diagnostic X-ray cameras and an optical tracking system. During CyberKnife treatment, the image processing system acquires X-ray images of the patient's body multiple times throughout the treatment, and the software compares the actual images with the images in a database to determine the direction and amount of any motion. The information regarding the new location is delivered to the robot, which corrects for the motion and then delivers radiation. Patients often receive fractionated treatments. Technical aspects of Gamma Knife and CyberKnife radiosurgery are compared in table 1.

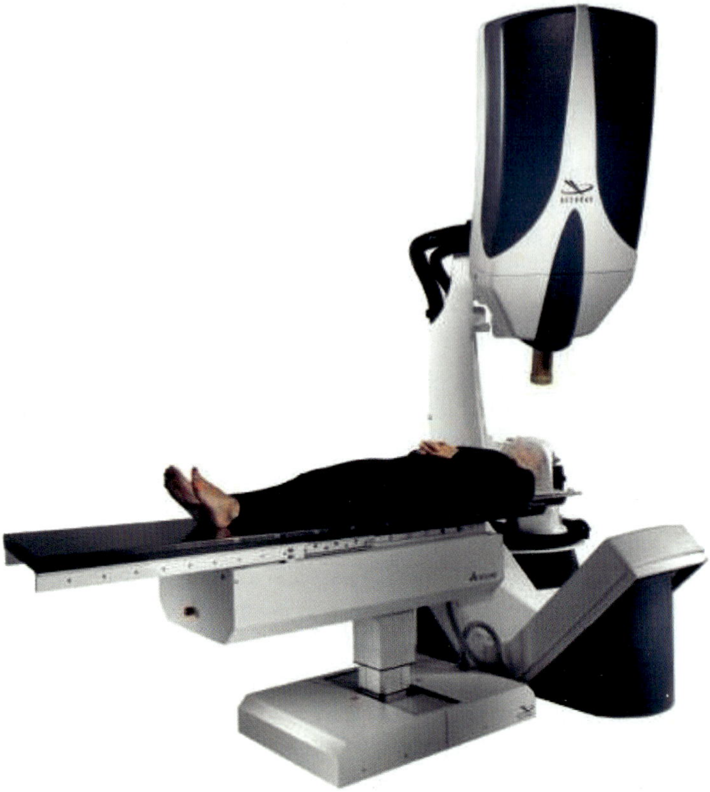

Fig. 3. CyberKnife.

Charged Particle Radiosurgery

This radiosurgery approach uses either the Bragg-peak method where charged particles stop within the target volume or the plateau-beam method in which deposition of the charged particles energy is spread across the target [24]. These facilities are only available at a limited number of centers due to the high cost of equipment and maintenance. The estimated cost of building a dedicated medical proton-beam treatment facility is approximately USD 40 million. In addition, significant maintenance costs and dedicated radiation physicists are required to assure continuous quality control. In the US, at present only few proton facilities are available (Loma Linda University Medical Center, Loma Linda, California and Northeast Proton Therapy Center,

Table 1. A comparison of Gamma Knife and CyberKnife radiosurgery

	Gamma Knife	CyberKnife
Patient selection	intracranial targets	intracranial and body targets
Target localization	rigid stereotactic frame	mask or fiducials
Imaging	MRI, CT, DSA, PET	CT
Target identification	by surgeon	by surgeon or oncologist
Dose planning	mostly by surgeon	mostly by physicist
Patient positioning	robotic positioning of head in a collimator helmet	robotic positioning of LINAC around the patient
Dose delivery	201 Co-60 beams	light-weight LINAC
Radiation	1.25-MeV photons	6-MV photons
Accuracy	0.3 mm	0.7 mm
Treatment time	single day procedure (frame placement, imaging, dose planning, radiation delivery)	multiple day procedure (fiducial placement or mask preparation, imaging, dose planning and treatment)

Massachusetts General Hospital, Boston). Most patients are treated with fractionated radiation therapy.

Spinal and Body Radiosurgery

Radiosurgery for spinal tumors and other body tumors is a relatively new concept. The movement of these targets with respiration has been the main concern for precise radiation delivery. In the last few years, researchers have developed spine and body stabilization systems. The indications of extracranial radiosurgery include spinal tumors, primary and secondary hepatic and thoracic tumors. Frameless stereotactic localization (used in CyberKnife) appears to be applicable to spine and body radiosurgery. At the University of Pittsburgh, more than 400 patients with spine and soft tissue tumors have been treated with the CyberKnife (fig. 3) [25, 26]. The concept of radiosurgery outside the brain and skull seems more promising with these developments [27–30]. Elekta Axesse® is a recent addition to the body radiosurgery systems. In Synergy, a LINAC is integrated with a suite of advanced imaging tools, specifically designed for image-guided radiation delivery. The intraoperative 3D CT imaging is used to visualize internal structures, including soft tissues within the reference frame of the treatment system at the time of treatment. This will eliminate the possibility of target movement between planning on a CT scanner and treatment on a LINAC as well as inter- or intra-fraction movement whilst the patient is undergoing treatment.

Radiosurgery Team

Radiosurgery is a multidisciplinary field, which involves coordinated input from neurosurgeons, radiation oncologists, medical physicists, and engineers. The knowledge of brain anatomy, understanding of brain pathologies, and the ability to choose among the available treatment options gives the neurosurgeon a decisive role as leader of the brain and spine radiosurgical team. The goal of radiosurgery differs from that of the conventional neurosurgery since the target is not physically removed after exposure to the radiation. The target is not destroyed immediately but instead is exposed to a single high dose of radiation, which ultimately translates into a specific (toxic) radiobiological response delivered to the target volume. Radiosurgery is based on the same fundamental principles that are used in stereotactic neurosurgery. For neurosurgeons, experienced in stereotactic surgery, radiosurgery is a logical addition to an arsenal of conventional surgical tools. Radiation oncologists also have an important role to play in patient selection as well as dose selection. Dose selection is based on many variables such as previous exposure to radiation, existing neurological deficits, and the functional significance of the surrounding tissue and its radiobiological tolerance. The medical physicist has an equally important role by assuming the responsibility of quality assurance of the technology, radiation delivery, verification of the dose planning system accuracy, dose planning, safety training and licensing issues inherent to radiosurgery. Strict quality control of the brain or body images is a crucial part of accurate targeting and regular checks of the imaging sets are necessary in order to maintain the accuracy of radiation delivery.

Terms Used for Radiosurgery

The evolution of new methods has contributed to significant confusion in the use of terminology. The term stereotactic radiosurgery (SRS) is used for stereotactically guided delivery of focused radiation to a defined target volume in a single surgical session. Radiosurgery is the application of the stereotactic frame followed by intraoperative imaging, dose planning, dose delivery, and frame removal, in such a way that the entire treatment is performed in a single session. SRS can be performed using Gamma Knife, LINAC-based systems, or Proton beam-based systems.

Some stereotactic radiosurgical procedures, in order to optimize results and reduce risks, are performed in a staged fashion, in a similar way that neurosurgical procedure sometimes is performed in two stages to remove, for example, a large skull base tumor. Staged SRS refers to stereotactically guided delivery of focused radiation to the defined target volume in a two or more sessions using rigid frame fixation. Prospectively staged (volume staging) radiosurgery may be used for large lesions where sufficient margin dose cannot be given in a single session due to large lesion volume. Staging often involves intervals of 3 or more months.

Although by definition 'radiosurgery' is a single radiation delivery procedure, some centers erroneously use the term 'fractionated stereotactic radiosurgery' loosely to include treatments involving radiation delivery in 5 or more consecutive sessions (dose staging). Stereotactic radiation therapy or fractionated stereotactic radiation therapy (FSRT) refers to the delivery of a standard fractionation scheme of radiation with a rigidly applied or relocatable stereotactic guiding device. The procedures are done in order to optimize the potential benefit of the radiobiology of certain tumors, or to reduce the risk to adjacent brain or critical structures. The principle of FSRT is quite different from radiosurgery. The rationale of using fractionation is that normal (late responding) tissues better tolerate many smaller radiation doses, but the tumor (fast-responding tissue) cannot due to rapid cell division. Normal tissues cannot tolerate single large treatments (unless the dose fall off in normal tissues is sharp). Fractionation seeks to take advantage of this difference between normal brain tissue and rapidly growing tumor cells. Whether done with LINACs, proton facilities, or other radiation dose delivery techniques, FSRT is performed in order to reduce the risks associated with radiation fall-off in surrounding normal tissues adjacent to the targeted tissue. The role of radiosurgical, hyperfractionated radiation therapy using image guidance, and conventional fractionated radiation, continue to be studied.

Radiosurgery Procedure

Following are the basic steps to the SRS procedure regardless of the method of delivery.

1. Daily quality assurance of radiosurgery system.
2. Application of the stereotactic guiding device to the patient's head.
3. Stereotactic brain imaging using an MRI, a CT scan, and/or an angiogram.
4. Quality assurance of images.
5. Determination of target volume(s).
6. Conformal radiosurgery dose planning by radiosurgery team.
7. Stereotactic delivery of radiation to the target volume by positioning the patient's head inside a collimator helmet (Gamma Knife), or on treatment couch (LINAC-based systems).

Although these steps are common to all the radiosurgery systems, there are specific procedures that are used with different systems. The specific techniques of SRS, fractionated stereotactic radiosurgery, or FSRT used with proton beam-based systems or LINAC-based systems, shaped beam radiosurgery, or CyberKnife radiosurgery are discussed in the appropriate chapters. In the following section, the techniques used with Gamma Knife radiosurgery are discussed.

Daily Quality Assurance of Radiosurgery System

Gamma Knife quality assurance testing is performed by an authorized medical physicist or his/her equivalent every morning. Medical physicist ensures that the system tests required by regulation are performed and functioning properly. These tests include the permanently mounted radiation monitor and its remote indicator, hand-held radiation monitor, patient viewing and communication systems, door interlock, timer termination of exposure, emergency stops, beam status indicators, availability of the release rods for the emergency removal of a patient, test run of the automatic patient positioning unit, microswitch test and function of the helmet hoist. Apart from daily quality assurance tests, monthly and annual quality assurance is also performed in addition to preventative maintenance of the Gamma Knife unit.

Application of the Stereotactic Guiding Device

For Gamma Knife radiosurgery, appropriate frame placement is the initial critical aspect of the procedure. Prior to frame placement, the radiosurgery team should review the preoperative images and discuss optimal frame placement strategy. The preoperative images should be kept in plain view while applying the head frame. An effort should be made to keep the lesion as close to the center of the frame as possible. The possibility of collision by the frame base ring, the post/pin assembly or the patient's scalp with the collimator helmet during treatment should also be considered prior to the frame application. Steps to avoid the possible collision should be taken during frame placement. The authors use the following strategies for optimal frame placement.

To target lower lesions (skull base tumors, acoustic tumors, cerebellar lesions), the frame is positioned lower by placing the ear bars in the top holes of the earpieces on the Leksell G frame. For higher lesions (sagittal sinus meningioma, metastases high in the frontal or parietal lobe), the frame is positioned higher by placing the ear bars in the bottom holes of the earpieces. For anterior targets (anterior frontal lobe tumors, cavernous sinus tumors, sellar lesion and lesion anterior to sella, anterior temporal lesion), the frame is shifted forward by placing ear pieces posteriorly on the base ring of the frame. The posterior edge of ear piece is kept at 90–75 mm on the Y-dimension of the head frame (instead of 95–100) depending upon the shift that is needed to bring the lesion closest to the center of the frame. Short posterior posts are preferred (to avoid collision of the posterior post/pin assembly with the collimator helmet). An extension gamma angle (e.g. 72°) is used during the radiation delivery. To target posterior-located lesions (occipital lobe tumors, transverse sinus tumor, cerebellar lesions), the frame is shifted backward by positioning the earpieces forward. The posterior edge of the ear-piece is kept at 110–125 mm instead of 95–100 mm. The anterior posts are positioned as low as possible on the supraorbital region to avoid collision of frontal post/pin assembly with the collimator helmet. For radiosurgery planning, a steeper gamma angle (120–140°) is used if a collision is detected at the default angle of 90°. To reach lateral targets (lateral metastases, convexity tumors, far lateral tumors), the frame is shifted laterally (right or left) toward the lesion. While shifting frame laterally, it is important to make sure that there is enough space on the contralateral side to allow positioning of the fiducial box on the base ring of the frame. The MRI fiducial should be tried on frame prior to sending the patient to the MRI unit. If the fiducial box does not fit on to the frame due to excessive shifting of the frame, the frame will have to be repositioned.

Techniques of Stereotactic Imaging

Aside from the frame application, the next most important aspect of radiosurgery is the imaging of the target. The accuracy of the procedure can only be as accurate as the least accurate aspect of all of the steps of the procedure. Generally, this occurs in the imaging phase. No matter which imaging method is used, the imaging (related to the pixel size of ~0.5 mm) accuracy is less than the accuracy of the Gamma Knife machine (≤0.4 mm).

Stereotactic MRI

The highlights of stereotactic imaging include optimal contrast between normal and abnormal tissues in addition to high spatial resolution, short scan time and thin slices so that accurate target localization can be achieved. The use of MRI in stereotactic planning has enhanced accurate targeting of lesions that are usually not adequately defined by any other imaging modality. Some physicians prefer the fusion of MR and CT images for stereotactic guidance as they believe that in certain type of scanners distortion may affect the accuracy of target localization in MR imaging. For the initial 2 years, authors used both MRI and CT for stereotactic planning. Significant target coordinate differences were not observed using the Leksell stereotactic system. Since 1993, MRI has been used for SRS planning in almost all eligible cases using a 1.5-tesla unit. In addition, arteriovenous malformations (AVMs) are imaged also by biplane angiography [31].

At our institution high-resolution, gadolinium-enhanced T_1-weighted sagittal scout images using spin echo pulse sequence are obtained first. These 3-mm-thick slices with 1-mm gap are used to localize ('Scout') the area of interest. The average time for this sequence is approximately 1.5 min. For stereotactic imaging of most lesions, a 3D-volume acquisition using Fast Spoiled-Gradient Recalled Acquisition in Steady State sequence at 512 × 256 matrix and 2 NEX (number of excitations) covering the entire lesion and surrounding critical structures is preferred. To define the radiosurgery target, this volume is displayed as 1- or 1.5-mm-thick axial slices. The field of view is kept at 25 × 25 cm in order to visualize all fiducials. The approximate imaging time for this sequence is 5–6 min.

We generally prefer Spoiled-Gradient Recalled Acquisition in Steady State sequence for most lesions. Additional sequences are performed when more information is needed. Pituitary lesions are particularly difficult to image especially if there has been prior surgery. A half dose of contrast is usually given to image pituitary adenomas. For residual pituitary tumors, after trans-sphenoid resection, a fat suppression SPGR sequence is recommended in order to differentiate tumor from the fat packed in the resection cavity. For cavernous malformations, an additional variable echo multiplaner imaging is obtained to define the hemosiderin rim. For thalamotomy planning, an additional fast inversion recovery sequence is performed to differentiate basal ganglia from white matter tracts. Brain metastases patients receive a double dose of contrast agent and the entire brain is imaged by 2-mm slices to identify all of the lesions. Before removing the patients from the MR scanner, the images must be checked for accuracy.

Stereotactic CT Imaging

When using CT imaging instead of MRI, it is advisable to use short posterior posts to avoid artifacts from the posts and pins. Care should also be taken in deciding the optimal place for the pins since they cause artifacts on CT. An effort should be made to keep the lesion away from the pin artifacts. With modern CT scanners, 1- or 2-mm-thick slices (depending upon the size of the lesion) without any gap can be obtained in 4–5 min. Before removing the patients from the CT table, accuracy checks are performed to make sure that images would be accepted by planning system and the lesions have coordinates that are achievable in the Gamma Knife unit.

Stereotactic Angiography

Angiography is the gold standard for AVM radiosurgery planning. It should be used in conjunction with MR or CT imaging to provide the third imaging dimension. The technique of angiography differs slightly from the conventional digital angiography as the stereotactic angiographic images are used not only for AVM nidus definition but also to guide radiation to the target. The orthogonal images (instead of oblique or rotated) are preferred but not necessary. For AVM nidi that are not properly visualized in orthogonal planes, a rotation of up to 10° in two dimensions or aspects can be used without compromising the accuracy of radiation delivery [32]. Before removing the angiography catheter, the images should be reviewed to make sure that all the fiducials are seen on the images. Digital subtraction techniques, despite a potential radial distortion error, have proven satisfactory.

Quality Assurance of Images

Regular quality control checks of the MRI unit are performed in order to maintain accuracy of images. With a properly shimmed magnet, regular servicing, and strict quality assurance on the unit as well as on the images, MRI provides high-resolution images with accurate target localization. A special frame holder is used in order to avoid head movement during MRI. Accuracy of images is checked for each image sequence by comparing the known frame measurement with image measurements in addition to the distance from the end fiducials to the middle fiducials. The images are exported from Imaging Suite via the Ethernet. Images are defined using GammaPlan software (LGP) after the images are transferred to the LGP computer. The measurements are again checked and compared with the known frame measurement and also the distance to the middle fiducial in order to check for any distortion during image transfer.

Determination of Target Volume

Target determination is an important step in order to make a conformal plan. Experienced surgeons can make conformal gamma plans without outlining the target. However, for new centers especially where the physicist has the responsibility of planning, target definition and outlining by surgeon or oncologist becomes an important step. Surgeon's input is especially helpful in defining radiosurgery targets for patients with AVMs and partially resected tumors. Defining the target volume also helps in calculating the conformality index. Treatment volume can be outlined using the GammaPlan software (manual or semiautomatic mode).

Techniques of Conformal Dose Planning

In the process of treatment planning, several strategies can be used. The Model C allows treatment using automatic patient positioning system (APS mode), manual positioning (trunnion mode) or mixed treatment (some isocenters in the APS mode and some in the trunnion mode). A different approach would be used if only a trunnion treatment plan was possible versus an APS treatment plan. Universally, in LGP (Leksell GammaPlan), one can start planning from the middle of the target and then move to the top and bottom of the target. Another approach is to start at the bottom or top and build from the starting point. Some physicians prefer to outline the target volume before planning the treatment volume. Beginners can also use the inverse dose planning algorithm (Wizard®) to create a plan and then optimize it manually. When planning a treatment using trunnions only, one might tend to use larger collimators (especially for larger lesions) to reduce the time and maximize coverage of the target. For example, for an acoustic tumor, in the trunnion mode, one might use a few 14-mm collimators for the majority of the tumor and few a 4-mm collimators for the intracanalicular portion of the tumor. In the APS mode, however, one would most likely use multiple 8-mm isocenters for the majority of the tumor and 4-mm isocenters for the intracanalicular portion since the total time spent would be less. There would be no need to go into the treatment room to set each isocenter. As long as the isocenters are in close proximity to one another, the software would automatically put them into the same treatment run and the patient would move from one set of coordinates to the next until all isocenters of one collimator size were treated. The conformal dose planning is enhanced by the use of multiple small collimators.

There are other tricks to use in planning such as using a steep (125°) gamma angle for posterior lesions (cerebellar or occipital). Another technique available for single isocenter lesions is to match the gamma angle to the angle of the target. This trick is only available for treatment using the trunnion mode should the angle of the target not match 72, 90, 110 or 125°. In the APS mode, during the setup phase of planning, the idea is to try to group as many isocenters in the same run as possible, even if it means changing all of the isocenters to high docking or a different gamma angle than the default of 90°. If a different gamma angle is used, the plan must be rechecked for accuracy and adjusted if necessary. In the current version of LGP, multiple targets (multiple tumors) can be treated using different isodose prescription and different central doses with the use of multiple matrices.

Techniques of Stereotactic Radiation Delivery Using Gamma Knife

The Model C Gamma Knife allows radiation delivery using the trunnion mode (manual patient positioning) or the APS mode (robotic positioning) or a combination of the two (mixed treatment). In trunnion treatment, the x, y, and z of each isocenter are set manually and double checked to avoid errors. The same coordinates and the time obtained from LGP are entered into the control console and treatment is administered. The APS plan is transferred directly from the planning computer to the control computer. The operator selects the run (a combination of isocenters of same beam diameter) that matches the collimator helmet on the gamma unit. The APS is moved to the dock position and the patient's head frame is fixed into the APS. The accuracy of the docking position is checked. The system prompts the user to perform clearance checks first for all those planned isocenters in which the pins, posts, frame or patient scalp would be less than 12 mm away from the inner surface of the collimator helmet (even though they may not match with the collimator size which is being used for the first run). The clearance check is performed moving the patient to those positions by using APS manual control and observing for the possibility of collision with the helmet. After the clearance check, the system prompts the user to carry out position checks. In the position checks, all the isocenters using the same helmet are checked, one by one, by moving the patient's head to these positions using APS manual control.

The team moves out after the position checks are completed, and the treatment is administered. The APS moves the patient to all the planned positions, one by one, until the treatment using that size collimator helmet is completed. The team monitors the patient and the coordinates of different isocenters on the control computer. If other treatment runs using a different gamma angle but using the same helmet are planned, then the patient is taken out, next run is selected, APS is moved to the dock position and the patient's head is again fixed in the APS using the planned angle (72, 90, 110, or 125°). Position checks are performed, and treatment is begun. Similarly, if additional treatment runs using different helmets are planned, the helmet is changed, patient's head is positioned in the APS, the position checks for all the isocenters for that helmet and gamma angle are performed and the treatment is begun. Performing all the planned treatment runs completes the treatment.

Conclusion

Great progress has been made in the past 15 years both in the hardware for SRS and in the software for all methods of delivery of the radiation prescribed. Available now are better image handling features including image fusion, faster more compact platforms that make the calculations almost real time, automated patient positioning, thus reducing the potential for human error, and the inception of inverse treatment planning. Expected in the future are better, more accurate imaging techniques and software handling of those images, and advances in inverse treatment planning for all modes of delivery in the hope that this progress will provide better treatment resulting in better patient outcomes.

References

1 Lunsford LD: Lars Leksell. Notes at the side of a raconteur. Stereotact Funct Neurosurg 1996;67:153–168.

2 Ammar A: Lars Leksell's vision – radiosurgery. Acta Neurochirurgica Suppl 1994;62:1–4.

3 Leksell L: Cerebral radiosurgery. I. Gammathalanotomy in two cases of intractable pain. Acta Chirurgica Scandinavica 1968;134:585–595.
4 Leksell L: Sterotaxic radiosurgery in trigeminal neuralgia. Acta Chirurgica Scandinavica 1971;137:311–314.
5 Niranjan A, Lunsford LD: Radiosurgery: where we were, are, and may be in the third millennium. Neurosurgery 2000;46:531–543 [see comment].
6 Fabrikant JI, Lyman JT, Hosobuchi Y: Stereotactic heavy-ion Bragg peak radiosurgery for intracranial vascular disorders: method for treatment of deep arteriovenous malformations. Br J Radiol 1984;57:479–490.
7 Fabrikant JI, Lyman JT, Frankel KA: Heavy charged-particle Bragg peak radiosurgery for intracranial vascular disorders. Radiat Res Suppl 1985;8:S244–S258.
8 Kjellberg RN: Stereotactic Bragg peak proton beam radiosurgery for cerebral arteriovenous malformations. Ann Clin Res 1986;18(suppl 47):17–19.
9 Lyman JT, Kanstein L, Yeater F, Fabrikant JI, Frankel KA: A helium-ion beam for stereotactic radiosurgery of central nervous system disorders. Med Phys 1986;13:695–699.
10 Griffin BR, Warcola SH, Mayberg MR, Eenmaa J, Eskridge J, Winn HR: Stereotactic neutron radiosurgery for arteriovenous malformations of the brain. Med Dosim 1988;13:179–182.
11 Colombo F, Benedetti A, Pozza F, Zanardo A, Avanzo RC, Chierego G, Marchetti C: Stereotactic radiosurgery utilizing a linear accelerator. Appl Neurophysiol 1985;48:133–145.
12 Lutz W, Winston KR, Maleki N: A system for stereotactic radiosurgery with a linear accelerator. Int J Radiat Oncol Biol Phys 1988;14:373–381.
13 Loeffler JS, Alexander E 3rd, Siddon RL, Saunders WM, Coleman CN, Winston KR: Stereotactic radiosurgery for intracranial arteriovenous malformations using a standard linear accelerator. Int J Radiat Oncol Biol Phys 1989;17:673–677.
14 Saunders WM, Winston KR, Siddon RL, Svensson GH, Kijewski PK, Rice RK, Hansen JL, Barth NH: Radiosurgery for arteriovenous malformations of the brain using a standard linear accelerator: rationale and technique. Int J Radiat Oncol Biol Phys 1988;15:441–447.
15 Betti OO, Munari C, Rosler R: Stereotactic radiosurgery with the linear accelerator: treatment of arteriovenous malformations. Neurosurgery 1989;24:311–321.
16 Colombo F: Linear accelerator radiosurgery. A clinical experience. J Neurosurg Sci 1989;33: 123–125.
17 Friedman WA, Bova FJ: The University of Florida radiosurgery system. Surg Neurol 1989;32:334–342.
18 Patil AA: Radiosurgery with the linear accelerator. Neurosurgery 1989;25:143.
19 Hamilton AJ, Lulu BA: A prototype device for linear accelerator-based extracranial radiosurgery. Acta Neurochirurgica Suppl 1995;63:40–43.
20 Winston KR, Lutz W: Linear accelerator as a neurosurgical tool for stereotactic radiosurgery. Neurosurgery 1988;22:454–464.
21 Lunsford LD, Flickinger J, Lindner G, Maitz A: Stereotactic radiosurgery of the brain using the first United States 201 cobalt-60 source gamma knife. Neurosurgery 1989;24:151–159.
22 Coffey RJ, Lunsford LD: Stereotactic radiosurgery using the 201 cobalt-60 source gamma knife. Neurosurg Clin N Am 1990;1:933–954.
23 Kondziolka D, Maitz AH, Niranjan A, Flickinger JC, Lunsford LD: An evaluation of the Model C gamma knife with automatic patient positioning. Neurosurgery 2002;50:429–431; discussion 431–422.
24 Harsh G, Loeffler JS, Thornton A, Smith A, Bussiere M, Chapman PH: Stereotactic proton radiosurgery. Neurosurg Clin N Am 1999;10:243–256.
25 Gerszten PC, Welch WC: Cyberknife radiosurgery for metastatic spine tumors. Neurosurg Clin N Am 2004;15:491–501.
26 Gerszten PC, Ozhasoglu C, Burton SA, Vogel WJ, Atkins BA, Kalnicki S, Welch WC: CyberKnife frameless stereotactic radiosurgery for spinal lesions: clinical experience in 125 cases. Neurosurgery 2004;55:89–98; discussion 98–89.
27 Adler JR Jr, Chang SD, Murphy MJ, Doty J, Geis P, Hancock SL: The Cyberknife: a frameless robotic system for radiosurgery. Stereotact Funct Neurosurg 1997;69(pt 2):124–128.
28 Ponsky LE, Crownover RL, Rosen MJ, Rodebaugh RF, Castilla EA, Brainard J, Cherullo EE, Novick AC: Initial evaluation of Cyberknife technology for extracorporeal renal tissue ablation. Urology 2003;61:498–501.

29 King CR, Lehmann J, Adler JR, Hai J: CyberKnife radiotherapy for localized prostate cancer: rationale and technical feasibility. Technol Cancer Res Treat 2003;2:25–30.
30 Whyte RI, Crownover R, Murphy MJ, Martin DP, Rice TW, DeCamp MM Jr, Rodebaugh R, Weinhous MS, Le QT: Stereotactic radiosurgery for lung tumors: preliminary report of a phase I trial. Ann Thorac Surg 2003;75:1097–1101.
31 Kondziolka D, Dempsey PK, Lunsford LD, Kestle JR, Dolan EJ, Kanal E, Tasker RR: A comparison between magnetic resonance imaging and computed tomography for stereotactic coordinate determination. Neurosurgery 1992;30:402–406; discussion 406–407.
32 Maitz AH, Niranjan A, Jungreis CA, Kondziolka D, Flickinger JC, Lunsford LD: Tube angulation improves angiographic targeting of arteriovenous malformations during stereotactic radiosurgery. Computer Aided Surgery 2001;6:225–229.

Ajay Niranjan, MD
Department of Neurological Surgery, Suite B-400
University of Pittsburgh Medical Center
200 Lothrop Street
Pittsburgh, PA 15213 (USA)
Tel. +1 412 647 9699, Fax +1 412 647 8447, E-Mail niranjana@upmc.edu

Szeifert GT, Kondziolka D, Levivier M, Lunsford LD (eds): Radiosurgery and Pathological Fundamentals. Prog Neurol Surg. Basel, Karger, 2007, vol 20, pp 68–81

6. Integration of Functional Imaging in Radiosurgery: The Example of PET Scan

Marc Levivier[a,b], *Nicolas Massager*[a,b], *David Wikler*[a,b], *Daniel Devriendt*[a,c], *Serge Goldman*[d]

[a]Gamma Knife Center, Université Libre de Bruxelles, [b]Department of Neurosurgery, Hôpital Erasme, Université Libre de Bruxelles, [c]Department of Radiation Therapy, Institut Jules Bordet, [d]PET/Biomedical Cyclotron Unit, Hôpital Erasme, Université Libre de Bruxelles, Brussels, Belgium

Abstract

Radiosurgery relies critically on the imaging modalities that are used for targeting. Leksell Gamma Knife (LGK) radiosurgery presents the highest requirements in terms of imaging accuracy as the treatment is applied in a single high-dose session with no other spatial control than medical imaging. The advent of functional imaging modalities opens new challenges for LGK planning strategies. The integration of stereotactic PET in LGK represents an example of such application of modern multimodality imaging in radiosurgery. Our experience consists of 130 patients treated with the combination of MR/CT and PET guidance. In order to analyze the specific contribution of PET, we developed a classification reflecting the strategy used to define the target volume. When combining PET and MR information, 149 target volumes were defined, because some patients presented with multiple lesions or multifocal tumor areas. Abnormal PET uptake was found in 88% of the lesions; using the classification, we found that the information provided by PET altered significantly the MR-based definition of the tumor in 73%. In conclusion, integration of PET in radiosurgery provides additional functional information opening new perspectives for the treatment of brain tumors. The use of a standardized classification allows to assess the relative role of PET. A similar approach could be useful and may serve as a template for the evaluation of the integration of other new imaging modalities in radiosurgery.

Radiosurgery treatment planning relies critically on medical imaging modalities. Medical images give the ability to define a treatment target volume as well as a geometric transformation from the image space to the stereotactic frame space. Each modality likely to be used for image-guided therapy planning has to be validated for its clinical relevance and accuracy in order to be compatible with the application requirements. Leksell Gamma Knife (LGK; Elekta Instruments AB, Stockholm, Sweden) radiosurgery presents the highest requirements in terms of imaging and registration accuracy as the treatment is applied in a single high-dose session with no other spatial control than medical imaging. Until recently, the only used and validated imaging modalities for Gamma Knife radiosurgery treatment planning were 2-D or 3-D morphological representations of the brain such as CT, MRI or digital subtraction angiography.

The advent of new functional imaging modalities such as PET, magnetic resonance spectroscopy, chemical shift imaging, diffusion- and perfusion-weighted MRI, task-based activation functional MRI maps, along with the demonstration of their value either for highly specific and prognostic delineation of brain tumors or eloquent functional areas, opens new challenges for Gamma Knife radiosurgery planning strategies.

As a first step toward the integration of new functional imaging modalities in LGK radiosurgery, our personal experience is based on the validation and evaluation of the integration of stereotactic PET in the dosimetry planning [13]. The background of this approach is based on the previous experience with the use of PET in stereotactic conditions for brain biopsy [15]. Briefly, it shows that PET uptake is an accurate expression of the extent and of the degree of anaplasia in brain tumors. Moreover, for patients harboring tumors with similar histology, PET uptake is a significant indicator of the degree of aggressiveness and of the prognosis of survival. Thus, further integration of PET in neurosurgical procedures may contribute to a better management of brain tumors, either in optimizing the delineation of their extension, or in defining the aggressive areas of heterogeneous large tumors. This strategy has been initiated with the integration of PET metabolic information in the neurosurgical planning of brain tumor resection using neuronavigation [14]. Accordingly, when we started with LGK radiosurgery, it was a logical step to also integrate PET in this therapeutic approach. In order to analyze the specific contribution of PET, we developed a classification reflecting the strategy used to define the target volume [11]. Its application is described here, together with our clinical experience with patients that have undergone LGK radiosurgery guided by the combination of MR/CT and PET stereotactic images.

Materials and Methods

Between December 1999 and April 2006, 130 patients had stereotactic PET as part of their image acquisition for the planning of LGK radiosurgery. Standard preparation was similar for all our patients undergoing LGK radiosurgery. Briefly, the Leksell G frame (Elekta Instruments AB) was attached to the patient's head under local anesthesia with mild sedation (except in the pediatric population, where the entire radiosurgical procedure is performed under general anesthesia). Stereotactic CT was always acquired as a standard quality control for MR distortion and PET threshold. Stereotactic MR was obtained using different image acquisition parameters, depending on the nature and the location of the lesion. T_1-weighted images before and after intravenous injection of gadolinium-diethylenetriaminepentaacetic acid were, however, obtained in all patients in this series with stereotactic PET, and were used as the primary reference for target definition on MR. In this particular group, the patients were then transferred to the PET/Biomedical Cyclotron Unit, which is directly connected to the main hospital building and to the Gamma Knife Center.

Stereotactic PET images were acquired with the Siemens/CTI ECAT 962 (HR+) 2-D and 3-D tomograph (Knoxville, Tenn., USA), allowing the simultaneous acquisition of 63 planes with a slice thickness of 2.4 mm. This high-precision PET imager is now used for all our stereotactic procedures. PET image acquisition with the Leksell G frame has been validated using a 3-D Lucite phantom containing spherical simulated targets that can be imaged in both PET and CT and provides submillimetric spatial accuracy [13]. The PET image files in the CTI ECAT 7 proprietary format are transferred to the Hewlett-Packard workstation used for the treatment planning with Leksell GammaPlan® (LGP; Elekta Instruments AB.). A custom software converting the PET data file format to the LGP file format is used to import PET images. The PET volume is then handled as a CT or MR volume in LGP, and therefore accessible only for visualization in a linear gray scale. To allow the analysis of PET images with a high-contrast pseudocolor lookup table (LUT), we replace the grayscale LUT file with our own PET color LUT file. The integration of PET image modality in LGP was part of a project in collaboration with Elekta R&D department, which has led to a new version of LPG that is integrated in the latest release of LGK (LGK 4C). In this version of LGK, which we use since September 2005, LGP includes a module (MultiView®) that allows visualization of color PET with various palettes, together with the other image modalities. Target volumes can be drawn in MultiView and then further used in LGP for treatment planning and dosimetry.

The stereotactic PET images are correlated with the other stereotactic image modalities of the same patient and used for the determination of the target volume. The planning always begins with a separate analysis of each stereotactic image modality. A 3-D volumetric contour is drawn on stereotactic MR on the basis of the neuroradiologic definition of the tumor on the diagnostic images; for radiosurgery, this mostly corresponds to the delineation of the area of gadolinium-diethylenetriaminepentaacetic acid enhancement. Then, the stereotactic PET images are analyzed independently from the MR images, jointly by the nuclear medicine physician, the neurosurgeon, and the radiation therapist. Both gray scale as well as pseudo-color LUT images are used. Abnormal metabolism suitable for target definition corresponds either to areas of increased tracer uptake as compared to the surrounding normal-appearing brain, or to foci of relative increase of the tracer in a hypometabolic lesion. A 3-D volumetric PET contour delineating these areas is drawn on a visual basis or using the software-based segmentation algorithm, and is projected onto the corresponding MR images. The final target volume is defined and drawn on the stereotactic MR, taking into account the respective contributions of PET and MR, as well as the anatomical location of the tumor and the functional areas at risk.

In order to analyze the specific contribution of PET, compared to MR, in the definition of the target volume, we have developed classification that reflects the strategy used to define the target volume [11]. Briefly, the description of the relative location of the projection of the PET and MR volumes is considered first, yielding 6 classes (class I: the PET-defined volume projects within the MR-defined volume; class II: the PET- and MR-defined volumes do not fully project in the same areas; class III: the MR-defined volume projects within the PET-defined volume; class IV: the PET- and MR-defined volumes are similar; class V: a PET volume can be defined, but MR is not contributive (no contrast enhancement or nonspecific signal changes); class VI: an MR volume can be defined, but PET is not contributive, because there is no specific uptake area that can be contoured). Based on these categories, a choice is made secondarily to define the target volume, when PET and MR volumes are different. Thus, in classes I, II and III, different subgroups (noted A, B, and C, respectively) can be defined if only PET-, only MR-, or a combination of the PET- and MR-defined volumes are used to define the target volume. For classes IV–VI, however, there is only one definition of target volume, and no subgroups are used. Based on this classification, the contribution of the PET findings may be quantified [11]. The contribution of PET is considered valuable (i.e. the target volume that was first defined on MR is significantly altered, based on PET information) in classes I.A. and I.B., II.A. and II.B., III.A. and III.B., and V. This classification is illustrated in figure 1.

Results

PET in stereotactic conditions was easily performed, within a 90-min period, and did not cause any major additional discomfort to the patient. Stereotactic PET images were successfully acquired, transferred to LGP and integrated in the dosimetry planning of all, but one patient in which the PET computer algorithm failed to reconstruct images that could be used in LGP. Out of the remaining 129 patients, 16 patients with metastases had stereotactic PET acquired as part of a prospective study on PET image segmentation, and are not included in this analysis.

For the 113 patients included, LGK radiosurgery with PET guidance (LGK-PET) was used because their tumor was ill-defined on MR, and we anticipated some limitation of target definition on MR alone. This represents more or less 10% of the total number of LGK radiosurgery procedures performed in our Center during the same period of time. LGK-PET was used in the following indications: 64 primary CNS lesions (57%), 24 recurrent metastases (21%), and 22 pituitary adenomas (19%), and 3% of other lesions (1 osteosarcoma and 2 choroid plexus carcinoma). When combining stereotactic PET and MR information in LGP, 147 target volumes were defined for the 113 patients, because some of them presented with multiple lesions or multifocal tumor areas. The analysis is based on the 147 target volumes (and not the 113 patients) because some targets in the same patient have different PET and MR characteristics, yielding different strategies in defining the target volumes.

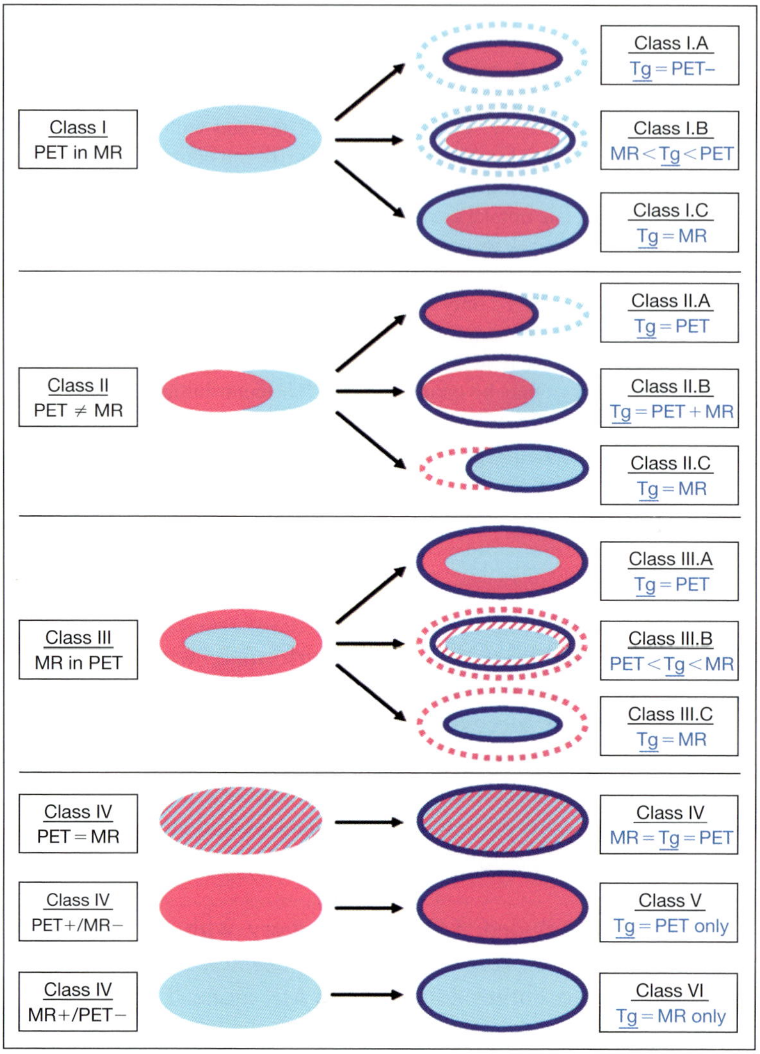

Fig. 1. Classification reflecting the strategy used to define the target volume.

Altogether, for the 147 targets, there were 84 target volumes in the primary CNS tumors, 36 in the metastases, and 22 in the pituitary adenomas. The volume of PET uptake projected within the MR-defined tumor (class I) in 42 targets (29% of all LGK-PET). In more than half of these cases, the target volume was based primarily on the PET information. Abnormal PET and MR areas projected, at least partially, in different regions (class II) for 37 targets (25% of all LGK-PET). The target volume was based primarily on PET information (useful PET) in 34 of the 37 targets, either because the target volume was restricted to the area of PET uptake, or because the target volume combined and included the entire PET and MR abnormal areas. The MR-defined volume was smaller and projected into a larger PET-defined volume (class III) in 10 targets (7% of all LGK-PET). The target volume was based on PET and included the entire PET volume in 8 of them. PET was not specifically used for target definition when PET- and MR-defined volumes were similar (class IV) in 12 targets (8% of all LGK-PET). Finally, the area of increased PET uptake was used as the sole information to define the target volume, because MR was considered not contributive (class V) in 29 targets (20% of all LGK-PET), and there was no specific PET uptake and the target volume has to be defined on MR only (class VI) in 17 targets (12%).

Altogether, abnormal PET uptake (all classes, except class VI) was found in 130 of the 147 lesions (88%). In these 130 lesions, the information obtained from stereotactic PET contributed to the definition of the target volume in altering significantly the MR-defined volume in 95 targets (73% of all positive PET). Representative examples are shown in figures 2–4. We have noticed differences in the contribution of PET among the different clinical indications. PET was considered contributive to target definition in 82% of the primary CNS tumors, in 59% of the metastases, and in 55% of the pituitary adenomas.

However, the usefulness of stereotactic PET was higher than only that of its contribution to target definition. Indeed, many cases in which PET information projected in the MR target volume (class I.C.) and in which PET information was equivalent to the MR target volume (class IV), PET was still useful for the dosimetry planning, because it helped to interpret difficult MR changes. This was especially the case when confirming tumor recurrence after surgery or after LGK. Representative examples are shown in figures 5 and 6. Thus altogether, stereotactic PET was useful 79% of the cases (84% in primary CNS lesions, 75% in metastases, 64% in pituitary adenomas).

Discussion

Both technically and clinically, the use of PET for radiosurgery is a continuation of our previous work on the integration of metabolic information in image-guided neurosurgery [14]. Here, the results also confirm that PET contains metabolic information that is independent of the morphological information provided by CT or MR, and that the integration of PET images in neurosurgical approaches, including radiosurgery, is useful for the management of brain tumors. Interestingly, similar approaches have been recently reported

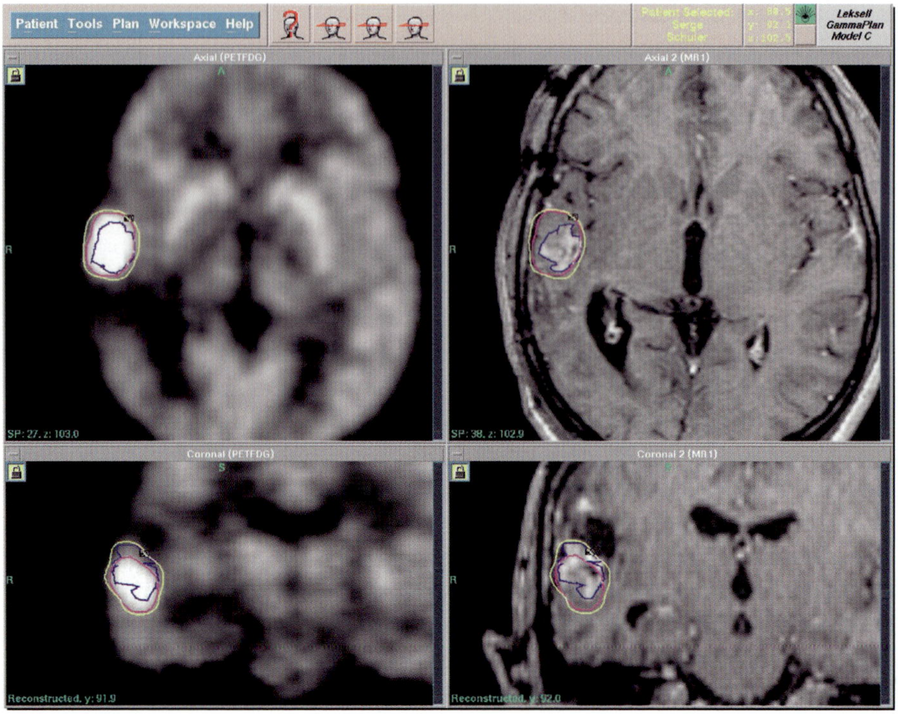

Fig. 2. Example of combined MR and PET guidance with ^{18}F-FDG in a patient with a recurrent and evolutive anaplastic astrocytoma, after multiple surgeries, radiation therapy, and chemotherapy. PET images (left side) allowed to define an area of hypermetabolism (purple line), which was larger than the tumor as defined by gadolinium enhancement (blue line), when projected on MR (right side). The entire area of PET uptake was used as the target volume and was included in the prescription isodose volume (yellow line). In this case, targeting on MR only would have resulted in undertreatment of the tumor, because the MR-defined volume projected entirely in the PET-defined volume (class III.A.).

for the radiotherapy planning of gliomas with ^{123}I-α-methyl-tyrosine-SPECT [7] and with PET with ^{18}F-FDG [19].

From a technical point of view, the registration of PET images to other modalities for the treatment of patients may be considered in the context of frame-based high-precision procedures, such as stereotactic biopsy, frame-based open surgery or radiosurgery, as well as in the context of frameless procedures, such as neuronavigation or radiotherapy. The choice of one or the other approach relies on a trade-off between accuracy and reliability against minimal invasiveness and clinical routine feasibility. For stereotactic PET, as it was used here for

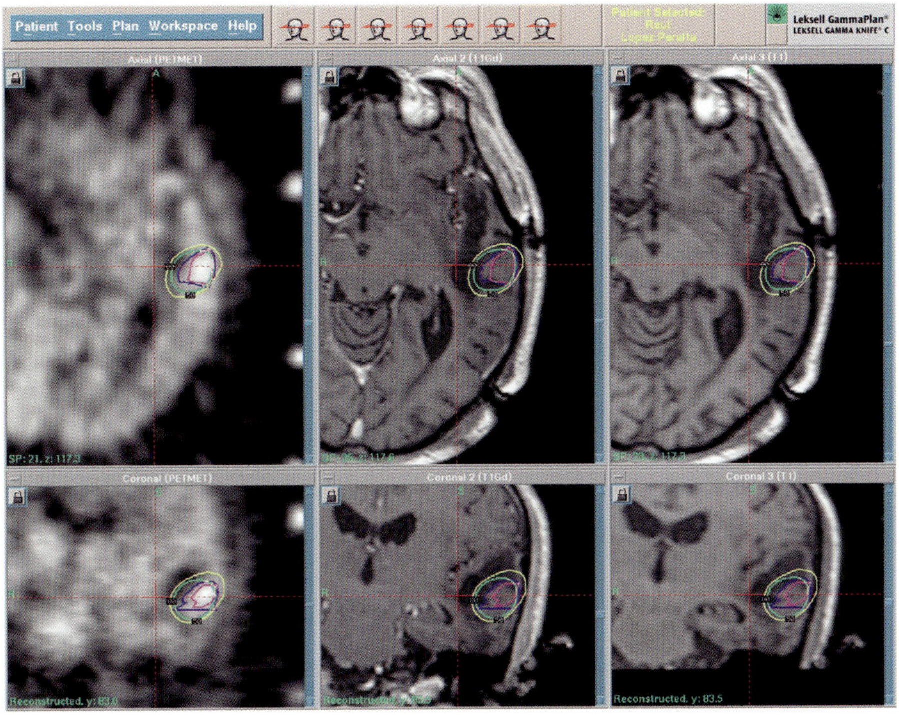

Fig. 3. Example of combined MR and PET guidance with ^{11}C-metionine in a patient with a recurrent low-grade astrocytoma after surgery and radiation therapy and chemotherapy. The patient suffers from intractable epilepsy and a new work-up showed an evolutive recurrent tumor on PET, while MR showed no lesion. PET images (left column) allowed to define an area of hypermetabolism (purple line), which was used as the target volume and was included in the prescription isodose volume (yellow line), after its projection on the corresponding MR with (middle column) and without (right column) gadolinium (class V).

LGK radiosurgery, an imaging fiducials system defining the stereotactic coordinate space of the frame attached to the patient is with no doubt the most accurate and reliable way of registering PET images with the patient treatment space. Nevertheless, this requires careful solutions in addressing the various technical challenges associated with PET acquisition, as discussed in detail elsewhere [12]. Phantom-based validation has been conducted to verify the application accuracy of the procedure [9], and the figures for mean and maximum fiducial registration error provide a valid indicator for stereotactic PET accuracy. In our experience, fiducial registration mean error is around 0.2 mm of mean for the volume, with a maximum value around 0.6 mm for higher error slice. Frameless PET should also be considered for the management of these patients, either in

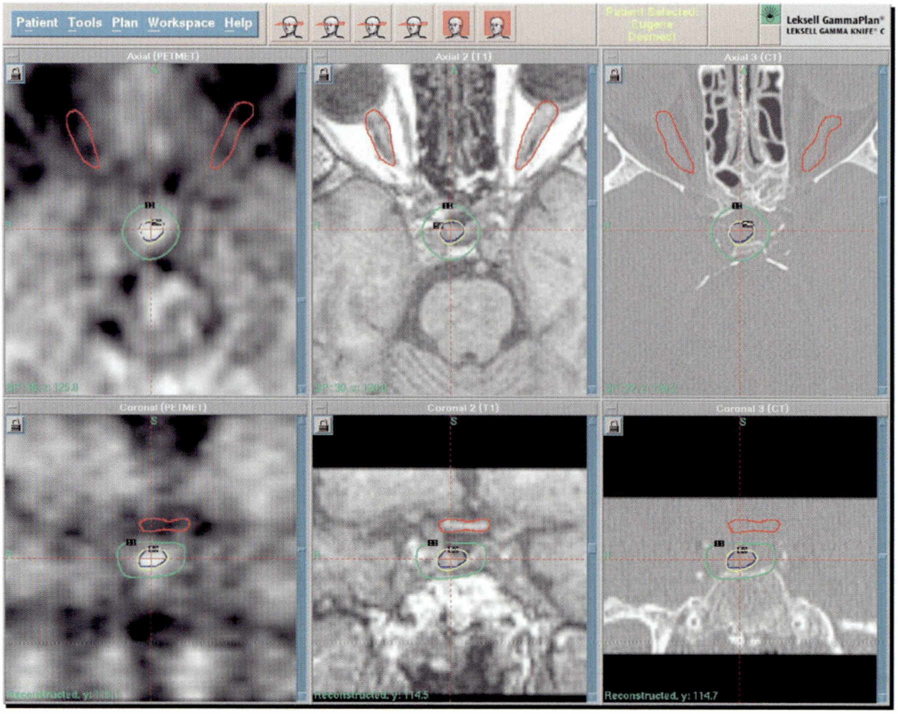

Fig. 4. Example of combined MR and PET guidance with ^{11}C-metionine in a patient with a residual pituitary adenoma after 2 transsphenoidal surgeries. PET images (left column) showed a high uptake of ^{11}C-metionine corresponding to the adenoma in the sella. This area of hypermetabolism was used as a target (blue line) and was included in the prescription isodose volume (yellow line), after its projection on the corresponding MR (middle column) and CT (right column) gadolinium. A target would have been difficult to define on MR, and the target volume was based on PET only (class V).

the context of a better evaluation of the follow-up PET examinations, or as a tentative alternative to stereotactic PET for the radiosurgery planning. The frameless approach may have the advantage to extend the accessibility to PET in radiosurgery to a larger number of centers. The comfort and planning flexibility would also benefit from the noninvasiveness of the procedure. This requires solutions to register PET without frame fiducials yet with high accuracy and reliability, and we currently perform studies to evaluate the feasibility and reliability of integrating frameless PET in LGK radiosurgery [21].

Compared to our experience with PET-guided stereotactic biopsy or neuronavigation, the use of LGK-PET has generated its own therapeutic challenges in

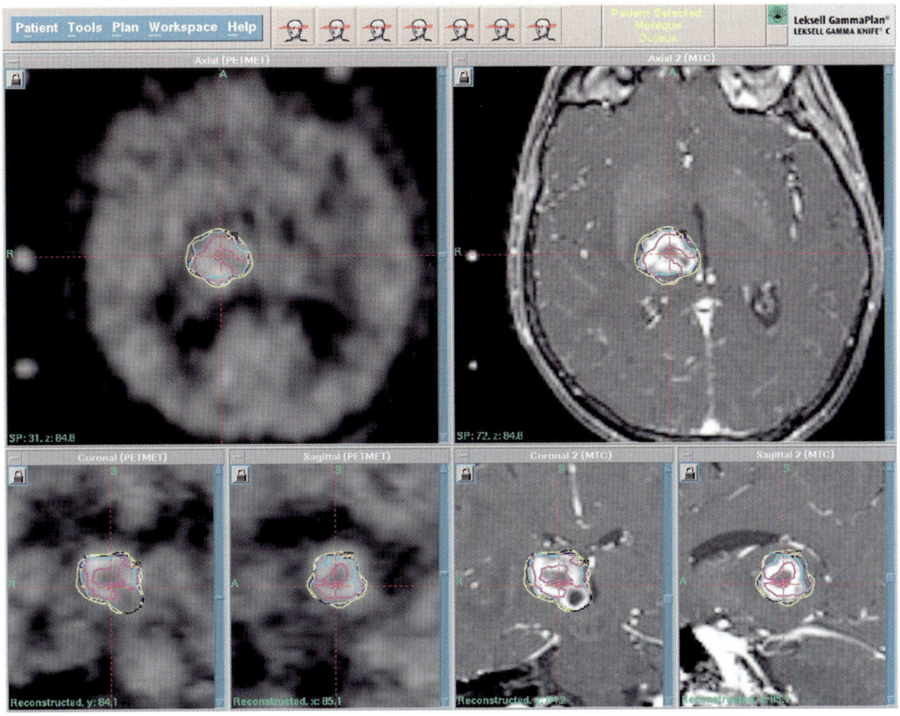

Fig. 5. Example of combined MR and PET guidance with ^{11}C-metionine in a patient with a recurrent thalamic metastasis after LGK radiosurgery. Although MR showed an evolutive area of contrast enhancement that was suggestive of tumor recurrence, PET was thought to be useful to differentiate areas of tumor recurrence and of radiation necrosis. PET images (left column) showed a area of high uptake of ^{11}C-metionine that was considered as active tumor (purple line), and projected on the corresponding MR images (right column). The final target volume on MR (blue line) was larger and included the entire PET-defined volume. Although using the classification a PET-defined volume included in the MR target (class I.C.) is not considered contributive, PET images were useful to differentiate tumor recurrence and radiation necrosis in target definition.

relation with the specific planning requirements of this approach. Stereotactic biopsy is a limited neurosurgical procedure in which stereotactic PET may be used for the selection of a discrete target [10]. Therefore, target selection will not be hindered by extensive PET abnormalities. On the contrary, stereotactic PET will help to optimize it, aiming at sampling the most representative area of the tumor [10, 16, 17]. Also with neuronavigation, even when stereotactic PET anomalies cannot be fully incorporated into the final target volume, standard cytoreductive surgery based on anatomical landmarks is the alternative, and the comparison between preoperative and postoperative PET will help to objectively

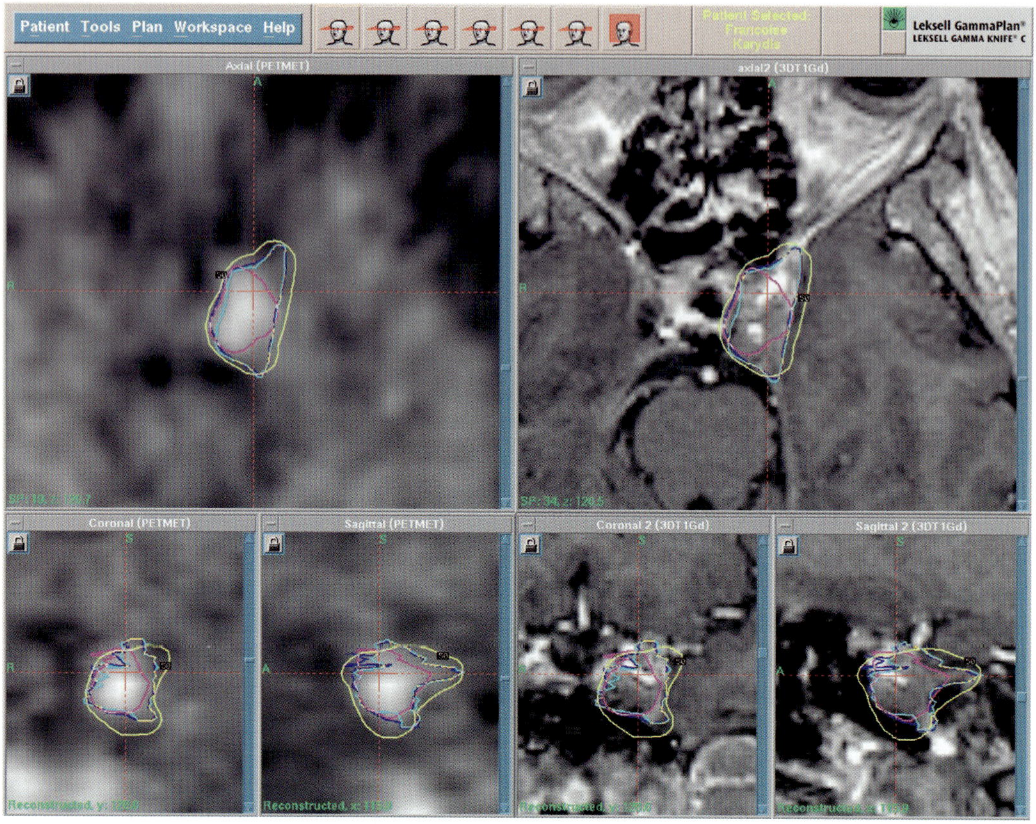

Fig. 6. Example of combined MR and PET guidance with ^{11}C-metionine in a patient with an ill-defined intracavernous residual pituitary adenoma after transsphenoidal surgery. PET images (left column) showed a area of high uptake of ^{11}C-metionine (purple line) which projected entirely in the cavernous sinus on the corresponding MR images (right column). The final target volume on MR (blue line) was larger and included the entire PET-defined volume. Although using the classification a PET-defined volume included in the MR target (class I.C.) is not considered contributive, PET images were useful to confirm that the recurrence was restricted to the cavernous sinus.

evaluate the extent of tumor resection [3]. Even in those cases, information provided by PET are used to further evaluate the prognosis and the need for adjuvant therapies [2, 4]. In radiosurgery, however, the limitation in the treatable target volume requires a strict strategy for the selection of the patients that may benefit from LGK-PET, as well as for the a priori choice of radiotracer and target definition. This is especially important when using LGK-PET in infiltrating brain tumors or for lesions that are not well defined on MR, in order to avoid circumstances where stereotactic PET images show an extended uptake of the radiotracer that is incompatible with radiosurgery, requiring to abort the procedure. Also, at the time of the planning, an assumption has to be made about the relevance of the presence of tumor tissue in the entire area of increased PET tracer uptake. Indeed, image-based radiosurgical planning does not allow documentation of histology to confirm that either PET- or MR-defined tumor volumes are correct. Such data, correlating MR findings with histology, have been obtained with stereotactic biopsies of brain tumors [8]. Along the same line, our long-term experience of the correlation of the pathology of stereotactic biopsy with its metabolic characteristics [5, 6], as well as the increased knowledge about PET in brain tumor in the literature [22] strengthen the valuable link between PET uptake and histology in brain tumors. Moreover, the clinical context, with most patients in our series harboring recurrent tumors (with known histology from previous surgery) or inoperable tumors (with known histology from stereotactic biopsy or from a primary tumor), also limits the risk of erroneous target selection using combined PET and MR data. Of course, one cannot rule out that some PET areas that have been included in target volumes could have contained necrotic nontumor tissue, especially when treating recurrent malignant gliomas after radiation therapy, or recurrent metastases after previous radiosurgery. Recent papers addressing this issue also support the use of PET in those conditions [1, 19, 20]. Also, we believe that complementary investigations, such as with MR spectroscopy, may be of important help in that respect [18].

The possibility to use and to integrate functional images, such as PET, in the dosimetry planning for LGK radiosurgery provides a unique opportunity to evaluate the benefit of such approach and its scope of application in radiosurgery. However, its real clinical advantage needs a comparative evaluation of local tumor control, functional results, and survival for the different clinical indications. For better objective evaluation of the benefits of such procedure, we developed a descriptive classification illustrating the relative information provided by PET and MR [11]. Two steps are used. Firstly, the description of the relative location of the projection of the PET and MR volumes is considered, yielding 6 classes. Secondly, the choice in defining the final target volume may yield 3 subgroups, depending on the amount of PET and MR volumes that are included. As this classification has been used to record and categorize the strategy of each treatment planning, it has proven to be useful for the assessment of the role of PET. Moreover, it allowed to group and identify classes corresponding to different planning strategies with PET. Indeed, in some instances, MR disclosed a large abnormal volume that was not compatible with LGK radiosurgery, and PET was used to focus the treatment on the metabolic active part of the tumor. Conversely, in some cases, the target volume was maximized thanks to the use of PET, and the delineation of the treated tumor would have been underestimated if MR only was used. Again, the real benefit for the patients will need further long-term analysis of the clinical results. We also believe that further accumulation of prospective data using this classification will allow to better distinguish the type of contribution PET provides in relation to the different clinical indications. Similarly, this approach could be useful and may serve as a template for the evaluation of the integration of other new functional imaging modalities in radiosurgery.

References

1 Belohlávek O, Simonova G, Kantorova I, Novotny J Jr, Liscák R: Brain metastases after stereotactic radiosurgery using the Leksell gamma knife: can FDG PET help to differentiate radionecrosis from tumour progression? Eur J Nucl Med 2003;30:96–100.

2 De Witte O, Goldberg I, Wikler D, Rorive S, Damhaut P, Monclus M, Salmon I, Brotchi J, Goldman S: Positron emission tomography with injection of methionine as a prognostic factor in glioma. J Neurosurg 2001;95:746–750.

3 De Witte O, Levivier M, Violon P, Brotchi J, Goldman S: Quantitative imaging study of extent of surgical resection and prognosis of malignant astocytomas. Neurosurgery 1998;43:398–399.

4 De Witte O, Levivier M, Violon P, Salmon I, Damhaut P, Wikler D Jr, Hildebrand J, Brotchi J, Goldman S: Prognostic value of positron emission tomography with [^{18}F]fluoro- 2-deoxy-D-glucose in the low-grade glioma. Neurosurgery 1996;39:470–476.

5 Goldman S, Levivier M, Pirotte B, Brucher JM, Wikler D, Damhaut P, Stanus E, Brotchi J, Hildebrand J: Regional glucose metabolism and histopathology of gliomas – a study based on positron emission tomography-guided stereotactic biopsy. Cancer 1996;78:1098–1106.

6 Goldman S, Levivier M, Pirotte B, Brucher J-M, Wikler D, Damhaut P, Dethy S, Brotchi J, Hildebrand J: Regional methionine and glucose metabolism in gliomas: a comparative study on PET-guided stereotactic biopsy. J Nucl Med 1997;38:1–4.

7 Grosu AL, Feldmann H, Dick S, Dzewas B, Nieder C, Gumprecht H, Frank A, Schwaiger M, Molls M, Weber WA: Implications of IMT-SPECT for postoperative radiotherapy planning in patients with gliomas. Int J Radiat Oncol Biol Phys 2002;54:842–854.

8 Kelly PJ, Daumas-Duport C, Scheithauer BW, Kall BA, Kispert DB: Stereotactic histologic correlations of computed tomography- and resonance imaging-defined abnormalities in patients with glial neoplasms. Mayo Clin Proc 1987;62:450–459.

9 Levivier M, Goldman S, Bidaut LM, Luxen A, Stanus E, Przedborski S, Balériaux D, Hildebrand J, Brotchi J: Positron emission tomography-guided stereotactic brain biopsy. Neurosurgery 1992;31:792–797.

10 Levivier M, Goldman S, Pirotte B, Brucher J-M, Balériaux D, Luxen A, Hildebrand J, Brotchi J: Diagnostic yield of stereotactic brain biopsy guided by positron emission tomography with [^{18}F]fluorodeoxyglucose. J Neurosurg 1995;82:445–452.

11 Levivier M, Massager N, Wikler D, Lorenzoni J, Ruiz S, Devriendt D, David P, Desmedt F, Simon S, Van Houtte P, Brotchi J, Goldman S: The use of stereotactic PET images in the dosimetry planning of radiosurgery for brain tumors: Clinical experience and proposed classification. J Nucl Med 2004;45:1146–1154.

12 Levivier M, Wikler D, De Witte O, Massager N, Goldman S, Brotchi J: Positron Emission Tomography (PET) for the Management of Brain Tumors; in Black PM, Loeffler J (eds): Cancer of the Nervous System, ed 2. Philadelphia, Lippincott William & Wilkins, 2004, pp 96–107.

13 Levivier M, Wikler D, Goldman S, David P, Metens T, Massager N, Gerosa M, Devriendt D, Desmedt F, Simon S, Van Houtte P, Brotchi J: Integration of the metabolic data of positron emission tomography in the dosimetry planning of radiosurgery with the gamma knife: early experience with brain tumors. J Neurosurg 2000;93(suppl 3):233–238.

14 Levivier M, Wikler D, Goldman S, Pirotte B, Brotchi J: Positron emission tomography in stereotactic conditions as a functional imaging technique for neurosurgical guidance; in Alexander III EB, Maciunas RM (eds): Advanced Neurosurgical Navigation. New York, Thieme Medical Publishers, 1999, pp 85–99.
15 Levivier M, Wikler D Jr, Massager N, David P, Devriendt D, Lorenzoni J, Pirotte B, Desmedt F, Simon S Jr, Goldman S, Van Houtte P, Brotchi J: The integration of metabolic imaging in stereotactic procedures including radiosurgery: a review. J Neurosurg 2002;97:542–550.
16 Massager N, David P, Goldman S, Pirotte B, Wikler D, Salmon I, Nagy N, Brotchi J, Levivier M: Combined magnetic resonance imaging- and positron emission tomography-guided stereotactic biopsy in brainstem mass lesions: diagnostic yield in a series of 30 patients. J Neurosurg 2000;93:951–957.
17 Pirotte B, Goldman S, Salzberg S, Wikler D, David P, Vandesteene A, Van Bogaert P, Salmon I, Brotchi J, Levivier M: Combined positron emission tomography and magnetic resonance imaging for the planning of stereotactic brain biopsies in children: Experience in 9 cases. Pediatr Neurosurg 2003;38:146–155.
18 Rock JP, Hearshen D, Scarpace L, Croteau D, Gutierrez J, Fisher JL, Rosenblum ML, Mikkelsen T: Correlations between magnetic resonance spectroscopy and image-guided histopathology, with special attention to radiation necrosis. Neurosurgery 2002;51:912–919.
19 Tralins KS, Douglas JG, Stelzer KJ, Mankoff DA, Silbergeld DL, Rostomilly R, Hummel S, Scharnhorst J, Krohn KA, Spence AM: Volumetric analysis of 18F-FDG PET in glioblastoma multiforme: prognostic information and possible role in definition of target volumes in radiation dose escalation. J Nucl Med 2002;43:1667–1673.
20 Tsuyuguchi N, Sunada I, Iwai Y, Yamanaka K, Tanaka K, Takami T, Otsuka Y, Sakamoto S, Ohata K, Goto T, Hara M: Methionine positron emission tomography of recurrent metastatic brain tumor and radiation necrosis after stereotactic radiosurgery: is a differential diagnosis possible? J Neurosurg 2003;98:1056–1064.
21 Wikler D, Sadeghi N, Goldman S, Massager N, Levivier M: Clinical validation methodology for the use of frameless PET in Leksell Gamma Knife® radiosurgery. Radiosurgery 2004;5:247–254.
22 Wong TZ, van der Westhuizen GJ, Coleman RE: Positron emission tomography imaging of brain tumors. Neuroimag Clin N Am 2002;12:615–626.

Marc Levivier, MD, PhD
Neurosurgery and Gamma Knife Center, U.L.B. – Hôpital Erasme
808, route de Lennik
BE–1070 Brussels (Belgium)
Tel. +32 2 555 31 74, Fax +32 2 555 31 76, E-Mail Marc.Levivier@ulb.ac.be

Szeifert GT, Kondziolka D, Levivier M, Lunsford LD (eds): Radiosurgery and Pathological Fundamentals. Prog Neurol Surg. Basel, Karger, 2007, vol 20, pp 82–90

7. The Role of Computer Technology in Radiosurgery

David Wikler, Olivier Coussaert, Frédéric Schoovaerts, Anthony Joly, Marc Levivier

Gamma Knife Center, Hôpital Erasme, Brussels, Belgium

Abstract

Stereotactic radiosurgery treatment principles and irradiation techniques have shown little evolution since its introduction in 1968. Conversely, technology progress linked to computers has produced a major impact on the methods used for treatment planning and dose delivery. In order to fully comprehend modern radiosurgery approaches, one has to acquire good insight of the underlying technology, specifically computer software. In this chapter, we describe the evolution from X-ray films to high-resolution digital imaging, the shift from simple trigonometric calculation to highly complex algorithms and new perspectives in patient follow-up. If these changes open new prospects, they also add complexity, which leads to new pitfalls and limits of the stereotactic radiosurgery method.

When Lars Leksell was performing the first Gamma Knife radiosurgery treatment in 1967, computers had already existed and the HAL 9000 was talking to Dave in Stanley Kubrick's *2001: A Space Odyssey*[1]. IBM was producing the System/360 and DEC was introducing the first minicomputer, PDP-8. However, computers were probably still science fiction and beyond finances for the Swedish neurosurgeon. During the next 5 years, computer research had been exploding. Intel launched the first commercial microprocessors, Bell Labs invented UNIX operating system and the US Department of Defense had been funding the first network Arpanet what led towards the Internet. These technological advance developed Gamma Knife radiosurgery planning with computer-assisted dose

[1] The HAL 9000 computer and the astronaut Dave were central characters in the science fiction film *2001: A Space Odyssey* by Stanley Kubrick and Arthur C. Clarke.

calculation tools in 1974. However, the most significant leap towards modern radiosurgery was probably the introduction of computer assisted tomography (CAT) scanner in 1972 for which Hounsfield and Cormack got the Nobel Prize of medicine in 1979. At the beginning of the 1980s, magnetic resonance imaging (MRI) systems were installed in hospitals providing even further improvements to Gamma Knife radiosurgery planning. In the same years, the advent of affordable and high-speed computing workstations with graphical capabilities led to a new revolution for dosimetry planning [1].

As a new treatment modality, Gamma Knife radiosurgery had to be assessed in terms of clinical outcome. The first statistical studies assessing results from the follow-up of a few hundreds of patients have been published from 1988. From that point, Gamma Knife installations spread throughout the whole world to reach over 320,000 treated patients today. In order to retrospectively and prospectively review Gamma Knife results, innovations in information technology on the field of database management systems have uttermost importance.

For both the treatment planning and follow-up perspective, we shall describe how computer technology may affect each stage of the radiosurgery practice and hence estimate the impact of Moore's law[2] on radiosurgery practice.

Medical Imaging

From Projections to Tomography

Gamma Knife treatments are dramatically dependent on medical imaging modalities as the prescribed isodose volume is solely defined on preoperative medical images. Before the introduction of CAT and MRI scanners, radiosurgery targets were chosen from X-ray projections of either radiograms, ventriculograms, pneumoencephalograms or cisternograms. AP and RL projections were imaged with stereotactic fiducial systems, and with the aid of these poorly contrasted images radiosurgeons and radiation physicists were able to define a target for dose delivery into the brain. For functional treatments, the method used was the localization of the AC-PC line (reference) onto X-ray projections and the definition of the target coordinates from the target to reference distance in an atlas. Lesions and normal brain structures were derived from restricted image information; functional targets were the result of an assumption of low individual variations of brain anatomy. These issues made the definition of the target volumes uncomfortable and probably quite inaccurate.

[2] Gordon Moore, cofounder of the Intel semiconductors company, forecasted that transistor density on integrated circuits would double every 2 years, this prediction is known as Moore's law.

By the advent of tomography modalities radiosurgery entered the arena of 3-D information, so radiosurgery equipments and software had to adapt to this novelty. Modifications were made for the fiducial system enabling accurate 3-D measurements of lesions and normal brain structures. However, if the first 3-D acquisition systems were able to measure volume information, the planning strategy remained fairly linked to planar data. Because of limitations of signal detection devices as well as the incapacity of the computers to handle large quantity of data, the output of the tomographs presented reduced resolution in the third axis. The lack of efficient and standard computer communication systems led to the output of sequences of image slices on films further used for treatment planning. An important consequence of these restrictions was the establishment of strict rules for the placement of the fiducial systems orthogonally to the imaging equipment geometry.

Radiosurgery Treatment Planning

From Rulers to Algorithms

The definition of the stereotactic coordinate system through the characterization of the geometric transformation between the patient imaging space and the stereotactic frame space was traditionally achieved with the help of a ruler system. When the computer workstation with graphic capabilities became available, the radiosurgery treatment planning platform was introduced. With the generalization of computer networks, a standard communication protocol for the transfer of medical images between software applications was established: the Digital Imaging and Communications in Medicine (DICOM®[3]) published in 1985 by the American College of Radiology and the National Electrical Manufacturers Association. The treatment planning software platform was then further enhanced to offer advanced 3-D visualization [2, 3] for real 3-D treatment planning methodology [4, 5] to the radiosurgery community. Algorithms replaced rulers and radiosurgeons were given the opportunity to outline their targets using features such as automatic fiducial extraction for stereotactic frame space definition, 3-D visualization [6], multimodal image fusion [7] as well as automatic segmentation of lesions and structures for the definition of volumes of interest.

[3] DICOM is the registered trademark of the National Electrical Manufacturers Association for its standards publications relating to digital communications of medical information.

From Pens to 3-D Models

Before the introduction of the treatment planning workstation, the optimization of a dose delivery plan was a time-consuming process. Shots coordinates had to be typed manually, computation of isodose volume were very slow and the results had to be drawn with pens on transparent paper in order to evaluate the conformality of the dose prescription. Using powerful computers, we have now the potential to prepare highly conformal treatment plans with automatic or interactive placement of dose delivery approaches, real-time computation and display of target and isodose volumes on 3-D models [8] as well as convenient measurements of dose-volume histograms.

Dose Delivery – From Screwdrivers to Robots

Even further, the technology enhancements in control systems and micromechanics automate the movements of positioning either the patient or the dose delivery equipment, allowing more complex dose application schemes with additional shots for better conformality or modulation of intensity.

If the development and the implementation of such complex algorithms by medical physicists and biomedical engineers raised new expectations and concerns in terms of accuracy and quality control, there is no doubt that radiosurgery principle of single and highly conformal dose application with very accurate delivery gained real establishment and acceptance thanks to these technological advances leveraged by the computer revolution. As reflected in the scientific literature and clinical practice, the evolution of clinical indications as well as clinical results of radiosurgery were significantly influenced by these various technological improvements.

Medical Data Management

Unlike conventional radiotherapy, where mathematical models, among which the well-known linear quadratic model [9, 10], could be derived to describe the radiobiological effects of low-dose ionizing radiation, predicting the biological response of radiosurgery is far more challenging. The use of high single-fraction dose induces vascular and antiproliferative effects that invalidate the common rules of fractionated radiotherapy [11]. Consequently, the radiosurgery community did deploy great effort to gather empirical data from well-designed statistical studies aimed at assessing guidelines for successful radiosurgery treatments in order to gain acceptance. The collection of patient, treatment and follow-up data has become a decisive element in the procedures of a radiosurgery center. The development of a radiosurgery information system for the management of the whole radiosurgery process including administrative tasks, treatment data collection, follow-up of the patient and generation of statistics is another benefit that radiosurgery can gain from the progress of computer technology. In the process of developing such an information system for the Gamma Knife Center of Erasme Hospital, Brussels, we were able to formulate some of the key features essential for this tool and to propose a proficient implementation [12].

Technology Platform

Any programming initiative needs first to rely on the selection of a technological platform to comply with a set of the application main requirements criteria. The design of an information system for radiosurgery practice has to meet constraints related to the multidisciplinary context of this treatment modality. Information has to be gathered from various sources: the hospital information system for patient identification and demographic data, from the radiology information systems for examination parameters and reports, the Pictures Archiving System (PACS) for images (Radiology Information System, pictures Archiving and Communication System) and the oncology, radio-oncology and neurosurgery departmental systems for patient clinical history and previous treatments. The other way around, the radio-surgery collected data must be available for review by the same range of clinical and scientific groups. These strong open connectivity requirements leveraged the conception of a solid networked and collaborative-based architecture relying on medical information system standards. Therefore, the platform shall be constructed around central servers aimed at (1) the transfer and archiving of imaging and treatment data (the file server with robust data redundancy and standard communication services), (2) the collection of patient and intervention data (the database server with relational data management capabilities) and (3) the interaction with the users (the application web server providing cross-platform front-end client interface).

In addition, we decided to base our developments solely on open-source and standardized software tools. The servers run the GNU/Linux operating system (http://www.gnu.org), the relational database management system is PostgreSQL (http://www.postgresql.org), the web server, the web application framework and other tools are projects of the Apache Software Foundation (http://www.apache.org) and all components are programmed in the Java (http://java.sun.com) object-oriented and cross-platform language.

Radiosurgical Intervention Administration

The application provides an agenda utility that allows the team members to schedule the interventions for patients. Patients are uniquely identified by their hospital number that includes a control code to assess its correctness and uniqueness. From that identifier, a unique intervention number is derived that will be used throughout the workflow of procedures and data management to guarantee consistency of information. As our system is web based, this intervention identifier can be copied and pasted to the patient ID text box of the treatment planning system when registering a new treatment. This procedure further reduces risks of error. The radiosurgical team and other actors of the hospital involved in the patient management access selected sections of the system with either read-only or read-write privileges according to their group and role defined by their system login information.

Data Archiving

Medical Imaging Data

A radiosurgery treatment is based on native imaging transferred from the radiology and nuclear medicine departments. During the whole management of the patient pathology, relevant images are selected either for the treatment decision, for target definition or for follow-up purpose. It is therefore very important to have constant access to this imaging information. Radiology PACS can provide this service, but centers without online archiving facility will have to care about that issue. We have built such a server system with the following specification: (1) implementation of DICOM 3.0 services in order to receive images from MRI, CT, DSA, CR and PET equipments through the network or CDROM; (2) sorting and labeling services in order to organize data on disks and build an image database; (3) forwarding services that send the images to the treatment planning workstation if required; (4) a web-based client application that offers the ability to search the image database, retrieve examination parameters and transfer the data to a DICOM viewing workstation for image reviewing or processing.

Treatment Data

The radiosurgery treatment planning and delivery process will produce data such as target definitions, dosimetry parameters and device settings. A standardization effort for the archiving and communication of the radiosurgery systems data has been completed within the DICOM 3.0 – Radiotherapy extensions. Unfortunately, not all manufacturers comply with this standard but rather stick to undisclosed proprietary formats for archiving radiosurgery data. In addition, proposed archiving solutions are sometimes cumbersome, leading to time-consuming operations and poor data security. In order to balance these deficiencies, our data management system provides solutions for automated data extraction, conversion as well secured transfer to online and offline archiving devices. Each night, the database server builds dedicated operating system commands scripts for several archiving tasks to be performed on new treatments data. The first task extracts data from proprietary formats and converts them to a documented data format (XML schema; http://www.w3.org/XML) that can be easily used by other applications. The second task backs up data to a local tape drive. The third task securely transfers data to a file server for online storage and offline writing to DVD media. Every step of these tasks is verified and logged to ensure maximum security of data integrity.

Data Collection

Treatment planning systems do not always provide tools to enter important data about radiosurgery treatment such as identification of indications, lesion identification and location, patient global treatment strategy or clinical nomenclatures. The web-based client of the database application that we developed offers a number of screen forms for user input of predefined data.

Report Generation

As all information related to patient treatment is gathered into the database, the system can easily generate printed reports. Reports for various purposes can be produced in Adobe PDF electronic documents for distribution inside and outside the radiosurgery center.

Treatment Follow-Up

We have already mentioned the critical aspect of patient follow-up in the radiosurgery area. Patient information will be collected from imaging reports, outpatient clinic visits, other physicians' letters or phone calls. The application provides forms to enter a follow-up record in the database. These records are organized chronologically and linked to the patient rather than to an intervention. Some lesion-specific data such as the evolution of tumor volume can be recorded and linked to the particular lesion.

Statistics

Of course, all these efforts to collect and archive radiosurgery data must be completed by a tool providing means to perform statistical analysis. Our system provides ways to extract data by simple and complex database queries. These queries can be built visually from the web-based application and saved for periodical use in the user profile. Results of these queries can be saved in text files organized in columns that can be imported in statistics software packages or data mining tools, hence establishing foundation of a valuable environment for scientific studies. As an example, we used this platform to analyze the results of metastases treatment which became a major indication of radiosurgery in recent years though still needs to be assessed in terms of clinical results compared to other treatment modalities. In order to evaluate clinical results according to the selection of the patients, oncologists recorded in the database stratification systems indices such as RPA, SIR, BS-BM [13]. They subsequently used our tool to collect the data and analyze survival data for each system. Once the database queries are saved and the data analysis is defined, the oncologists are able to analyze their results with a few clicks of a button.

From a Knowledge Base to an Expert System

Beyond clinical research studies to assess and control the validity of radiosurgery treatments, a radiosurgery data management system could be used as a tool to build a knowledge base of treatment parameters and results. Using valuable published methods, the database system could be used to compute dose-response data [14] according to several factors such as the treated volume, nature of tissue, target location, follow-up time or patient selection criteria. With such online computation, a radiosurgery center would be able to compare its own results with standardized or published data to evaluate and eventually adapt their treatment strategy. The sharing of such data among centers for treatments with sufficiently standardized treatment and result evaluation protocols would generate enough data to build a common and dynamically evolving radiosurgery knowledge base that could be used to assist radiosurgery physicians and physicists in the planning of a treatment in terms of dose selection. Such a multicentric database system would pave the way for the development of an expert system for radiosurgery planning.

Conclusion

This overview of the variety of aspects where computer technology adds value to the field of radiosurgery shows how radiosurgery is closely coupled to the evolution of information technology in both hardware and software developments. From medical imaging to robotics, from dose computations to large database systems, the computer is not anymore a tool to assist radiosurgery staff to plan a treatment; it is now one of the core elements of the radiosurgery technique. As the pace of current developments in the field of computing is even higher than expected by optimistic previsions, the radiosurgery community can anticipate new progress along with new challenges in their treatment strategies.

References

1 McShan L, Silverman A, Lanza DM, Reinstein LE, Glicksman AS: A computerized three-dimensional treatment planning system utilizing interactive colour graphics. Br J Radiol 1979;52: 478–481.

2 Herman GT: A survey of 3D medical imaging technologies. IEEE Eng Med Biol Mag 1990;9: 15–17.

3 Robb RA, Barillot C: Interactive display and analysis of 3-D medical images. IEEE Trans Med Imaging, 1989;8:217–226.

4 Flickinger JC, Lunsford LD, Wu A, Maitz AH, Kalend AM: Treatment planning for gamma knife radiosurgery with multiple isocenters: Int J Radiat Oncol Biol Phys 1990;18:1495–1501.

5 Kooy HM, Nedzi LA, Loeffler JS, Alexander E 3rd, Cheng CW, Mannarino EG, Holupka EJ, Siddon RL: Treatment planning for stereotactic radiosurgery of intra-cranial lesions. Int J Radiat Oncol Biol Phys 1991;21:683–693.

6 Barillot C: Surface and volume rendering techniques to display 3-D data. IEEE Eng Med Biol Mag, 1993;12:111–119.

7 Kooy HM, van Herk M, Barnes PD, Alexander E 3rd, Dunbar SF, Tarbell NJ, Mulkern RV, Holupka EJ, Loeffler JS: Image fusion for stereotactic radiotherapy and radiosurgery treatment planning. Int J Radiat Oncol Biol Phys 1994;28:1229–1234.

8 Smith V, Verhey L, Wara W, Harsh GT, Larson D: Beta test site report: gamma plan. Stereotact Funct Neurosurg 1998;61(suppl 1):116–123.

9 Barendsen GW: Dose fractionation, dose rate and ISO-effect relationships for normal tissue responses. Int J Radiat Oncol Biol Phys 1982;8:1981–1997.

10 Dale R, Carabe-Fernandez A: The radiobiology of conventional radiotherapy and its application to radionuclide therapy. Cancer Biother Radiopharm 2005;20:47–51.

11 Gross MW, Engenhart-Cabillic R: Normal tissue reactions after linac-based radiosurgery and stereotactic radiotherapy. Front Radiat Ther Oncol 2002;37:140–150.

12 Coussaert O, Schoovaerts F, Joly A, Levivier M, Wikler D: Computer-aided interventions information system. Presented at 4th International IEEE EMBS Special Topic Conference on Information Technology Applications in Biomedicine, 2003.

13 Lorenzoni J, Devriendt D, Massager N, David P, Ruiz S, Vanderlinden B, Van Houtte P, Brotchi J, Levivier M: Radiosurgery for treatment of brain metastases: estimation of patient eligibility using three stratification systems. Int J Radiat Oncol Biol Phys 2004;60:218–224.

14 Flickinger JC, Lunsford LD, Wu A, Kalend A: Predicted dose-volume isoeffect curves for stereotactic radiosurgery with the 60Co gamma unit. Acta Oncol 1991;30:363–367.

David Wikler
Gamma Knife Center, Hôpital Erasme
Route de Lennik, 808
BE–1070 Brussels (Belgium)
Tel. +32 2 555 31 74, Fax +32 2 555 31 76, E-Mail David.Wikler@ulb.ac.be

Szeifert GT, Kondziolka D, Levivier M, Lunsford LD (eds): Radiosurgery and Pathological Fundamentals. Prog Neurol Surg. Basel, Karger, 2007, vol 20, pp 91–105

8. Radiosurgical Pathology of Brain Tumors: Metastases, Schwannomas, Meningiomas, Astrocytomas, Hemangioblastomas

György T. Szeifert[a], *Douglas Kondziolka*[b], *Dave S. Atteberry*[b], *Isabelle Salmon*[c], *Sandrine Rorive*[c], *Marc Levivier*[c], *L. Dade Lunsford*[b]

[a]National Institute of Neurosurgery and Department of Neurological Surgery, Semmelweis University, Budapest, Hungary; [b]Center for Image-Guided Neurosurgery, Department of Neurological Surgery, UPMC Presbyterian Hospital, University of Pittsburgh, Pittsburgh, Pa., USA; [c]Centre Gamma Knife, Hôpital Académique Erasme, Université Libre de Bruxelles, Brussels, Belgium

Abstract

Systematic human pathological background to brain tumor radiosurgery explaining biological and pathophysiological effects of focused irradiation barely exists. The goal of this study was to explore histopathological changes evoked by single high-dose irradiation in a set of different brain tumors following Gamma Knife radiosurgery (GKRS). Light microscopy revealed that GKRS evokes degenerative and proliferative pathological changes in the parenchyma, stroma and vessels of the irradiated tumors. Three main histological types of gamma radiolesions, that is acute, subacute and chronic variants of tissue reactions were recognized in different neoplasms irrespective of their ontogenetic nature. Acute type gamma radiolesions were characterized mainly with necrotic changes and appeared either early or in a delayed time interval. Subacute type gamma radiolesions expressed resorptive activity also with early or delayed chronology. Chronic type lesions showed a reparative tendency but presented only at the delayed stage. These changes seem to follow each other consecutively. There was no significant relation between morphological characteristics of the generated tissue reaction and the time interval elapsed after GKRS. This relative time and environment autonomy of the developed pathological lesions with similar histological picture in different neoplasms suggests either a vascular mechanism or/and a genetically directed origin presumably induced by the ionizing energy of high-dose irradiation.

During the past 4 decades, radiosurgery has become an effective and widespread treatment modality in the neurosurgical realm [1–4] for the management of intracranial neoplasms with a variety of histological types, including traditionally radioresistant ones as well [5–14]. The first pituitary adenoma was treated by Leksell on January 27, 1968 in the Sophiahemmet Hospital, Stockholm, Sweden, with the prototype Gamma Knife (GK), a dedicated neurosurgical tool to perform stereotactic radiosurgery for predetermined intracranial targets [2, 15–17]. The first vestibular schwannoma was treated also by Leksell in June 1968 and the first meningioma by Backlund in 1971 [17, 18]. Since then, it has been widely accepted either as a primary alternative intervention, or as a supplementary tool to microsurgery especially for high-risk cases with difficult surgical access in critical locations [19–34]. Complications related to GK radiosurgery (GKRS), which are usually temporary, are rare and the risk for permanent neurological deficit following irradiation is low [35–39].

Although radiosurgical treatment methods have become quite straightforward and well elaborated for brain tumors [40–48], the radiobiological effect of focused single high-dose gamma irradiation on neoplastic tissue is still not fully understood [49, 50]. More than 200,000 patients with benign and malignant intracranial neoplasms have already been treated worldwide with the GK, but the pathophysiological mechanism by which radiosurgery can control or stop tumor progression has not been elucidated completely. Apart from sporadic neuropathological reports [51–55], systematic comprehensive pathological background to brain tumor radiosurgery basically does not exist. Therefore the purpose of this study was to analyze histopathological changes in cases where a GK treatment had been performed as a first step and then the patient underwent an open conventional craniotomy-related surgery for some reason.

Patients and Methods

Out of a series of 7,500 patients who had Leksell GKRS at two centers (Université Libre de Bruxelles, n = 1,000, and University of Pittsburgh, n = 6,500), 5,776 patients harbored cerebral tumors with a variety of histological types. We selected 38 patients who underwent later craniotomy for lesion resection (n = 47) after radiosurgery because of radiological and clinical progression. Histopathological review revealed 26 metastases, 5 astrocytomas grade III, 1 astrocytoma grade II, 5 meningiomas, 3 atypical meningiomas, 3 sporadic vestibular schwannomas, 2 NF-2 vestibular schwannomas, 1 jugular bulb schwannoma and 1 hemangioblastoma among the resected tumors. Radiosurgery was carried out using the Leksell GK Models U, B or C (Elekta Instruments AB, Stockholm, Sweden). Dose planning was based on MR and CT imaging. Treated volumes ranged between 266 and 25.600 mm^3 (median 4.700 mm^3). Tumors received 12–20 Gy as a marginal dose (median 16 Gy) at 30–60% isodose line (median 50%), with 24–40 Gy maximal dose (median 32 Gy).

Histopathological investigations were performed on surgical pathology materials. Resected specimens were fixed in 10% neutral buffered formaldehyde, processed routinely, and embedded in paraffin. Besides routine hematoxylin-eosin and Masson's trichrome staining, immunohistochemical reactions were carried out for GFAP, vimentin, S100, neurofilament, synaptophysin, EMA, pankeratin, CK7, CK20, CAM5.2, CD3, CD20, CD31 and CD68 (PGM1) antigens to characterize phenotypic nature of tumor cells and the reactive cell population around/or infiltrating neoplastic tissues. Ki67 and p53 reactions were used to assess proliferative activity of tumor cells. Biotin-streptavidin-peroxidase complex methods were performed according to standard protocols on 5-μm paraffin sections.

Results

The morphological appearance of various lesions suggestive of radiation effect in different tumors was neither significantly related with the histopathological type of the irradiated neoplasm nor with the time interval between radiosurgery and craniotomy. Considering the temporal development of radiation-induced tissue and organ reactions, there are immediate (milliseconds to hours), early (days to weeks) and delayed (months to years after exposure) responses. However, the morphological and clinical types can be described as acute, subacute or chronic. The acute type histological reaction may develop early or during the delayed period, but chronic type tissue response evolves only in a delayed manner [56].

Histopathological changes attributable to radiosurgery were observed within the tumor parenchyma, connective tissue stroma and vessels. These changes were either degenerative or proliferative. The main histopathological characteristics are summarized in table 1. Degenerative alterations occurred mostly in the parenchyma of different tumors, while proliferative processes took place first of all in the connective tissue stroma and vessels of neoplasms. The basic histopathological alteration evoked by the ionizing energy of high-dose radiation was recognized as a well-circumscribed lesion with sharp demarcation towards surrounding tissues according to the steep radiation fall-off (fig. 1a). Regarding the histological and cellular composition of these gamma radiolesions, three main types were obtained following GK treatment. In the *acute type* reaction, coagulation necrosis constituted the center with a network of acidophilic fibrinoid material and amorphous homogeneous tissue or cellular debris (fig. 1b). No cellular reaction, or scanty basophilic hyperchromatic apoptotic cells characterized by nuclear fragmentation and pyknosis intermingled with scattered polymorphonuclear leukocytes and some dilated postcapillary venules surrounded this necrotic core (fig. 1c). There was no prominent macrophage or lymphocytic infiltration, reactive gliosis or scar tissue formation. The necrosis in this targeted volume was usually circumscribed, homogeneous and sharply

Table 1. Histopathological characteristics of gamma radiolesions

Type	Parenchymal changes	Stromal alterations	Vasculopathy	Temporal development
Acute	sharply demarcated coagulation necrosis	no cellular reaction or scattered apoptotic cells and polymorphonuclear leukocytes around the necrosis	dilated small venules; endothelial destruction, undulation of internal elastic membrane, fibrinoid changes in vessels' wall, vacuolar degeneration	early or delayed
Subacute	well-circumscribed coagulation necrosis	macrophage reaction around the necrosis; granulation tissue; reactive gliosis	proliferative vasculopathy with narrowing of the lumen	early or delayed
Chronic	replaced by scar tissue	focal lymphocytic infiltration; hyaline degenerated scar tissue, calcification	subendothelial cell proliferation; subtotal or complete lumen obliteration; hyaline degeneration in the wall	delayed

demarcated from surrounding remaining tumor tissue (fig. 1a) as compared to other necrotic tumor areas outside of the focused irradiation which had an irregular multifocal appearance and entrapped tumor islands (fig. 1d). A similar histological picture of the acute type lesion could be observed either at an early or a delayed time interval after radiosurgery. These parenchymal changes were accompanied with alterations of stromal vessels around the necrotic core characterized by endothelial destruction, fibrinoid necrosis, undulation of the internal elastic membrane, and vacuolation and accumulation of eosinophilic material (transudation) in the vessel wall (fig. 1e, f).

The second group of gamma radiolesions had the characteristics of *subacute type* pathological reactions that were observed several months to years after radiosurgery. The main histological feature of these lesions was an inflammatory tissue response. The central coagulation necrotic core was surrounded by a macrophage rim (fig. 2a). These macrophages revealed phagocytotic activity and mainly CD68 (PGM1) but sometimes CD31 immunohistochemical reactivity as well (fig. 2b). A granulation tissue zone was situated outside of the macrophage layer containing abundant small vessels, capillaries, arterioles and venules accompanied by inflammatory cells, fibrocytes and fibroblasts expressing vimentin positivity (fig. 2c, d). Postirradiation vasculopathy was

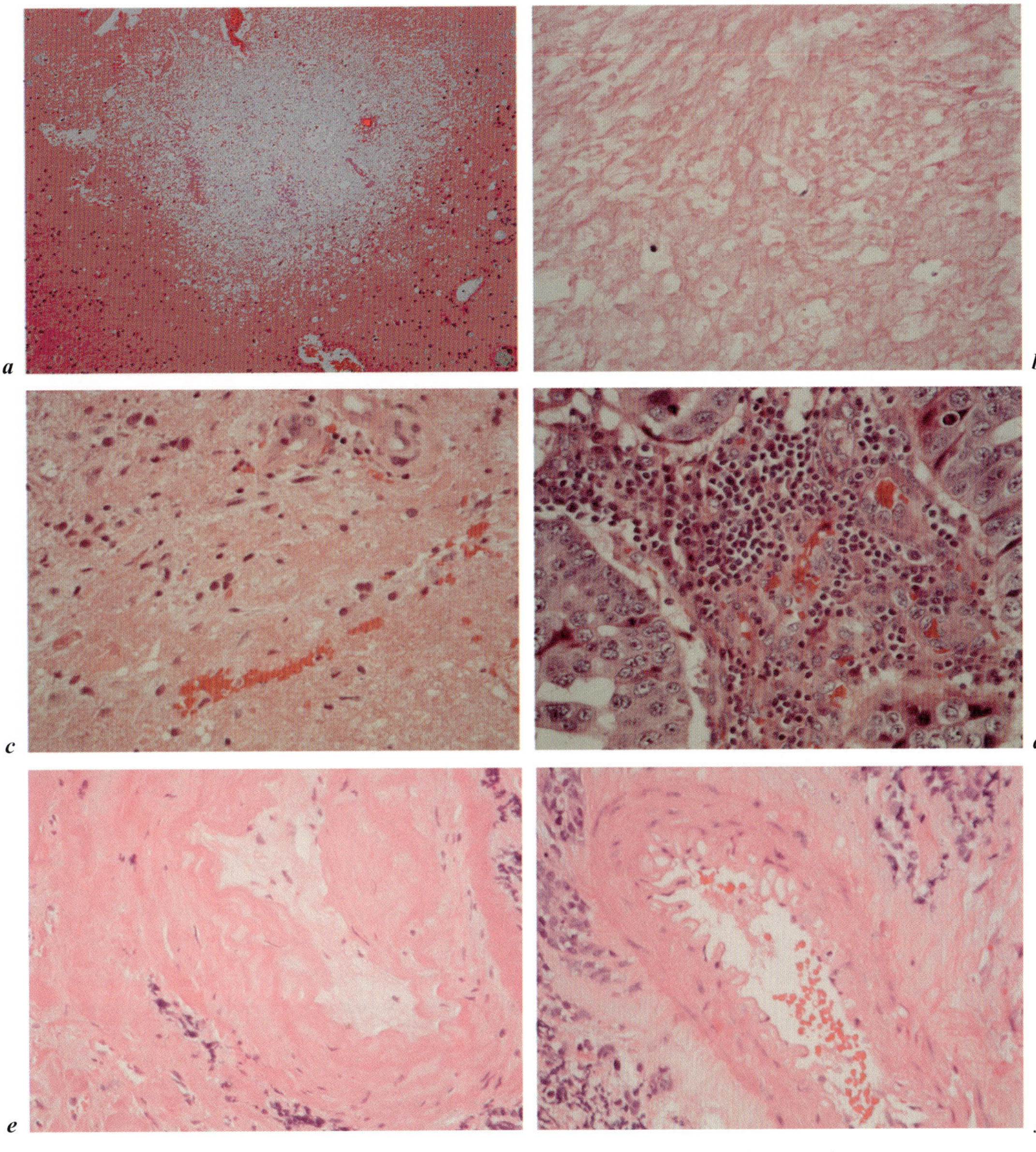

Fig. 1. Histological characteristics of acute type gamma radiolesions. ***a–d*** Metastatic non-small cell carcinoma 4 months after GKRS. ***a*** Sharply demarcated coagulation necrosis in tumor parenchyma (HE, ×100). ***b*** Fibrinoid mesh in the center of the radiolesion (HE, ×300). ***c*** Scattered pyknotic cells at the periphery of the lesion (HE, ×300). ***d*** Irregular tumor necrosis outside of the irradiated target volume (HE, ×300). ***e, f*** Metastatic small cell lung carcinoma 3 months following GKRS. ***e*** Fibrinoid necrosis in vessel's wall (HE, ×300). ***f*** Endothelial destruction, undulation of internal elastic membrane, vacuolar degeneration of vessel's wall (HE, ×300).

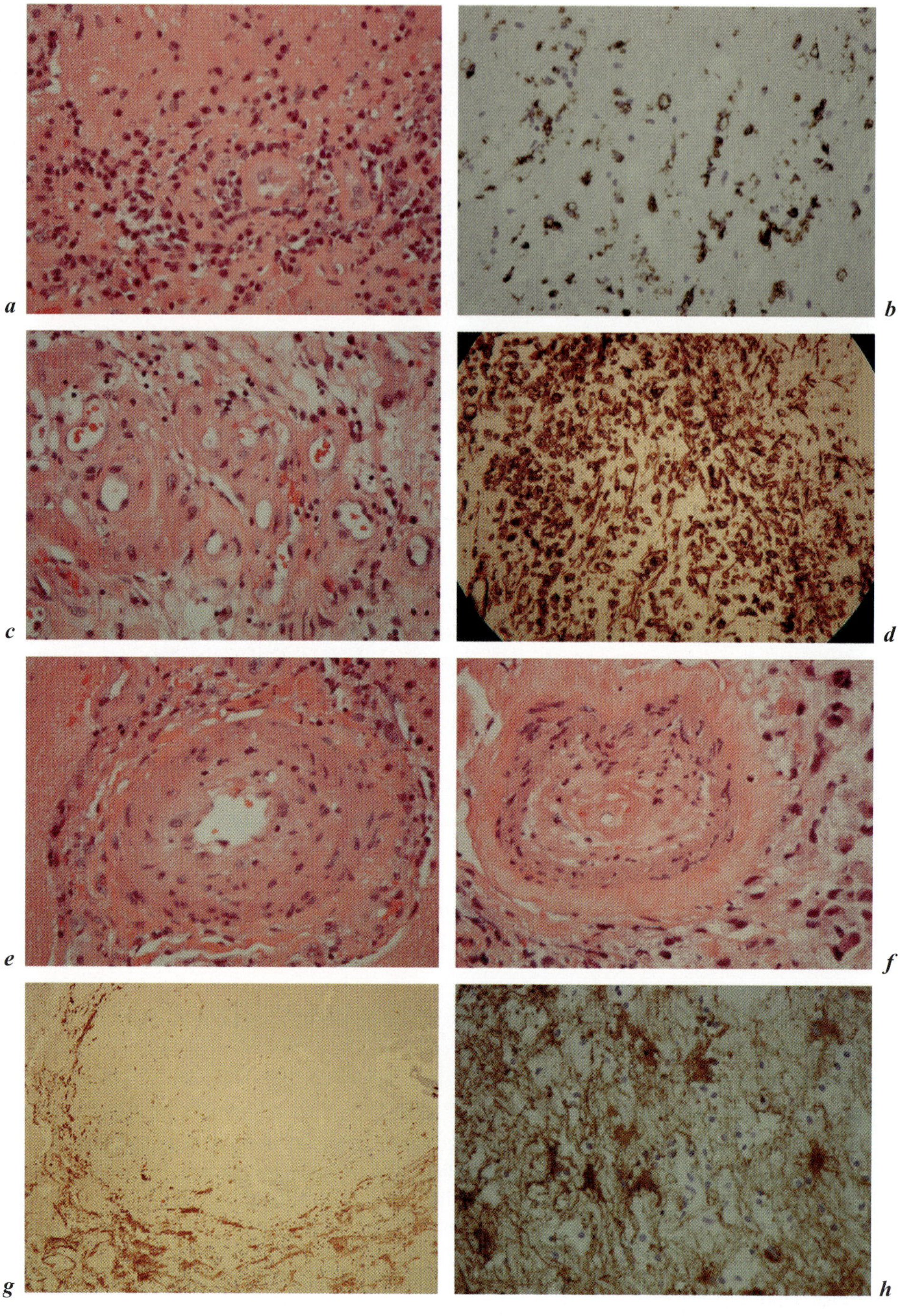
a
b
c
d
e
f
g
h

also observed at the periphery of the central necrotic region (fig. 2e, f). A reactive gliotic scar mantle formed by astrocytic elements and abundant glial filaments coated and constituted the outer border of the radiolesion as it was demonstrated by GFAP immune reaction (fig. 2g, h).

The third, so-called *chronic type* or 'end-stage' pathological reaction appeared several years after radiosurgery. The central part of the radiolesion was replaced by hypocellular scar tissue with degenerative changes that included hyaline deposition and/or focal calcification that demarcated sharply towards remaining surrounding tumor tissue (fig. 3a). Scattered fibrocytes, fibroblasts and sporadic focal lymphocytic infiltration were disclosed around dense collagen bundles (fig. 3b). Immunohistochemical markers for tumor antigens like S100 or neurofilament reactions demonstrated considerable decrease in these areas (fig. 3c, d). Advanced postirradiation vasculopathy with subendothelial spindle-shaped cell proliferation and hyaline degeneration resulted in subtotal or even complete luminal obliteration (fig. 3e, f).

Acute type histological changes were found in 8 tumors (2 anaplastic astrocytomas, 1 nonsmall cell lung metastasis, 1 small cell lung metastasis, 1 breast carcinoma metastasis, 1 meningioma, 1 atypical meningioma and 1 hemangioblastoma) at 2–17 months (median, 11 months) following radiosurgery. The subacute type histological reaction developed in 12 tumors (8 nonsmall cell metastases, 2 renal cell metastases, 1 metastatic breast carcinoma and 1 metastatic melanoma). These alterations were observed at 4–59 months (median 16 months) after the GK procedure. The chronic type tissue response occurred in 5 neoplasms (1 sporadic vestibular schwannoma, 1 NF2 vestibular schwannoma, 1 jugular foramen schwannoma, 1 atypical meningioma, and 1 metastatic breast carcinoma). These were noted 18–82 months (median, 32 months) following radiosurgery.

Fig. 2. Subacute type histological changes in gamma radiolesions. ***a–d*** Metastatic renal cell carcinoma 10 months after GKRS. ***a*** Intense macrophage reaction at the periphery of the necrotic core (HE, ×300). ***b*** CD68 (PGM1) immune reactivity demonstrates active macrophages (×300). ***c*** Granulation tissue with inflammatory cells surrounding and organizing necrosis (HE, ×300). ***d*** Vimentin positivity indicates fibroblasts and fibrocytes in granulation tissue (×300). ***e–h*** Metastatic renal cell carcinoma 7 months following GKRS. ***e*** Proliferative vasculopathy in the stroma (HE, ×300). ***f*** Vasculopathy combined with newly formed fibrin thrombus (HE, ×300). ***g*** Reactive gliosis demarcating the radiolesion (GFAP immunohistochemistry, ×100). ***h*** Astrocytic cells with processes and fiber production (GFAP, ×300).

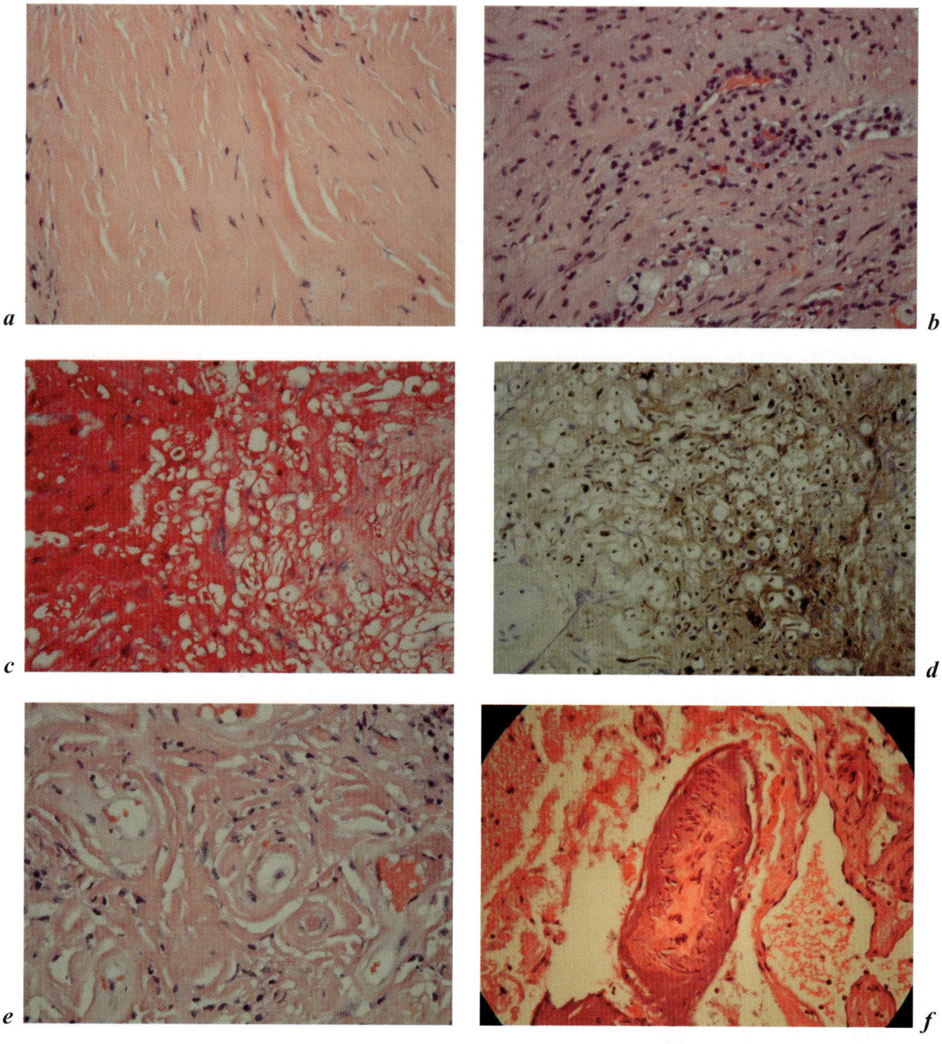

Fig. 3. Chronic type histological findings in gamma radiolesions. ***a–d*** Vestibular schwannoma 18 months after GKRS. ***a*** Hypocellular hyaline degenerated collagen bundles replacing necrotic tissue in the targeted volume (HE, ×300). ***b*** Focal lymphocytic infiltration in scar tissue (HE, ×300). S100 immunoreactivity (***c***) and neurofilament positivity (***d***) at the periphery of the treated volume, decreasing towards the center, indicating recurrent or residual tumor tissue at the edge of the lesion (×300). ***e, f*** Atypical meningioma 33 months following GKRS. ***e*** Fibrotic changes around and in the vessels' wall narrowing the lumina (HE, ×300). ***f*** Complete lumen occlusion by spindle-shaped cell proliferation in a larger artery (HE, ×100).

Discussion

Although a large clinical experience has been accumulated in brain tumor radiosurgery during the past 4 decades, a comprehensive human pathology study has not yet been performed. This is partly due to the high success rate of radiosurgery, but also due to the paucity of postmortem examinations. The term of radiosurgery signifies the application of ionizing radiation energy, in experimental biology or clinical medicine, aiming at the precise and complete destruction of chosen target structures containing healthy and/or pathological cells, without significant concomitant or late radiation damage to adjacent tissues [57]. Therefore, the goal of radiosurgical pathology and experimental studies should be to investigate short-, and long-term effects of high-dose ionizing radiation on neural tissue and its pathologies with histological tissue culture and biochemical methods. The experimental basis for brain tumor radiosurgery is well established and provides evidence of the effectiveness of high-dose irradiation [58–65]. Sporadic human pathological case reports [51–55, 66–68] and a recent study on vestibular schwannomas have been published [69]. The purpose of the present comprehensive study was to evaluate comparatively the effect of GKRS in a series of brain tumors with a variety of histological types and different time intervals after irradiation.

Initial Studies

The basic histopathological lesion, created by high-energy ionizing radiation in neural tissue is coagulation necrosis within the target volume, surrounded by a distinct boundary between the necrosis and the surrounding normal structures, according to the sharp radiation fall-off [1, 70–72]. Whereas target necrosis was the goal with maximum doses above 100 Gy, almost all tumors are radiated at lower, more cytostatic doses. In 1958, Larsson et al. [1] reported in *Nature* that in animal experiments 'with high-energy protons a sharply delimited lesion can be made at any desired site in the central nervous system'. Early lesions appeared in the spinal cord following irradiation with doses of 400 and 200 Gy on the 3rd and 9th day, respectively. They were sharply defined and had about the same width as the beam.

In the cerebral hemispheres, the earliest alterations were observed 14 days after irradiation with 200 Gy, and the changes between 2 and 8 weeks were similar. A striking feature of these lesions was the paucity of cellular reaction at the periphery of necrosis, and that tissue further away from the lesion appeared undamaged. However, irradiation with about 400 Gy produced a very different lesion [70]. The irradiated hemisphere of the animal was markedly swollen, the midline structures were displaced. The affected region surrounding the necrosis was at least the size of the necrotic area itself. Other parts of the brain showed no pathological changes.

These were the early experimental changes after single high-dose irradiation. This phase of postirradiation changes was also called the *necrotic stage* [72]. The next period of postradiosurgery changes was the *stage of resorbtion.* This stage was characterized by resorbtion of cellular debris and beginning glial scar formation. These changes were observed in goat experiments between 18 and 28 months following high-dose irradiation. The *late stage* was characterized histologically by prominent glial scar formation surrounding a cavity.

Human Tissue Responses

In the human brain, the morphology of radiolesions appeared to be similar. The temporal development of radiation lesions are divided into three phases in human oncology practice [56]. The *immediate* response occurs milliseconds to hours after initiation of exposure, usually less than 24 h. Witham et al. [73] noted immediate apoptotic responses in brain tumors following experimental radiosurgery. Histologically and clinically, the lesions are regarded as the acute type. The *early* reaction develops days to weeks after initial exposure, most frequently 24 h to 2 months. Morphologically and clinically the lesions may be acute or subacute. The *delayed* response presents months to years after exposure, often 2 months to many years, and could even occur beyond a decade [74, 75]. Pathologically and clinically the lesions may be acute, subacute, or chronic.

The first available pathological report about the morphology of a human radiolesion observed in the brain of a patient operated on with 200 Gy proton beam radiosurgery for intractable pain due to metastasizing carcinoma was published by Larsson et al. in 1963 [76]. At autopsy 2 months after radiosurgery, the radiolesion macroscopically demonstrated a well-demarcated necrotic area surrounded by a zone of slight cellular reaction. The necrosis measured about 2–4 mm along the three major axes. Microscopically there was a complete destruction of axons, myelin and glial cells. In the marginal zone of the lesion, nuclear debris and macrophages had collected. In the belief that the synchrocyclotron-produced high-energy proton beams had proved to be too complicated for general neurosurgical practice, the GK was designed specifically for brain radiosurgery and incorporated within the array of stereotactic tools developed by Leksell in 1967 [15]. The radiolesions investigated in two autopsy cases (with 3 lesions) created with 200- or 250-Gy gamma thalamotomies for intractable cancer pain expressed similar morphological characteristics as the proton radiolesion. Macroscopically there were well-defined lesions in the targeted areas. Histological examinations revealed sharply demarcated areas from the surrounding brain tissue 10, 14 and 20 weeks after the operation. The lesions consisted mainly of dense necrosis with few distinguishable cellular components. There was a narrow region of astrocytic gliosis, about 0.3 mm thick, surrounding the lesion. Outside this gliosis, the brain parenchyma had a normal appearance. The blood vessels in the center of the lesions were thrombotic and had necrotic walls, while at the periphery of the lesions the vessel walls were somewhat fibrotic but their lumen remained patent. There was virtually no histological difference among the three gamma radiolesions. In 1970, a histopathological review was reported on 9 patients managed with a dose of 180–250 Gy for intractable pain and in which autopsies were performed 3 weeks to 7.5 months after irradiation [71]. The histopathological changes were fairly uniform in all cases in spite of the differences in the age of the lesions. They were well demarcated from the undamaged surrounding tissues. The lesions were necrotic and in them thrombosed vessels with necrotic walls could be identified, sometimes surrounded by small hemorrhages. In lesions older than 3 weeks, necrosis was also infiltrated by macrophages and some round cells. Immediately around the necrotic tissue was a spongy zone, 0.3–0.5 mm wide, which presented a moderate increase in the number of vessels, which were often congested and had a thickened intima. The tissue around this zone appeared normal. Steiner et al. [77] demonstrated that at least 140 Gy was necessary to produce a stable lesion in the human brain after radiosurgery. Higher doses up to 250 Gy did not change the physical characteristics of the lesion, which was due to the sharp dose gradient. The nature of these lesions provided confidence for the widespread use of radiosurgery.

Human Tumors

The present study found that ionizing energy from high-dose irradiation evoked either degenerative or proliferative histopathological changes in the investigated brain tumors. Among degenerative changes, necrosis and apoptosis occurred in the parenchyma of neoplasms contributing to tumor cell destruction, while hyaline, fibrinoid and calcium deposition appeared mostly in the connective tissue stroma and vessel wall. On the other hand, proliferative processes like granulation tissue formation, inflammatory reaction, macrophage invasion, fibrocyte-fibroblast proliferation and scar tissue production were found in the stroma and vasculature of tumors. They have a scavenger function and their contribution to the radiosurgery effect is to remove destroyed neoplastic tissue (necrotic debris) and eventually replace the defect with scar tissue. Scar tissue consists of hyaline degenerated collagen bundles and glial fibrils that have a certain propensity for contraction.

This contraction of scar tissue might play a role in the volumetric regression of the tumor as noted frequently on follow-up imaging studies.

Three main histopathological types of gamma radiolesions were delineated in the present study (table 1). Acute gamma radiolesions were characterized mainly by necrotic changes and appeared at either the early or the delayed stage; subacute type gamma radiolesion expressed resorptive activity at the early or the delayed stage, and chronic type lesions showed a reparative tendency but only at the delayed stage. These changes seem to follow each other consecutively without any significant relationship between tumor type or time after irradiation, and the type of the evoked radiolesion. The only consistent observation was that chronic type lesions were noted only at the delayed stage, which is in accordance with the idea that these are end-stage alterations. The similar morphological appearance of the target effects in different tumors and different patients suggests that the evoked histopathological reaction is likely related to the biologic effect of radiosurgery. We believe these responses represent both direct cellular effects and vascular mechanisms induced by the radiation energy. The acute effects indicate a direct cellular response, mediated by cytokines released at the time of injury. Subacute and chronic effects appear to be mediated by the inflammatory cascade induced at the time of injury. Research into radiation protection has focused on modulating this inflammation effect [78, 79].

References

1 Larsson B, Leksell L, Rexed B, Sourander P, Mair W, Andersson B: The high-energy proton beam as a neurosurgical tool. Nature 1958;182:1222–1223.

2 Leksell L: The stereotaxic method and radiosurgery of the brain. Acta Chir Scand 1951;102: 316–319.

3 Leksell L: Stereotaxis and Radiosurgery. An Operative System. Springfield, Thomas, 1971.

4 Kondziolka D, Lunsford LD, Witt TC, Flickinger JC: The future of radiosurgery: radiobiology, technology, and applications. Surg Neurol 2000;54:406–414.

5 Kondziolka D, Lunsford LD, McLaughlin MR, Flickinger JC: Long-term outcomes after radiosurgery for acoustic neuromas. N Engl J Med 1998;339:1426–1433.

6 Lunsford LD, Kondziolka D, Flickinger JC: Stereotactic radiosurgery: current spectrum and results. Clin Neurosurg 1992;38:405–444.

7 Niranjan A, Lunsford LD, Gobbel GT, Kondziolka D, Maitz A, Flickinger JC: Brain tumor radiosurgery: current status and strategies to enhance the effect of radiosurgery. Brain Tumor Pathol 2000;17:89–96.

8 Niranjan A, Lunsford LD: Radiosurgery: where we were, are, and may be in the third millennium. Neurosurgery 2000;46:531–543.

9 Lunsford LD, Maitz A, Lindner G: First United States 201 source cobalt-60 gamma unit for radiosurgery. Appl Neurophysiol 1987;50:253–256.

10 Lunsford LD, Kondziolka D, Flickinger JC: Stereotactic radiosurgery for benign intracranial tumors. Clin Neurosurg 1993;40:475–497.

11 Payne BR, Prasad D, Szeifert G, Steiner M, Steiner L: Gamma surgery for intracranial metastases from renal cell carcinoma. J Neurosurg 2000;92:760–765.

12 Friedman WA, Foote KD: Linear accelerator radiosurgery in the management of brain tumours. Ann Med 2000;32:64–80.

13 Flickinger JC: Radiosurgery of brain metastases from renal cell carcinoma: how can you improve on results like this? Cancer J 2000;6:360–361.

14 Flickinger JC, Kondziolka D, Lunsford LD, Coffey RJ, Goodman ML, Shaw EG, et al: A multi-institutional experience with stereotactic radiosurgery for solitary brain metastasis. Int J Radiat Oncol Biol Phys 1994;28:797–802.

15 Leksell L: Cerebral radiosurgery. I. Gammathalamotomy in two cases of intractable pain. Acta Chir Scand 1968;134:585–595.

16 Leksell L: Stereotactic radiosurgery. J Neurol Neurosurg Psychiatry 1983;46:797–803.
17 Karlsson B: Gamma Knife surgery in a historic perspective. Gamma Knife Surgery of Cerebral Arteriovenous Malformations. Thesis. Department of Neurosurgery, Neuroradiology and Radiation Physics, Karolinska Hospital Stockholm: Karolinska, 1996.
18 Leksell L: A note on the treatment of acoustic tumors. Acta Chir Scand 1971;137:763–765.
19 Pendl G, Schrottner O, Eustacchio S, Ganz JC, Feichtinger K: Cavernous sinus meningiomas–what is the strategy: upfront or adjuvant gamma knife surgery? Stereotact Funct Neurosurg 1998;70(suppl 1):33–40.
20 Liscak R, Vladyka V, Wowra B, Kemeny A, Forster D, Burzaco JA, et al: Gamma Knife radiosurgery of the glomus jugulare tumour – early multicentre experience. Acta Neurochir (Wien) 1999;141:1141–1146.
21 Prasad D, Steiner M, Steiner L: Gamma surgery for vestibular schwannoma. J Neurosurg 2000;92:745–759.
22 Lunsford LD, Kondziolka D, Flickinger JC: Radiosurgery as an alternative to microsurgery of acoustic tumors. Clin Neurosurg 1992;38:619–634.
23 Lunsford LD, Flickinger J, Coffey RJ: Stereotactic gamma knife radiosurgery. Initial North American experience in 207 patients. Arch Neurol 1990;47:169–175.
24 Lunsford LD, Flickinger J, Lindner G, Maitz A: Stereotactic radiosurgery of the brain using the first United States 201 cobalt-60 source gamma knife. Neurosurgery 1989;24:151–159.
25 Kondziolka D, Lunsford LD, Flickinger JC: Acoustic tumors: operation versus radiation–making sense of opposing viewpoints. Part II. Acoustic neuromas: sorting out management options. Clin Neurosurg 2003;50:313–328.
26 Regis J, Pellet W, Delsanti C, Dufour H, Roche PH, Thomassin JM, et al: Functional outcome after gamma knife surgery or microsurgery for vestibular schwannomas. J Neurosurg 2002;97:1091–1100.
27 Flickinger JC, Kondziolka D, Pollock BE, Lunsford LD: Evolution in technique for vestibular schwannoma radiosurgery and effect on outcome. Int J Radiat Oncol Biol Phys 1996;36:275–280.
28 Flickinger JC, Kondziolka D, Niranjan A, Lunsford LD: Results of acoustic neuroma radiosurgery: an analysis of 5 years' experience using current methods. J Neurosurg 2001;94:1–6.
29 Yamakami I, Uchino Y, Kobayashi E, Yamaura A: Conservative management, gamma-knife radiosurgery, and microsurgery for acoustic neurinomas: a systematic review of outcome and risk of three therapeutic options. Neurol Res 2003;25:682–690.
30 Liscak R, Simonova G, Vymazal J, Janouskova L, Vladyka V: Gamma knife radiosurgery of meningiomas in the cavernous sinus region. Acta Neurochir (Wien) 1999;141:473–480.
31 Pendl G, Eustacchio S, Unger F: Radiosurgery as alternative treatment for skull base meningiomas. J Clin Neurosci 2001;8(suppl 1):12–14.
32 Kondziolka D, Hadjipanayis CG, Flickinger JC, Lunsford LD: The role of radiosurgery for the treatment of pineal parenchymal tumors. Neurosurgery 2002;51:880–889.
33 Kondziolka D, Lunsford LD, Flickinger JC: Intraparenchymal brain stem radiosurgery. Neurosurg Clin N Am 1993;4:469–479.
34 Fedorcsak I, Sipos L, Horvath A, Kontra G, Bognar L, Osztie E: Multiple intracranial melanoma metastases treated with surgery and radiosurgery with long term control. A case report. J Neurooncol 1993;16:173–176.
35 Flickinger JC, Kondziolka D, Lunsford LD, Kassam A, Phuong LK, Liscak R, et al: Development of a model to predict permanent symptomatic postradiosurgery injury for arteriovenous malformation patients. Arteriovenous Malformation Radiosurgery Study Group. Int J Radiat Oncol Biol Phys 2000;46:1143–1148.
36 Chin LS, Ma L, DiBiase S: Radiation necrosis following gamma knife surgery: a case-controlled comparison of treatment parameters and long-term clinical follow up. J Neurosurg 2001;94:899–904.
37 Chin LS, Lazio BE, Biggins T, Amin P: Acute complications following gamma knife radiosurgery are rare. Surg Neurol 2000;53:498–502; discussion 02.
38 Flickinger JC, Kondziolka D, Lunsford LD, Pollock BE, Yamamoto M, Gorman DA, et al: A multi-institutional analysis of complication outcomes after arteriovenous malformation radiosurgery. Int J Radiat Oncol Biol Phys 1999;44:67–74.

39 Flickinger JC, Kondziolka D, Lunsford LD: Radiobiological analysis of tissue responses following radiosurgery. Technol Cancer Res Treat 2003;2:87–92.
40 Levivier M, Wikier D, Goldman S, David P, Metens T, Massager N, et al: Integration of the metabolic data of positron emission tomography in the dosimetry planning of radiosurgery with the gamma knife: early experience with brain tumors. Technical note. J Neurosurg 2000;93(suppl 3): 233–238.
41 Flickinger JC, Kondziolka D, Lunsford LD: Radiosurgery of Benign Lesions. Semin Radiat Oncol 1995;5:220–224.
42 Kondziolka D, Nathoo N, Flickinger JC, Niranjan A, Maitz AH, Lunsford LD: Long-term results after radiosurgery for benign intracranial tumors. Neurosurgery 2003;53:815–821; discussion 21–22.
43 Flickinger JC, Kondziolka D: Radiosurgery instead of resection for solitary brain metastasis: the gold standard redefined. Int J Radiat Oncol Biol Phys 1996;35:185–186.
44 Yamamoto M, Ide M, Nishio S, Urakawa Y: Gamma Knife radiosurgery for numerous brain metastases: is this a safe treatment? Int J Radiat Oncol Biol Phys 2002;53:1279–1283.
45 Pendl G, Unger F, Papaefthymiou G, Eustacchio S: Staged radiosurgical treatment for large benign cerebral lesions. J Neurosurg 2000;93(suppl 3):107–112.
46 Levivier M, Wikler D Jr, Massager N, David P, Devriendt D, Lorenzoni J, et al: The integration of metabolic imaging in stereotactic procedures including radiosurgery: a review. J Neurosurg 2002;97(suppl):542–550.
47 Kondziolka D, Flickinger JC, Perez B: Judicious resection and/or radiosurgery for parasagittal meningiomas: outcomes from a multicenter review. Gamma Knife Meningioma Study Group. Neurosurgery 1998;43:405–413; discussion 13–14.
48 Duma CM, Lunsford LD, Kondziolka D, Harsh GRt, Flickinger JC: Stereotactic radiosurgery of cavernous sinus meningiomas as an addition or alternative to microsurgery. Neurosurgery 1993;32:699–704; discussion 04–05.
49 Yamamoto M: Gamma Knife radiosurgery: technology, applications, and future directions. Neurosurg Clin N Am 1999;10:181–202.
50 Kondziolka D, Lunsford LD, Flickinger JC: The radiobiology of radiosurgery. Neurosurg Clin N Am 1999;10:157–166.
51 Szeifert GT, Massager N, DeVriendt D, David P, De Smedt F, Rorive S, et al: Observations of intracranial neoplasms treated with gamma knife radiosurgery. J Neurosurg 2002;97 (suppl):623–626.
52 Thompson BG, Coffey RJ, Flickinger JC, Lunsford LD: Stereotactic radiosurgery of small intracranial tumors: neuropathological correlation in three patients. Surg Neurol 1990;33:96–104.
53 Hirato M, Hirato J, Zama A, Inoue H, Ohye C, Shibazaki T, et al: Radiobiological effects of gamma knife radiosurgery on brain tumors studied in autopsy and surgical specimens. Stereotact Funct Neurosurg 1996;66(suppl 1):4–16.
54 Szeifert GT, Massager N, Brotchi J, Levivier M: Morphological redifferentiation in a malignant astrocytic tumor after gamma knife radiosurgery. J Neurosurg 2002;97(suppl):627–630.
55 Szeifert GT, Salmon I, David P, Devriendt D, De Smedt F, Rorive S, Brotchi J, Levivier M: Tumor control and growth in a patient with two cerebral metastases treated with the leksell gamma knife; in Kondziolka D (ed): Radiosurgery. Basel, Karger, 2002, vol. 4, pp 152–161.
56 Fajardo L-GLF, Berthrong M, Anderson RE: Radiation Pathology. New York: Oxford University Press, Inc., 2001.
57 Larsson B: Radiobiological fundamentals in radiosurgery; in Steiner L (ed): Radiosurgery: Baseline and Trends. New York, Raven Press, 1992, pp 3–15.
58 Lunsford LD, Altschuler EM, Flickinger JC, Wu A, Martinez AJ: In vivo biological effects of stereotactic radiosurgery: a primate model. Neurosurgery 1990;27:373–382.
59 Kondziolka D, Lunsford LD, Claassen D, Pandalai S, Maitz AH, Flickinger JC: Radiobiology of radiosurgery: Part II. The rat C6 glioma model. Neurosurgery 1992;31:280–287; discussion 87–88.
60 Blatt DR, Friedman WA, Bova FJ, Theele DP, Mickle JP: Temporal characteristics of radiosurgical lesions in an animal model. J Neurosurg 1994;80:1046–1055.
61 Inoue HK, Kohga H, Hirato M, Nakamura M, Ohye C: Neurobiologic effects of radiosurgery: histologic, immunohistochemical and electron-microscopic studies of a rat model. Stereotact Funct Neurosurg 1994;63:280–285.

62 Linskey ME, Martinez AJ, Kondziolka D, Flickinger JC, Maitz AH, Whiteside T, et al: The radiobiology of human acoustic schwannoma xenografts after stereotactic radiosurgery evaluated in the subrenal capsule of athymic mice. J Neurosurg 1993;78:645–653.

63 Niranjan A, Wolfe D, Tamura M, Soares MK, Krisky DM, Lunsford LD, et al: Treatment of rat gliosarcoma brain tumors by HSV-based multigene therapy combined with radiosurgery. Mol Ther 2003;8:530–542.

64 Niranjan A, Wolfe D, Fellows W, Goins WF, Glorioso JC, Kondziolka D, et al: Gene transfer to glial tumors using herpes simplex virus. Methods Mol Biol 2004;246:323–337.

65 Niranjan A, Moriuchi S, Lunsford LD, Kondziolka D, Flickinger JC, Fellows W, et al: Effective treatment of experimental glioblastoma by HSV vector-mediated TNF alpha and HSV-tk gene transfer in combination with radiosurgery and ganciclovir administration. Mol Ther 2000;2:114–120.

66 Kwon Y, Khang SK, Kim CJ, Lee DJ, Lee JK, Kwun BD: Radiologic and histopathologic changes after Gamma Knife radiosurgery for acoustic schwannoma. Stereotact Funct Neurosurg 1999;72(suppl 1):2–10.

67 Noren G, Arndt J, Hindmarsh T: Stereotactic radiosurgery in cases of acoustic neurinoma: further experiences. Neurosurgery 1983;13:12–22.

68 Nielsen SL, Kjellberg RN, Asbury AK, Koehler AM: Neuropathologic effect of proton-beam irradiation in man. I. Dose-response relationship after treatment of intracranial neoplasms. Acta Neuropathol (Berl) 1972;20:348–356.

69 Szeifert GT, Figarella-Branger D, Roche PH, Régis J: Histopathological observations on vestibular schwannomas after gamma knife radiosurgery: the Marseille experience. Neurochirurgie 2004;50:327–337.

70 Leksell L, Larsson B, Andersson B, Rexed B, Sourander P, Mair W: Lesions in the depth of the brain produced by a beam of high energy protons. Acad Radiol 1960;54:251–264.

71 Wennerstrand J, Ungerstedt U: Cerebral radiosurgery. II. An anatomical study of gamma radiolesions. Acta Chir Scand 1970;136:133–137.

72 Andersson B, Larsson B, Leksell L, Mair W, Rexed B, Sourander P, et al: Histopathology of late local radiolesions in the goat brain. Acta Radiologica Therapy Physics Biology 1970;9:385–394.

73 Witham T, Okada H, Fellows W, Hamilton R, Flickinger J, Chambers WH, Pollack IF, Watkins SC, Kondziolka D: The characterization of tumor apoptosis after experimental radiosurgery. Stereotact Funct Neurosurg 2005;83:17–24.

74 Adams RD: The neuropathology of radiosurgery. Stereotact Funct Neurosurg 1991;57:82–86.

75 Julow J, Slowik F, Kelemen J: Late post-irradiation necrosis of the brain. Acta Neurochir (Wien) 1979;46:135–150.

76 Larsson B, Leksell L, Rexed B: The use of high energy protons for cerebral surgery in man. Acta Chir Scand 1963;125:1–7.

77 Steiner L, Forster D, Leksell L, Meyerson BA, Boethius J: Gammathalamotomy in intractable pain. Acta Neurochir (Wien) 1980;52:173–184.

78 Kondziolka D, Somaza S, Martinez AJ, Jacobsohn J, Maitz A, Lunsford LD, et al: Radioprotective effects of the 21-aminosteroid U-74389G for stereotactic radiosurgery. Neurosurgery 1997;41:203–208.

79 Kondziolka D, Mori Y, Martinez AJ, McLaughlin M, Flickinger JC, Lunsford LD: Beneficial effects of the radioprotectant 21-aminosteroid U-74389G in a radiosurgery rat malignant glioma model. Int J Radiat Oncol Biol Phys 1999;44:179–184.

György T. Szeifert, MD, PhD
National Institute of Neurosurgery and Department of Neurological Surgery
Semmelweis University
Amerikai út 57
HU–1145 Budapest (Hungary)
Tel. +36 1 2512999, Fax +36 1 2515678, E-Mail gyorgyszeifert@yahoo.com

Szeifert GT, Kondziolka D, Levivier M, Lunsford LD (eds): Radiosurgery and Pathological Fundamentals. Prog Neurol Surg. Basel, Karger, 2007, vol 20, pp 106–128

9.1. Radiosurgery for Metastatic Brain Tumors

Masaaki Yamamoto

Katsuta Hospital Mito GammaHouse, Hitachi-Naka, Japan

Abstract

New, not yet widely known concepts pertaining to Gamma Knife (GK) radiosurgery for brain metastases are reviewed. In the author's experience, GK is a safe and effective treatment. Though lesion size is a limitation, high tumor control rates are possible when 1–4 lesions are irradiated with ≥20 Gy. Recurrence is rare in such cases, as are radiosurgical complications. Symptomatic complications, i.e. radionecrosis of normal brain tissues, are slightly more common in long-surviving patients. However, since most patients die of causes other than metastatic brain disease, i.e. before long-term complications manifest, good brain function is usually maintained till death. Factors predicting longer survival are youth, better performance status and absence of active nonbrain disease. Although some studies found retreatment for new lesions to be less frequent when whole brain radiotherapy (WBRT) is combined with surgery or GK radiosurgery, in our experience neither survival nor local recurrence rates improve significantly with WBRT. Advantages of GK over WBRT include brief hospitalization, higher control rates, better symptom palliation, all MRI-detected lesions can be treated, other treatments (e.g. radiotherapy) need not be postponed, irradiation can be repeated, the incidence of dementia (due to radionecrosis) is far lower and more tumors (30+) can be treated in one session. We advocate meticulous MRI follow-up to detect recurrence and assess tumor necrosis. All detectable tumors should be irradiated, so long as the patient wishes to continue treatment.

Successful application of Gamma Knife (GK) radiosurgery to the treatment of brain metastasis (MET), from a recurrent hypernephroma, was first reported by Lindquist in 1989 [1]. Stereotactic radiosurgery with a GK or a LINAC system is now being used as primary management or booster treatment with whole brain radiation therapy (WBRT), in an increasing number of patients with metastatic cancers, both radiosensitive and radioresistant, single and multiple [2–20]. Early data from patients undergoing GK treatment, accumulated through 1994, include 4,383 (16.4% of 26,717) patients with brain

Table 1. 1,165 patients with brain METs treated with GK by one neurosurgeon (Nov., 1991 through Oct., 2004)

Gender:	434 females, 731 males			
Mean age:	63 years (range 19–92)			
GK procedures:	One	850 (73.0%)		
	Two	242 (20.8%)		
	Three	56 (4.8%)		
	Four	14 (1.2%)		
	Five	3 (0.3%)		
Total		1572 (10,321 tumors)		
Primary tumors:	Lung	717 (61.5%)	Ad.	392 (54.7%)
	Breast	118 (10.1%)	SCC	114 (15.9%)
	Kidney	59 (5.1%)	Sq.	70 (9.8%)
	Colon	55 (4.7%)	Others	54 (7.3%)
	Rectum	47 (4.0%)	Unknown	87 (12.1%)
	Gastrium	34 (2.9%)		
	Esophagus	15 (1.3%)		
	Ovarium	11 (0.9%)		
	Uterus	10 (0.9%)		
	Others	50 (4.3%)		
	Unknown	34 (2.9%)		

METs worldwide and 935 (19.6% of 4,764) in Japan. GK treatment percentages had risen to 32.5% (81,595 of 251,681) worldwide and 52.2% (34,199 of 65,462) in Japan by 2003; most notably, the patient number for 2003 was 7,681 (65.3% of 11,761) in Japan. Although no data are available as to numbers of patients treated with LINAC systems, it is reasonable to assume that the number is several times that treated with GK worldwide. Thus, radiosurgery has become relatively routine, rather than the special, 'high-tech' treatment that it was regarded as less than a decade ago.

In this review, relatively new, not yet widely known concepts, including the pathological background of radiosurgery for brain METs, will be described.

What We Have Already Learned

Numerous publications focusing on radiosurgery for brain METs have been comprehensively reviewed by Boyd and Mehta [21] and Pollock and Brown [22]. Though a comprehensive review is beyond the scope of the present article, the author's personal experience with 1,167 patients (1,572 procedures, table 1) who

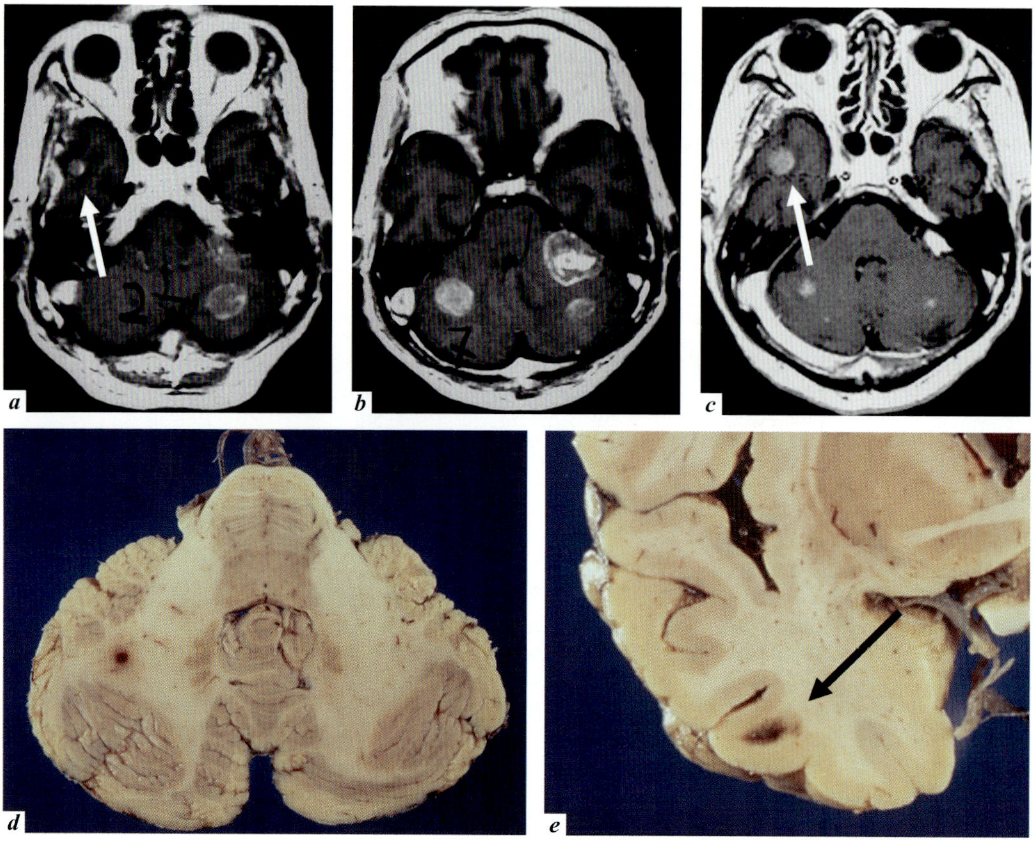

Fig. 1. This 69-year-old man with small-cell lung cancer underwent GK radiosurgery for multiple brain METs on October 30, 1998. Each tumor was irradiated with 15.0 Gy at the tumor margin. The irradiated tumors seen on MR images obtained before radiosurgery (***a***, ***b***) had undergone remarkable shrinkage or disappeared on MR images obtained 4 weeks after treatment (***c***). One lesion located in the right temporal lobe was missed and was not irradiated (arrow). This unirradiated lesion showed significant growth. An autopsy study performed on December 17, 1998, revealed the treated lesions to have nearly or completely disappeared (***d***) while the untreated lesion persisted (***e***).

underwent GK radiosurgery for brain METs (10,321 tumors) during the 13-year period from November 1991 through October 2004 will be summarized along with much of what we have learned from a wealth of already published data.

Although the size limitation on treatable lesions is crucial in radiosurgery, tumor control rates of 90%, or even slightly better, can be expected if 1–4 lesions are irradiated with a peripheral dose of 20 Gy or more. In such cases, true recurrence is extremely rare. As shown in figure 1, postradiosurgical MR images reveal immediate disappearance of tumors and complete cure, as confirmed by autopsy, can be expected in most cases. In contrast, the one untreated lesion in this case continued to grow.

The incidence of radiosurgery-related complications, i.e. symptomatic radionecrosis of the normal brain, is no more than 3.0%. As expected, however, in the special group of patients surviving for 3–5 years or more after radiosurgery, the complication incidence exceeds 5.0%.

Prolonged survival cannot be expected because survival duration depends primarily on the state of nonbrain lesions (including the primary tumor). It merits emphasis that 80–90% of patients die of causes other than brain tumor progression. Thus, most patients can maintain good brain function until death.

Known factors predictive of longer survival are younger age, better performance status and absence of active nonbrain diseases.

Controversy persists as to whether radiosurgery should be combined with WBRT. For patients undergoing radiosurgery, although some reports have supported combining treatment with WBRT to achieve optimal tumor control rates as well as survival periods [23, 24], others have questioned the usefulness of WBRT [17, 25–27]. The majority of studies have found the only merit of combining radiosurgery with WBRT to be that re-treatment necessitated by new lesions is significantly reduced. In the author's experience, neither the survival rate nor the local tumor recurrence rate differs significantly between groups with vs. without WBRT.

Detectability of Small METs on MR Images

The recent development of MR imaging has unquestionably made an enormous contribution to improving the results of radiosurgery for brain METs. Figure 2 presents a patient the author treated in 1997. This patient had one metastatic lesion with a diameter of 4 mm which was demonstrated using an old 0.5-tesla MR unit. The patient died a few weeks after this MR image was obtained. However, the lesion could not be found in a routine macroscopic postmortem examination with a slice thickness of 5 mm. Only a microscopic study of sequential slices revealed the existence of a cell cluster. According to a recent analysis conducted at the author's facility, using a more advanced 1.5-tesla MR unit allows even lesion volumes as small as 0.004 cm^3 to be detected by routine examination with a 5-mm slice thickness and a single dose of gadolinium (fig. 3). In contrast, the minimum volume detectable with 1.0-tesla MR imaging was 0.012 cm^3. It can be concluded that the detectability of metastatic lesions by MR imaging far exceeds that achieved in routine macroscopic autopsy studies. Textbooks giving incidences of brain METs from various primary tumors,

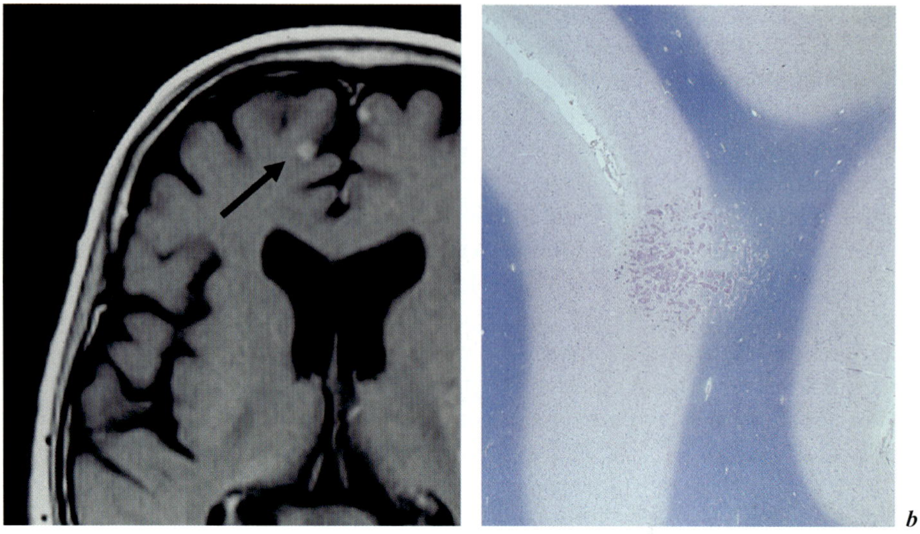

a b

Fig. 2. This 59-year-old man had lung adenocarcinoma. ***a*** One metastatic lesion (arrow) with a diameter of 4 mm was demonstrated using an old 0.5-tesla MR unit. The patient died a few weeks after this examination and the author, with two pathologists, performed a postmortem examination. However, the lesion could not be found in a routine macroscopic postmortem examination with a slice thickness of 5 mm. ***b*** Only a microscopic study of sequential slices revealed the existence of a cell cluster (LFB, ×2.5).

e.g. 34% for lung cancer, 30% for breast cancer, 72% for melanoma, and so on, are based on macroscopic autopsy studies [28]. Such texts should perhaps be rewritten based on MR imaging data. It is unfortunately not feasible for microscopic analyses covering the whole brain to be performed in routine autopsy studies.

How Many Lesions Can Be Treated?

'How many tumors can and should be treated?' has long been a central question in the field of radiosurgery for brain METs. With a LINAC system, the upper tumor number limit is generally considered to be 4–5 lesions in a single session due mainly to the prolonged procedure time. In GK radiosurgery, the maximum number of lesions that can be treated in a 1-day session is 30 or even slightly more, the prolonged procedure time again accounting for the limitation in tumor numbers. If a patient has more than 40 lesions, the author recommends that the procedure be divided into two sessions, 1 day apart, with the patient keeping the stereotactic head frame on overnight.

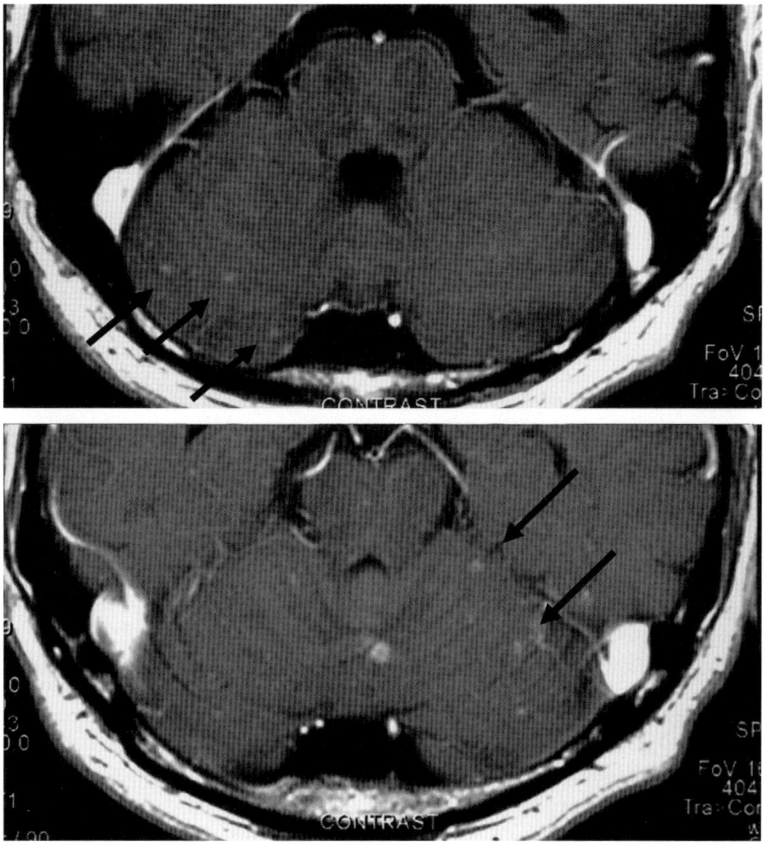

Fig. 3. A more advanced 1.5-tesla MR unit allows even lesion volumes as small as 0.004 cm^3 to be detected by routine examination with a 5-mm slice thickness and a single dose of gadolinium (arrows).

GK radiosurgery for multiple METs reportedly produces survival rates similar to those achieved using this technique for single METs [16, 29–31]. A comprehensive review found no correlation between lesion number, even in patients with eight or more lesions, and survival [21]. Presently, even among patients with metastatic lesions scattered throughout the brain, most can be treated using a GK in one frame position, without replacing the frame, as was previously required (fig. 4). This improvement in treatment stems from three technical advances; application of long Z slides, treatment in the lateral position and a specially designed Y-Z slide. The author's group and others have demonstrated radiosurgery to be beneficial for carefully selected end-stage patients with 10 or more brain METs [29, 30, 32, 33]. Even a patient with 10 or more such tumors

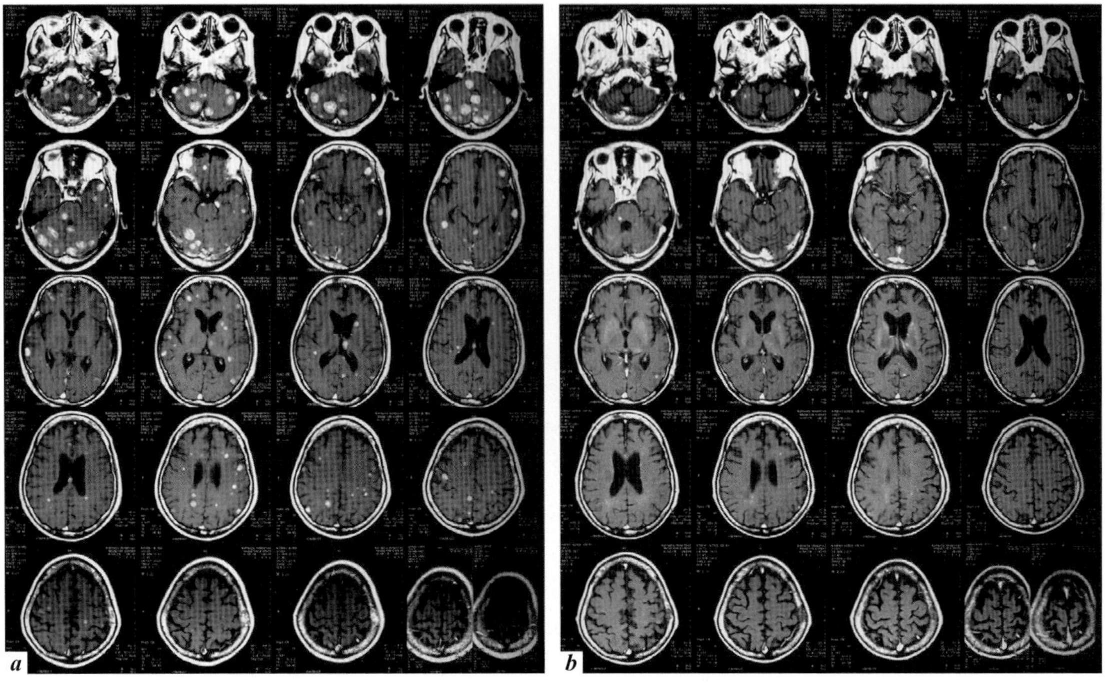

Fig. 4. ***a*** This 63-year-old woman with breast cancer underwent GK radiosurgery for 48 METs on October 19, 2000. ***b*** MR images obtained 6 months after radiosurgery demonstrated disappearance of most tumors, remarkable shrinkage of others.

can maintain good performance status for a major portion of his/her remaining life. In the author's personal experience, the number of tumors treated with GK radiosurgery markedly influences the survival period, as shown in figure 5. However, approximately 80% of patients with brain METs died of causes other than brain disease progression, regardless of tumor number (fig. 6).

Is GK Radiosurgery More Advantageous than WBRT?

The author is absolutely convinced that GK radiosurgery is superior to WBRT for several reasons: (1) Only a brief hospital stay is necessary. This allows the patient to maximize any remaining time with his/her family. (2) Higher control rates and earlier symptom palliation can be achieved. (3) All observable lesions on MR images can be treated, even if such lesions are radioresistant. (4) Other treatments, such as radiation therapy for other parts of

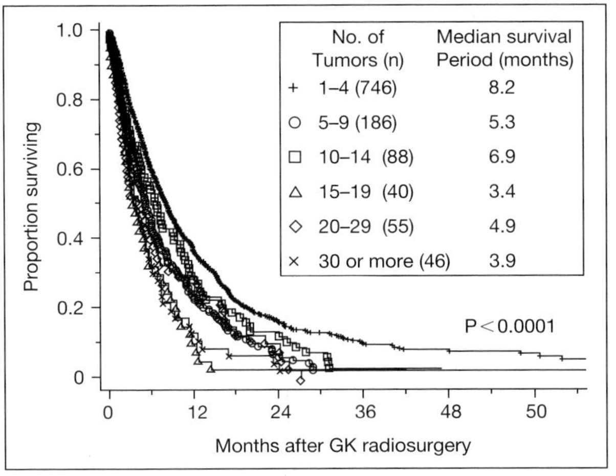

Fig. 5. Median survival according to tumor number.

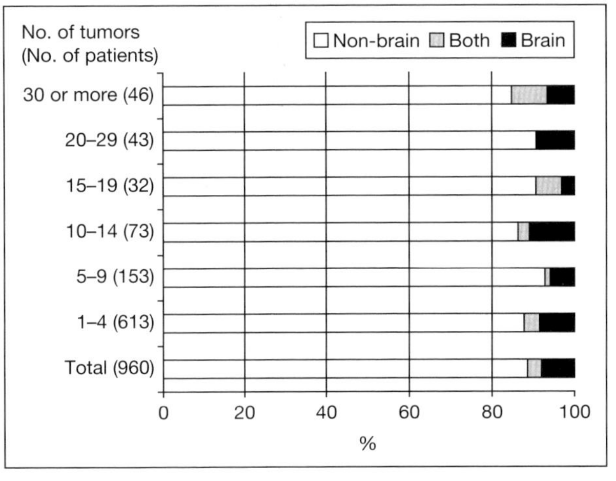

Fig. 6. Causes of death according to tumor number.

the body, surgery and chemotherapy, need not be interrupted. The availability of an alternative treatment for brain METs allows WBRT to be reserved for subsequent treatment attempts, or to be postponed relative to the courses of other management strategies, such as extensive chemotherapy and/or radiation therapy for spinal lesions or other organ involvement, which are also urgent. (5) Procedures can be repeated, even after WBRT. WBRT usually cannot be repeated. Therefore, WBRT should be postponed until it is absolutely necessary, e.g. in cases with miliary or meningeal dissemination that cannot be treated with GK radiosurgery. (6) Patients never lose all of their hair, though there may be a small area of transient hair loss if a treated lesion is located superficially. (7) A very low incidence of dementia can reasonably be expected; this issue is discussed in detail below.

Is GK Treatment for Multiple METs Safe?

As the author described elsewhere, a Rand phantom experiment based on an actual treatment protocol, in which 48 lesions were treated in 1 patient, yielded estimated cumulative irradiation doses to the normal brain of 8.85–13.4 Gy in areas close to the lesions and 2.60–3.55 Gy in areas at some distance from the lesions [32]. The cumulative irradiation doses to the normal brain were also calculated based on the treatment protocols for 92 patients who underwent GK radiosurgery for 10 or more METs, as reported elsewhere [34]. The integral doses to the whole normal brain were estimated to be 4.0–6.0 J in most patients (range 2.2–11.9 J). These estimates confirm theoretically that cumulative irradiation doses for patients with numerous radiosurgical targets do not exceed the threshold level associated with necrosis of normal brain tissue. In fact, the symptomatic complication rate is very low, 1% (2 of 200 patients who underwent GK radiosurgery for 10 or more METs) in the author's personal experience. However, two thirds of these 200 patients died less than 12 months after treatment, i.e. one third of patients lived long enough to possibly experience radiation-induced complications. This incidence of such complications was 3% in the latter special patient group.

Can the Risk of Mental Changes Often Seen after WBRT Be Reduced?

It is well known that a considerable number of patients undergoing WBRT, if they survive for some years after treatment, will experience mental state deterioration [35]. In such patients, T_2-weighted MR images revealed diffuse hyperintense changes in the white matter, as shown in figures 7 and 8. Figure 9 presents a patient, with lung adenocarcinoma, who underwent WBRT for brain METs. GK radiosurgery was performed for a small recurrent tumor 10 months after WBRT. This patient experienced severe deterioration of mental status 3 years after treatment, and eventually died of malnutrition caused by severe dementia, 61 months after GK radiosurgery. An autopsy study demonstrated severe global demyelination of the white matter; this can be regarded as radiation-induced leukoencephalopathy. The author's recent analyses are based

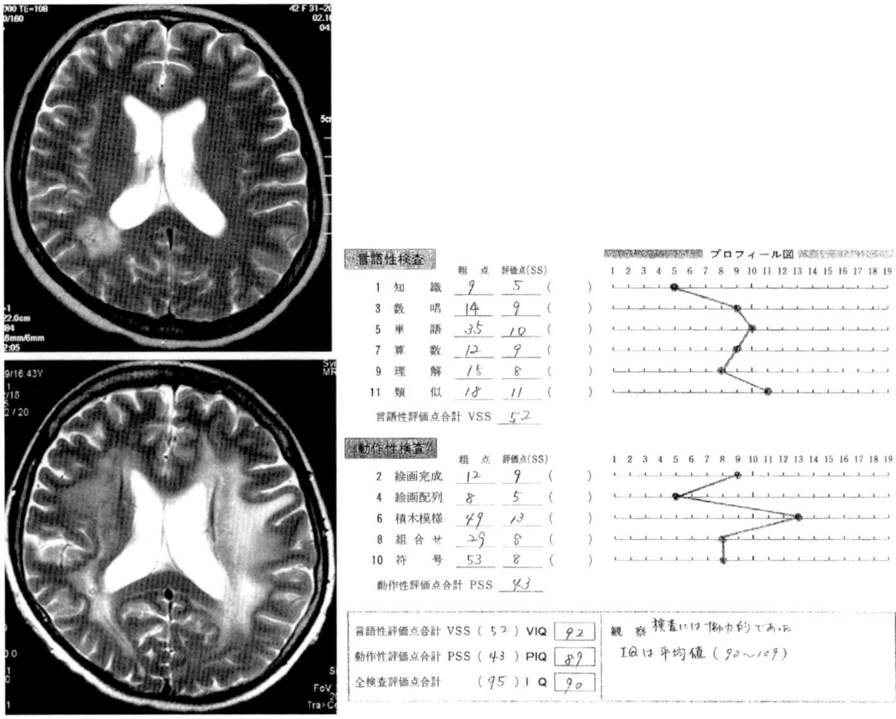

a b c

Fig. 7. ***a*** This 43-year-old woman with breast cancer underwent WBRT with a total dose of 44 Gy for multiple brain METs. ***b*** MR images obtained 12 months after WBRT demonstrated significant diffuse increases in white matter intensity. ***c*** Her IQ, determined by the WAIS method, was within the low normal range, 91, but there were significant decreases in several of the 11 subscores; the technician reported that the pattern seen in this patient was very similar to that of the initial stage of diseases causing dementia such as Alzheimer's disease.

on 45 referred patients who had previously undergone WBRT. MR images obtained 6–42 (mean, 16) months after WBRT demonstrated diffuse white matter change in 21 (47%) of these 45 patients. This change occurred in 8, 50, 63 and 84% of the patients, 6, 12, 18 and 24 months after WBRT, respectively. In a considerable number of patients with MR-demonstrated diffuse white matter changes, mental state was subnormal or worse, as shown in figures 7–9. Therefore, this change is considered to be associated with a possible risk of future dementia. In contrast, the author recently analyzed 60 patients with five or more lesions who received only GK radiosurgery. Follow-up MR images were obtained more than 6 months after treatment in all 60. Images obtained 7–56 (mean; 14) months after treatment demonstrated no white matter changes in any of the 60 patients. It can be tentatively concluded that the risk of mental

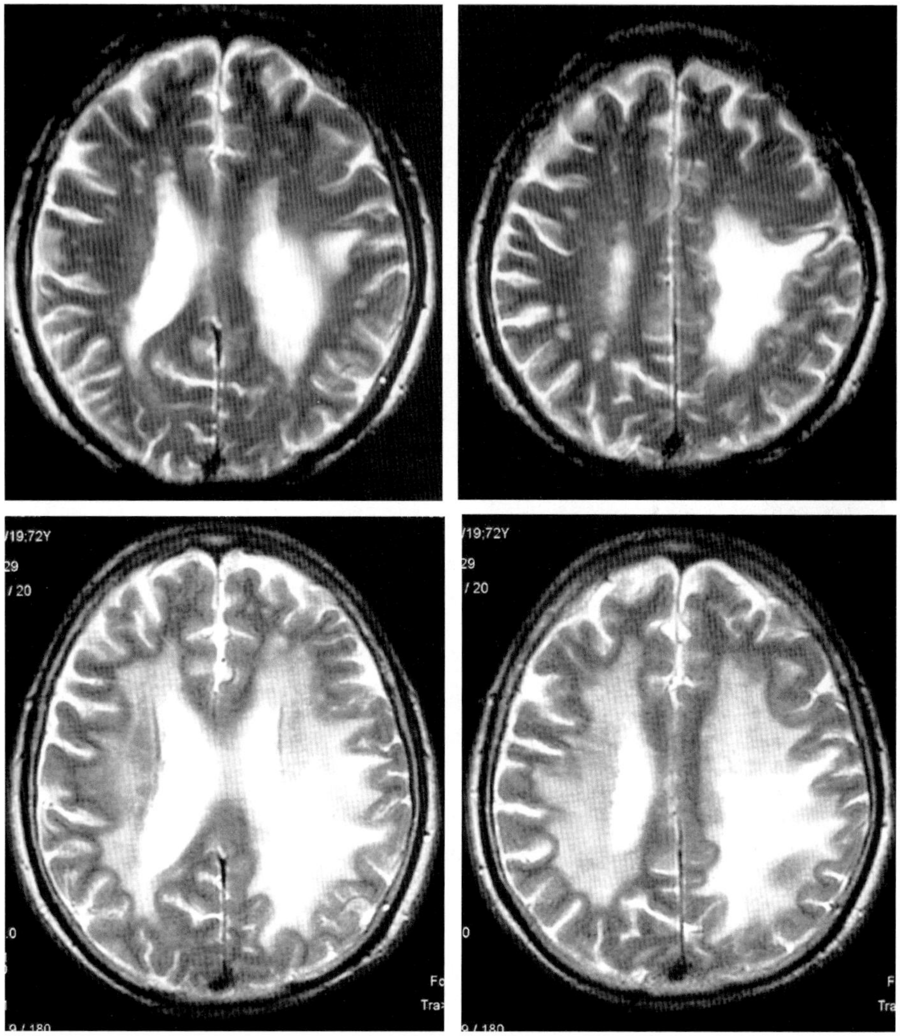

Fig. 8. ***a*** This 72-year-old man with lung adenocarcinoma underwent WBRT with a total dose of 30 Gy for multiple brain METs. ***b*** MR images obtained 16 months after WBRT demonstrated significant diffuse increases in white matter intensity. The WAIS examination was not performed in this patient, but his mental capacity was clearly diminished.

changes, often seen after WBRT, is minimal even when GK radiosurgery is performed for patients with numerous brain METs. Rather than attempting to obliterate invisible brain METs with WBRT (prophylactic WBRT for brain METs from small cell lung cancer, for example), the author advocates meticulous MR imaging examinations repeated at intervals of no more than

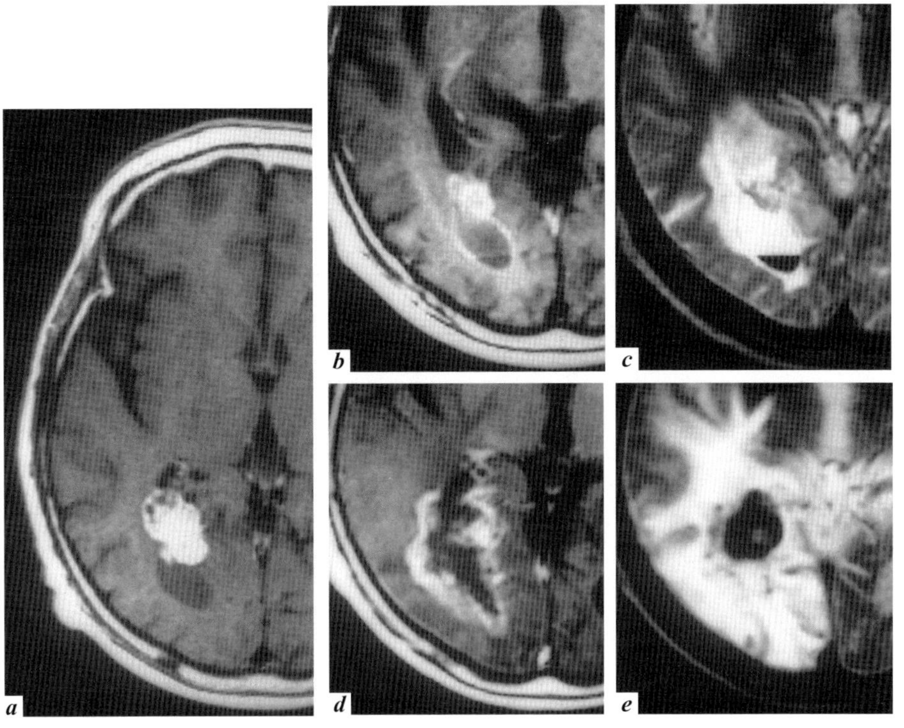

Fig. 9. This 64-year-old woman with lung adenocarcinoma underwent WBRT for brain METs. ***a*** GK radiosurgery was performed for a small recurrent tumor 10 months after WBRT on November 21, 1991. MR images obtained 6 months after GK radiosurgery showed good tumor control (T_1-weighted image with gadolinium enhancement, ***b***; T_2-weighted image, ***c***). This patient experienced severe deterioration of mental status 3 years after treatment. She eventually died due to malnutrition, associated with severe dementia, 61 months after GK radiosurgery. MR images obtained 47 months after GK radiosurgery showed an irregularly shaped area of enhancement and white matter hyperintensity (T_1-weighted image with gadolinium enhancement, ***d***; T_2-weighted image, ***e***). An autopsy study demonstrated severe global demyelination of the white matter; this can be regarded as radiation-induced leukoencephalopathy (HE, ×1, ***f***; Kliiver-Barrel (K-B), ×1, ***g***; K-B, ×2.5, ***h***; K-B, ×50, ***i***). ***j*** There were no tumor cells in the enhanced area (HE, ×1) on the MR image obtained 47 months after treatment.

3 months. If new small lesions appear, radiosurgery should be repeated. As shown in figure 10, if GK radiosurgery is repeated for multiple brain METs, it appears that MR-demonstrated diffuse white matter changes may not occur and, therefore, long-surviving patients would possibly not experience significant mental status deterioration.

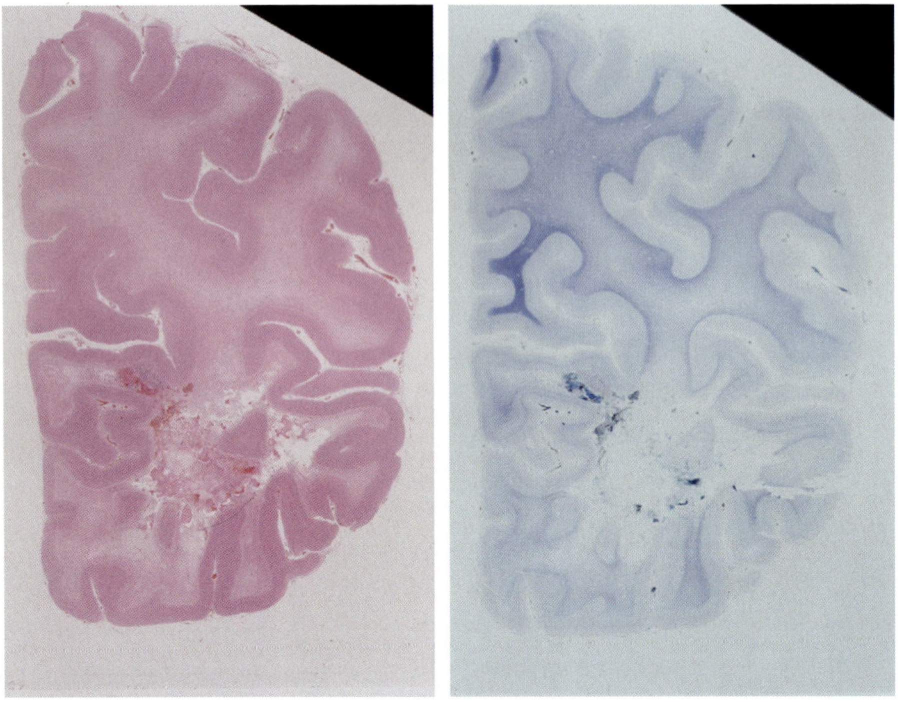

f g

Fig. 9. (continued)

Radiosurgery as Postoperative Irradiation

Postoperative WBRT is widely accepted as significantly reducing the incidence of tumor recurrence as compared with surgery alone [36, 37]. Very little information is available however on radiosurgery as an alternative to fractionated radiotherapy for postoperative irradiation. The author recently reviewed 23 patients who underwent surgical removal followed by GK radiosurgery, with a mean interval of 34 days (range 12–67). GK irradiation was delivered to the cavity remaining after operative tumor removal. The local tumor control rate, 78.3% (18 of the 23 patients), was comparable to the reported rates of local control achieved with surgery followed by WBRT. However, one or more GK procedures were required for new lesions which appeared in areas at some distance from the treated lesion in 14 (60.9%) of the 23 patients; this remote tumor recurrence rate was significantly higher than those reported after surgery and WBRT or the rate of re-GK treatment (27.2% of 1,165 patients) at the author's facility. It is noteworthy, however, that 16 of the 23 patients had had one or more

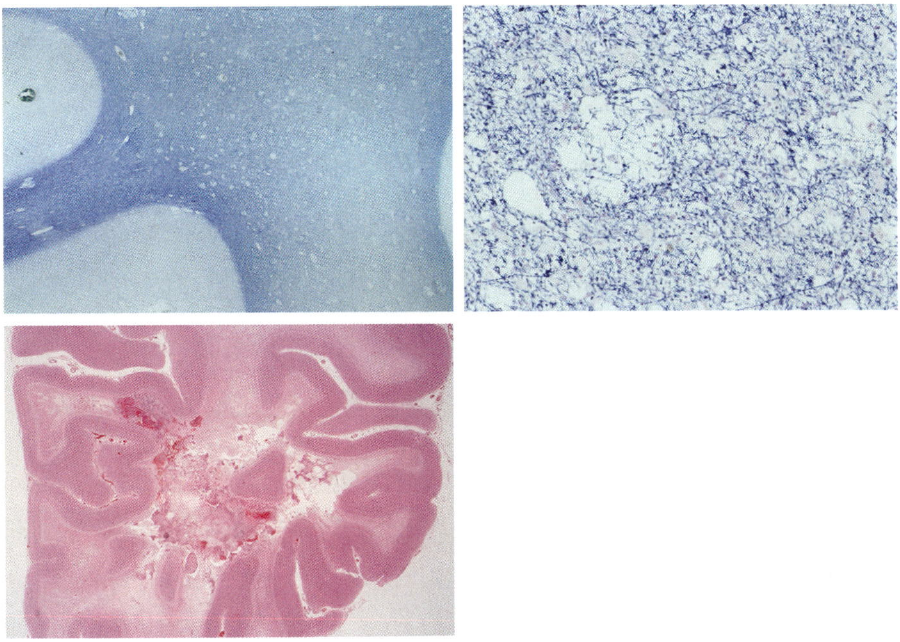

h i j

Fig. 9. (continued)

known metastatic lesions at the time of surgery; thus, these patients were at relatively high risk of developing new lesions. Even if the incidence of remote recurrence is expected to be high, radiosurgery can be safely repeated. Therefore, radiosurgery can be used as postoperative irradiation instead of WBRT, which has several disadvantages, as described above.

A Pitfall in Follow-Up after Radiosurgery

As described earlier in this chapter, most radiosurgically treated tumors showed gradual shrinkage and ultimately disappeared from follow-up MR images. However, in considerable numbers of patients undergoing radiosurgery for brain METs, tumor necrosis occurs 3–12 months after irradiation and persists for several months. Typical MR findings of tumor necrosis are (1) the tumor shows less enhancement after irradiation, (2) a ring-like enhanced area surrounding the irradiated tumor that usually appears following significant shrinkage of the enhanced tumor. This ring-like enhancement is considered to represent increased exudation of tumor fluid, (3) perilesional T_2-hyperintense

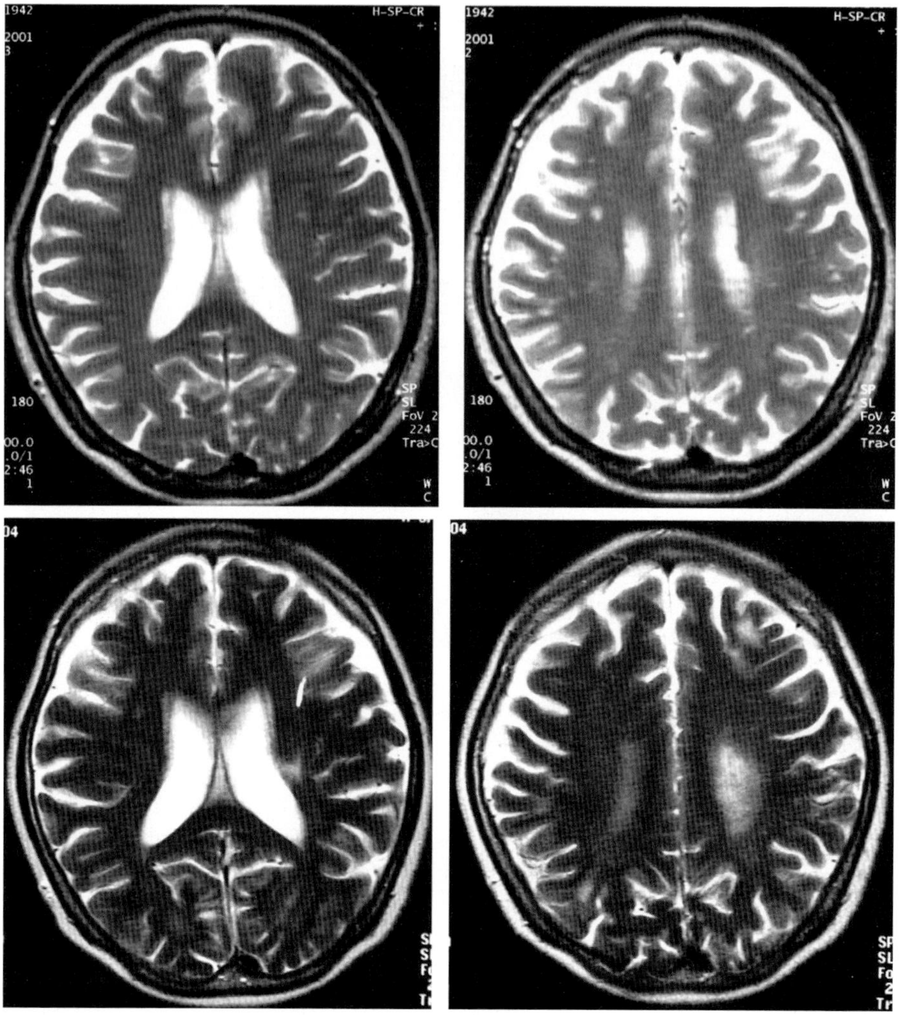

Fig. 10. This 59-year-old woman underwent two GK radiosurgical procedures. At the first treatment, 13 lesions were irradiated with 20 Gy at the tumor margin. All irradiated tumors were well controlled but 22 new lesions demonstrated on MR images necessitated a second treatment. All 22 were irradiated with 15 Gy at the tumor margin. ***a***, ***b*** MR images obtained at the time of the first radiosurgery showed few signal changes within the white matter. ***c***, ***d*** No diffuse white matter changes were demonstrated on MR images obtained 28 months after the first radiosurgery.

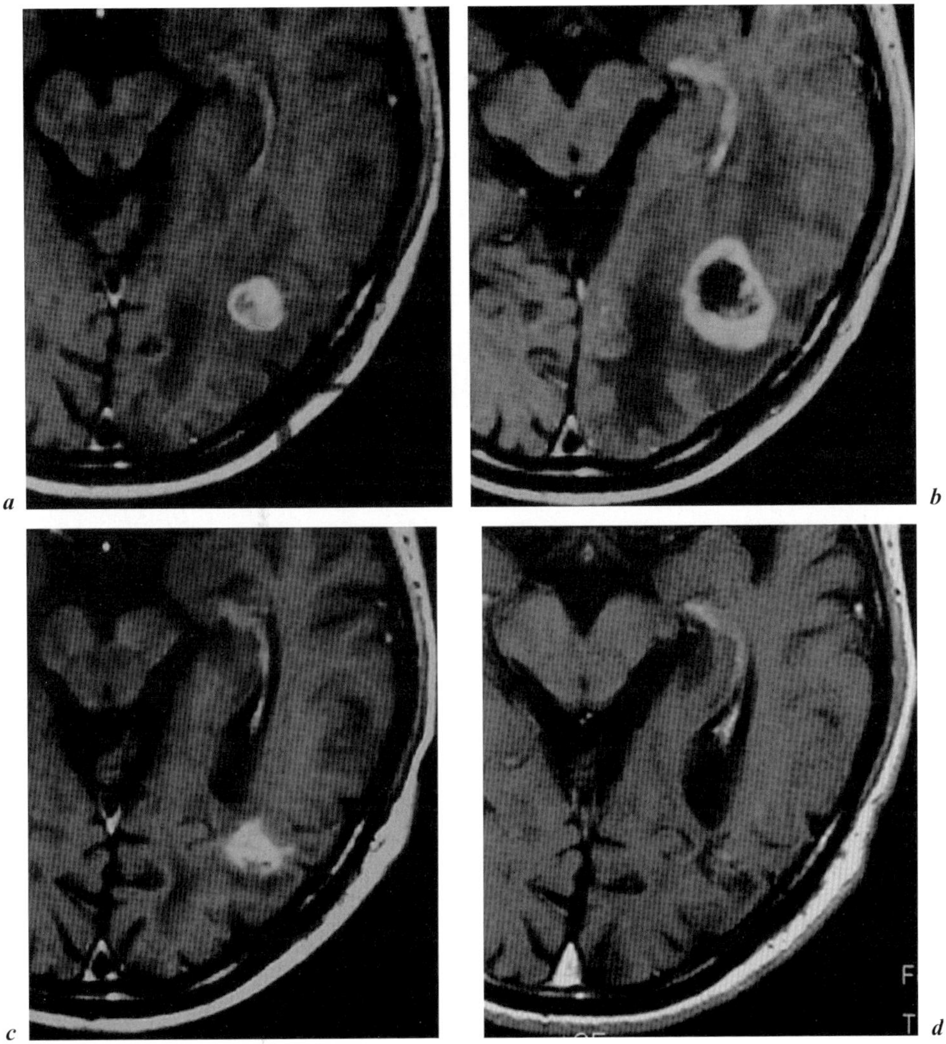

Fig. 11. ***a*** This 56-year-old man with lung adenocarcinoma underwent GK radiosurgery for one brain MET. Follow-up MR studies demonstrated typical findings of tumor necrosis (see text; ***b****:* 4 months, ***c****:* 7 months, and ***d****:* 36 months after radiosurgery).

edema with a smaller mass effect, as compared with a large volume, than is usually seen in untreated or recurrent metastatic tumors (fig. 11). In some patients, tumor necrosis produces severe neurological impairments and long-term steroid therapy or a surgical procedure is required. An autopsy case is presented in figure 12. This patient underwent GK radiosurgery for a cerebellar

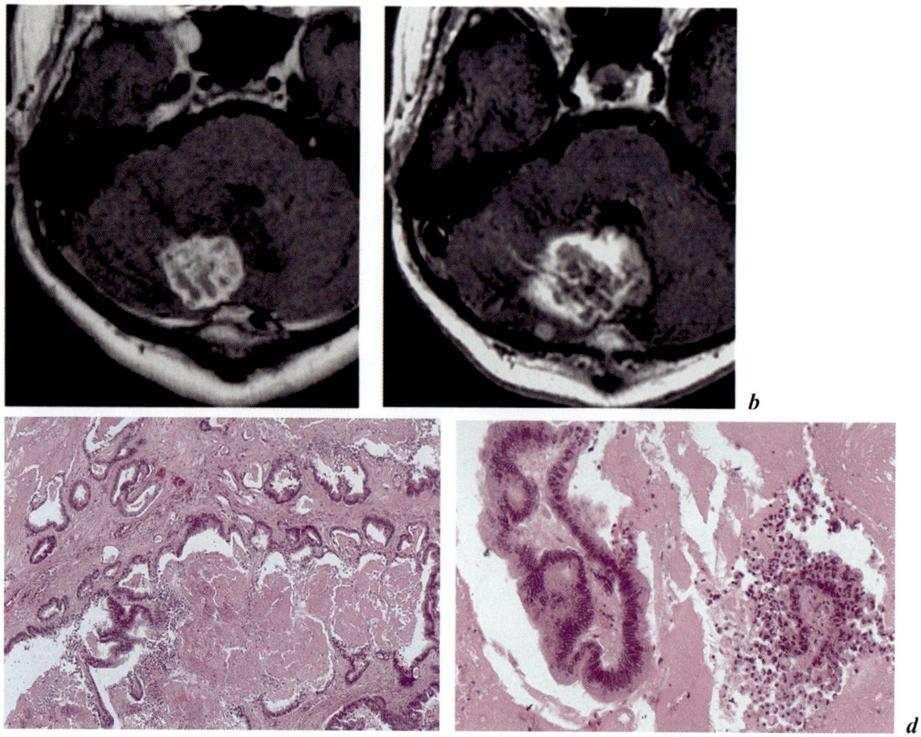

a b c d

Fig. 12. ***a*** This 58-year-old man with colon cancer underwent GK radiosurgery for a cerebellar MET and died 16 weeks after radiosurgery due to systemic disease. ***b*** An MR image obtained 2 weeks before death (3 months after radiosurgery) demonstrated typical findings of tumor necrosis. The autopsy study yielded very important information; there is a wide spectrum of changes encompassing liquefaction necrosis, clusters of cells showing significant degeneration (pyknosis) and seemingly vital malignant cells (HE, ×16, ***c***; HE, ×50, ***d***).

MET and died 16 weeks after radiosurgery due to systemic disease. MR images obtained 2 weeks before death demonstrated typical findings of tumor necrosis. Due to this patient's early death, further follow-up MR images could not be obtained. Therefore, it is unknown whether the lesion was tumor necrosis and would eventually have subsided. The autopsy study yielded very important information; there is a wide spectrum of changes encompassing liquefaction necrosis, clusters of cells showing marked degenerative change (pyknosis) and seemingly vital malignant cells. Interestingly, these three components were stratified in many layers, such that, even if malignant cells are irradiated with a similar dose, the response varies widely from area to area and radiosurgery-induced degenerative changes do not proceed simultaneously within a tumor and can even continue for several months after irradiation. Although there were many clusters of seemingly vital cells facing an area of liquefaction necrosis, these cells showed some degeneration as compared with unirradiated, newly appearing tumor cells and could, therefore, be considered to possibly be undergoing pyknosis and, eventually, liquefaction necrosis.

The author recently evaluated 226 patients in whom follow-up MR images were obtained more than 3 months after radiosurgery for brain METs. Tumor necrosis was demonstrated in 33 (14.6%) of the 226 patients, 14 symptomatic and 19 nonsymptomatic. Tumor necrosis occurred between 2.5 and 12 (median 5.5) months after radiosurgery and varied in duration from 6 to 12 (median, 9) months. Steroid therapy was required in 19 (8.4%) and surgical removal in 3 (1.3%) of the 33 patients. Pathological findings of excised specimens were consistent with necrosis in most areas, with small areas of seemingly vital tumor cells, in all 3 surgical patients. The author analyzed factors possibly influencing tumor necrosis: gender, primary tumor pathology, Karnofsky performance score (KPS), previous treatment (radiotherapy or surgery), tumor volume and number, radiosurgical doses, and so on. Only a well-controlled primary tumor (18.5 vs. 9.3%, $p = 0.0462$) was a statistically significant favorable predictor of tumor necrosis, i.e. a patient with a high KPS receiving meticulous MR follow-up will have a better chance of showing documentable tumor necrosis. In other words, the incidence of tumor necrosis may be higher if all patients, including those with relatively low KPS, undergo meticulous MR follow-up studies.

There has been considerable confusion regarding the terminology used to describe radiation necrosis. Radiation necrosis occurs within the irradiated normal brain, usually a year or more after irradiation. Tumor necrosis that occurs within the irradiated tumor itself is quite different from radiation necrosis involving the normal brain. Either ring-like enhancement or peritumoral edema may be attributable to increased infiltration of tumor fluid. Another important issue is areas of the normal brain surrounding the tumor that receive a dose of 15–25 Gy. Brain tissues irradiated at such doses have been suggested to be a major cause of pathology, but the author's experience to date does not support this speculation. If the normal brain irradiated with a dose of 15–25 Gy is the source of the ring-like enhancement surrounding the lesion, similar observations would be made in patients with arteriovenous malformations that are generally irradiated with very similar doses. However, although T_2-hyperintensity is seen in some cases, ring-like enhancement due to infiltration of lesion fluid is rare within 12 months of irradiation in arteriovenous malformation patients. This type of gadolinium infiltration is occasionally seen after radiosurgery for meningiomas in which irradiation doses at the tumor margin are approximately 12 Gy in most cases. A dose as low as 12 Gy cannot be considered to produce changes in the normal brain, such as the aforementioned ring-like enhancement, within 1 year after irradiation. This type of enhancement is attributable to hyper-exudation of tumor fluid from an irradiated tumor.

As described above, given that all factors predicting tumor necrosis have not as yet been identified, close MR follow-up after GK radiosurgery for brain METs is crucial for both detecting such tumor necrosis and ruling out true recurrence. For precise diagnosis, FDG-PET is tentatively recommended. There is no question that PET using methionine or other amines is the most reliable examination for ruling out true recurrence. Unfortunately, this examination, is currently available at only a very limited number of facilities. Also, although proton MR spectrography is useful in some cases, in the author's experience a weakness of this technique is the lack of reproducibility of results. SPECT is reportedly applicable to making a precise diagnosis. However, the author stopped using this technique several years ago, again due to the lack of reproducibility in the results.

Another problem encountered in following patients with MR imaging is that a long-standing area of enhancement is not always a tumor remnant. As shown in figure 13, despite ring-like enhancement persisting for 9 months after radiosurgery in this case, autopsy revealed only fibrous tissue. There were no tumor cells. Figure 9 shows another case in whom ring-like enhancement persisted for almost 5 years after radiosurgery. Again, there were no tumor cells in the enhanced area at autopsy.

Interpretation

Finally, we would all be well advised to keep in mind the words of Lindquist and Steiner [38], 'Although effective, it must be realized that radiosurgery at best only kills intracranial tumor cells. Suffering should not be prolonged by treatment of terminal patients. Which tumors should be treated? How many tumors can and should be treated?' A gradual decrease in consciousness level due to progression of intracranial METs, which occurs sooner or later, might be nature's way of relieving the suffering of terminal patients. Recent advances in multidisciplinary management strategies have, however, allowed physicians to relieve much of the suffering of end-stage patients. Furthermore, we believe that as physicians we should not shrink from the challenge of treating patients with very difficult to manage disorders, provided that the patient wants to continue living and being treated. Therefore, the author advocates treating all detectable, if sufficiently small, tumors, however time-consuming and laborious the treatment procedure may be. This commitment demands a considerable effort on the part of all members of the radiosurgical treatment team.

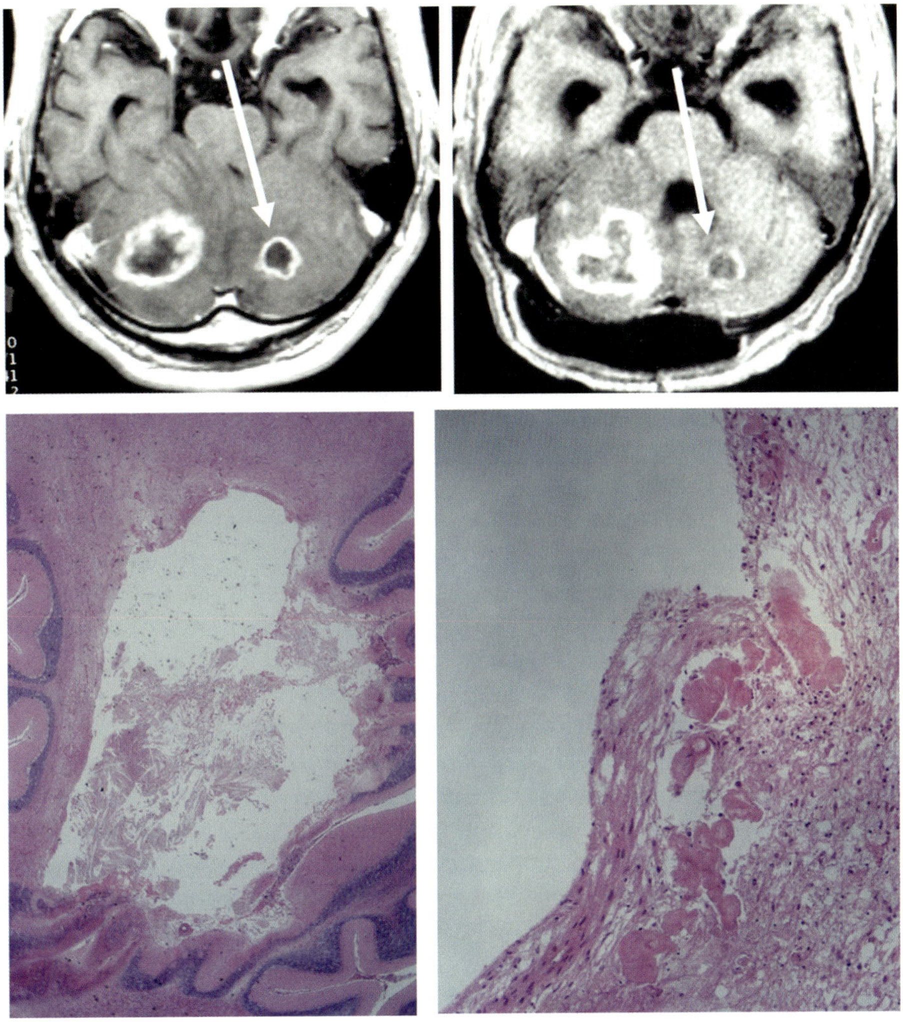

a *b* *c* *d*

Fig. 13. ***a*** This 73-year-old man with lung adenocarcinoma underwent GK radiosurgery for a cerebellar MET (arrow). A large tumor located in the right cerebellum was removed surgically. ***b*** An MR image obtained 9 months after radiosurgery demonstrated persistent ring-like enhancement. The patient died a month after this examination and autopsy revealed only fibrous tissue at the enhanced area seen on the MR image (HE, ×2, ***c***; HE, ×20, ***d***). There were no tumor cells.

Acknowledgement

The author would like to thank Bierta E. Barfod, MD, Katsuta Hospital Mito GammaHouse, for her assistance in the preparation of the manuscript.

References

1 Lindquist C: Gamma knife surgery for recurrent solitary metastasis of a cerebral hypernephroma: case report. Neurosurgery 1989;25:802–804.
2 Adler JR, Cox RS, Kaplan I, Martin DP: Stereotactic radiosurgical treatment of brain metastases. J Neurosurg 1992;76:444–449.
3 Alexander E III, Moriarty TM, Davis RB, Wen PY, Fine HA, Black PM, Kooy HM, Loeffler JS: Stereotactic radiosurgery for the definitive, noninvasive treatment of brain metastases. J Natl Cancer Inst 1995;87:34–40.
4 Buatti JM, Friedman WA, Bova FJ, Mendenhall WM: Treatment selection factors for stereotactic radiosurgery of intracranial metastases. Int J Radiat Oncol Biol Phys 1995;32:1161–1166.
5 Coffey RJ, Flickinger JC, Bissonette DJ, Lunsford LD: Radiosurgery for solitary brain metastases using the cobalt-60 gamma unit: methods and results in 24 patients. Int J Radiat Oncol Biol Phys 1991;20:1287–1295.
6 Engenhart-Cabillic R, Kimming BN, Höver KH, Wowra B, Romahn J, Lorenz WJ, van Kaick G, Wannenmacher M: Long-term follow-up for brain metastases treated by percutaneous stereotactic single high-dose irradiation. Cancer 1993;71:1353–1361.
7 Fuller BG, Kaplan ID, Adler J, Cox RS, Bagshaw MA: Stereotaxic radiosurgery for brain metastases: the importance of adjuvant whole brain irradiation. Int J Radiat Oncol Biol Phys 1992;23:413–418.
8 Jokura H, Takahashi K, Kayama T, Yoshimoto T: Gamma knife radiosurgery of a series of only minimally selected metastatic brain tumours. Acta Neurochir 1994;62(suppl):77–82.
9 Kida Y, Kobayashi T, Tanaka T: Radiosurgery of the metastatic brain tumours with gamma-knife. Acta Neurochir 1995;63(suppl):89–94.
10 Kihlström L, Karlsson B, Lindquist C: Gamma knife surgery in brain metastases; in Lunsford LD (ed): Stereotactic Radiosurgery Update. Amsterdam, Elsevier, 1992, pp 429–434.
11 Kihlström L, Karlsson B, Lindquist C: Gamma knife surgery for cerebral metastases: implications for survival based on 16 years' experience. Stereotact Funct Neurosurg 1993;61(suppl): 45–60.
12 Loeffler JS, Alexander E III: Radiosurgery for the treatment of intracranial metastases; in Alexander E III, Loeffler JS, Lunsford LD (eds): Sterotactic Radiosurgery. New York, McGraw-Hill, 1993, pp 197–206.
13 Loeffler JS, Kooy HM, Wen PY, Fine HA, Cheng CW, Mannarino EG, Tsai JS, Alexander E III: The treatment of recurrent brain metastases with stereotactic radiosurgery. J Clin Oncol 1990;8:576–582.
14 Martens F, Verbeke L: Stereotactic radiosurgery of cerebral metastases: preliminary results. Acta Clin Belg 1993;48:228–233.
15 Mehta MP, Rozental JM, Levin AB, Mackie TR, Kubsad SS, Gehring MA, Kinsella TJ: Defining the role of radiosurgery in the management of brain metastases. Int J Radiot Oncol Biol Phys 1992;24:619–625.
16 Moriarty TM, Loeffler JS, Black PMcL, Shrieve DS, Wen PY, Fine HA, Kooy HM, Alexander E III: Long-term follow-up of patients treated with stereotactic radiosurgery for single or multiple brain metastases; in Kondziolka D (ed): Radiosurgery 1995. Basel, Karger, 1996, pp 83–91.
17 Muacevic A, Kreth FW, Horstmann GA, Schmid-Elsaesser R, Wowra B, Steiger HJ, Reulen HJ: Surgery and radiotherapy compared with gamma knife radiosurgery in the treatment of solitary cerebral metastases of small diameter. J Neurosurg 1999;91:35–43.

18 Serizawa T, Iuchi T, Ono J, Saeki N, Osato K, Odaira M, Ushikubo O, Hirai S, Sato M, Matsuda S: Gamma knife treatment for multiple metastatic brain tumors compared with whole-brain radiation therapy. J Neurosurg 2000;93(suppl 3):32–36.
19 Somaza S, Kondziolka D, Lunsford LD, Kirkwood JM, Flickinger JC: Stereotactic radiosurgery for cerebral metastatic melanoma. J Neurosurg 1993;79:661–666.
20 Sturm V, Kober B, Höver KH, Schlegel W, Boesecke R, Pastyr O, Hartmann GH, Schabbert S, Winkel K, Kunze S, Lorenz WJ: Stereotactic percutaneous single dose irradiation of brain metastases with a linear accelerator. Int J Radiat Oncol Biol Phys 1987;13:279–282.
21 Boyd TS, Mehta MP: A comprehensive review of the role of radiosurgery in patients with intracranial metastases; in Kondziolka D (ed): Radiosurgery 1997. Basel, Karger, 1998, pp 31–50.
22 Pollock BE, Brown PD: Stereotactic radiosurgery for brain metastases; in Pollock BE (ed): Contemporary Stereotactic Radiosurgery: Technique and Evaluation. Armonk, Futura, 2002, pp 245–261.
23 Kondziolka D, Patel A, Lunsford LD, Kassam A, Flichinger J: Stereotactic radiosurgery plus whole brain radiotherapy versus radiotherapy alone for patients with multiple brain metastases. Int J Radiat Oncol Biol Phys 1999;45:427–434.
24 Chidel MA, Suh JH, Reddy CA, et al: Application of recursive partitioning analysis and evaluation of the use of whole brain radiation among patients treated with stereotactic radiosurgery for newly diagnosed brain metastases. Int J Radiat Oncol Biol Phys 2000;47:993–999.
25 Pirzkall A, Debus J, Lohr F, Fuss M, Rhein B, Engenhart-Cabillic R, Wannenmacher M: Radiosurgery alone or in conjunction with whole-brain radiotherapy for brain metastases. J Clin Oncol 1998;16:3563–3569.
26 Sneed PK, Lamborn KR, Forstner JM, McDermott MW, Chang S, Park E, Gutin PH, Phillips TL, Wara WM, Larson DA: Radiosurgery for brain metastases: is whole brain radiotherapy necessary? Int J Radiat Oncol Biol Phys 1999;43:549–558.
27 Sneed PK, Suh JH, Goetsch SJ, Sanghavi SN, Chappell R, Buatti JM, Regine WF, Weltman E, King VJ, Breneman JC, Sperduto PW, Mehta MP: A multi-institutional review of radiosurgery alone vs. radiosurgery with whole brain radiotherapy as the initial management of brain metastases. Int J Radiat Oncol Biol Phys 2002;53:519–526.
28 Bender Al, Posner JB: Current treatment of brain metastases; in Maciunas RJ (ed): Advanced Techniques in Central Nervous System Metastases. Parkridge, American Association of Neurological Surgeons, 1998, pp 1–15.
29 Serizawa T, Iuchi T, Ono J, Saeki N, Osato K, Odaira M, Ushikubo O, Hirai S, Sato M, Matsuda S: Gamma knife treatment for multiple metastatic brain tumors compared with whole-brain radiation therapy. J Neurosurg 2000;93(suppl 3):32–36.
30 Suzuki S, Omagari J, Nishio S, Nishiye E, Fukui M: Gamma knife radiosurgery for simultaneous multiple metastatic tumors. J Neurosurg 2000;3(suppl 3):30–31.
31 Young RF, Jacques DB, Duma C, Rand RW, Henderson J, Vermeulen SS, Grimm P, Blasko JC, Posewitz A, Copcutt B, Bolles GE, Breeze RE, Pribil SG, Winston K, Johnson SD: Gamma knife radiosurgery for treatment of multiple brain metastases; in Kondziolka D (ed): Radiosurgery 1995. Basel, Karger, 1996, pp 92–101.
32 Yamamoto M, Ide M, Jimbo M, Aiba M, Ito M, Hirai H, Usukura M: Gamma knife radiosurgery with numerous target points for intracranially disseminated metastases: early experience in three patients and experimental analysis of whole brain irradiation doses; in Kondziolka D (ed): Radiosurgery 1997. Basel, Karger, 1998, vol 2, pp 94–109.
33 Yamamoto M, Kamiryo T, Ide M, Barfod BE, Urakawa Y: Gamma knife radiosurgery for 551 patients with brain metastases: tumor number impacts survival period but not cause of death. 2003 Annu Meet AANS, San Diego, April 2003; abstract in J Neurosurg 2003;98:685.
34 Yamamoto M, Ide M, Nishio S, Urakawa Y: Gamma knife radiosurgery for numerous brain metastases: is this a safe treatment? Int J Radiat Oncol Biol Phys 2002;53:1279–1283.
35 DeAngelis LK, Delattre JY, Posner JB: Radiation-induced dementia in patients cured of brain metastases. Neurology 1989;39:789–796.
36 Patchell RA, Tibbs PA, Walsh JW, Dempsey RJ, Maruyama Y, Kryscio RJ, Markesbery WR, MacDonald JS, Young B: A randomized trial of surgery in the treatment of single metastases to the brain. N Engl J Med 1990;322:494–500.

37 Patchell RA, Tibbs PA, Regine WF, Dempsey RJ, Mohinddin M, Kryscio RJ, Markesbery WR, Foon KA, Young B: Postoperative radiotherapy in the treatment of single metastasis: a randomized trial. JAMA 1998;280:1485–1489.
38 Lindquist C, Steiner L: Radiosurgery for tumors; in Wilkins RH, Rengachary SS (eds): Neurosurgery, ed 2. New York, McGraw-Hill, 1996, pp 1887–1907.

Masaaki Yamamoto, MD
Katsuta Hospital Mito GammaHouse
5125-2 Nakane, Hitachi-naka
Ibaraki 312–0011 (Japan)
Tel. +81 29 271 0011, Fax +81 29 274 1475, E-Mail BCD06275@nifty.com

Szeifert GT, Kondziolka D, Levivier M, Lunsford LD (eds): Radiosurgery and Pathological Fundamentals. Prog Neurol Surg. Basel, Karger, 2007, vol 20, pp 129–141

9.2. Modern Management of Vestibular Schwannomas

Jean Régis, Pierre Hughes Roche, Christine Delsanti, Jean Marc Thomassin, Maurice Ouaknine, Karin Gabert, William Pellet

Departments of Functional Neurosurgery and ENT Surgery, Timone University Hospital, and Skull Base Neurosurgery Department, Sainte Marguerite, Marseille, France

Abstract

Within the last 3 decades, microsurgery and stereotactic radiosurgery (SRS) have become well-established management options for vestibular schwannomas (VSs). Advancement in the management of VSs can be separated into three periods: the microsurgical pioneer period, the demonstration of SRS as a first-line therapy for small and medium-sized VSs, and currently, a period of SRS maturity based on a large worldwide patient accrual. The Marseille SRS experience includes 1,500 patients, with 1,000 patients having follow-up longer than 3 years. A long-term tumor control rate of 97%, transient facial palsy lower than 1%, and a probability of functional hearing preservation between 50 and 95% was achieved in this large series of patients treated with state-of-the-art SRS.

The Swedish Experience

Vestibular schwannomas (VSs), initially termed acoustic neurinomas, arise from the Schwann cells of the vestibular nerve instead of the cochlear nerve [7]. These benign tumors are surgically challenging lesions. The neurosurgical management of VSs began in the 20th century. Pioneers such as Dr. Harvy Cushing, operated on VS patients for survival enhancement. These patients had large tumors, presenting with cerebellopontine angle clinical manifestations, and were diagnosed by internal auditory canal enlargement on radiography. The surgical approach performed was a retrosigmoid suboccipital approach. Between 1925 and 1950, other pioneers such as Dr. Walter Dandy were able to rely on ventriculography, angiography and pneumencephalography for radical removal of these tumors.

In the second half of the 20th century, microsurgery and stereotactic radiosurgery (SRS) were introduced in the management of VSs. The microotoneurosurgical experience began in 1962 with surgeons such as Dr. W. House, who developed a translabyrinthine approach for preservation of facial nerve function. The availability of auditory evoked potentials (1970), CT scan (1973), and MRI (1982) have been major advances during this period. A shift to functional hearing and facial nerve preservation were the goals of surgical removal of VSs after these advances.

Gamma Knife SRS was first used in 1969 by Dr. Lars Leksell to treat VS [8]. Between 1968 and 1974 [9], the first prototype of the Gamma Knife unit was initially designed for functional targeting. This unit was used to treat 9 patients with a VS, including one neurofibromatosis type 2 (NF2) patient. Stereotactic fixation and imaging localization (pneumoencephalography) were crude methods at this time. Dosimetry was manually calculated and the central maximum dose was high (50–100 Gy), while the minimum dose was very low. None of the patients developed facial weakness and 1 patient experienced transient facial hypoesthesia. Tumor control was achieved in 4 patients with a marginal tumor dose between 2 and 35 Gy (<1 Gy for failed cases) [12].

A second Gamma Knife unit (Elekta Model U) was designed specifically for tumors (spherical focus; 2 collimators of 8 and 14 mm) and used between 1974 and 1987. CT was incorporated into the first SRS computerized dose planning system in 1975. The first 11 patients treated with this system were administered high tumor marginal radiation doses (20–70 Gy). Postoperatively, these patients developed a high rate of facial weakness (45%) and hypoesthesia (80%). Consequently, marginal doses were decreased to 8 Gy. Unfortunately, patients failed treatment at this lower dose. A higher radiation dose between 10 and 20 Gy (mean 16.5) was then used through 1987. No patient developed a facial palsy and a high rate of tumor control (92%) was achieved.

The powerful Elekta Model B Gamma Knife was introduced in 1988 along with the Elekta G stereotactic frame (1987). MRI was coupled to SRS planning in 1989. Freshly loaded with new cobalt sources, the B unit was able to achieve a much higher dose rate than prior units. Despite using the same marginal dose as before, the rate of facial palsy increased to 27%. As a result, in 1989 the tumor marginal dose was lowered by Noren [12] to 12 Gy (10 Gy for large and 14 Gy for small lesions). A high level of functional hearing preservation (75%), absent facial palsy, and a high rate of tumor control (97%) was achieved.

The Pittsburgh Experience

No group has contributed more to the evaluation and administration of SRS in the management of VSs than Drs. L. Dade Lunsford, Douglas

Kondziolka and John Flickinger from the University of Pittsburgh. Since 1987, when the University of Pittsburgh acquired the first Gamma Knife unit in North America, this team has treated thousands of patients and published numerous manuscripts on the management of VSs. This group has established optimal treatment parameters for tumor control of VSs in combination with hearing and facial nerve preservation. Flickinger et al. [3] have confirmed the importance of G. Noren's policy of 'low irradiation doses which are therapeutically effective'. They have demonstrated the impact of technical advances in the improvement of clinical results [5]. Flickinger et al. [4] recently reviewed their series of 313 patients presenting with previously untreated unilateral VSs who underwent SRS (with 12- to 13-Gy margin) between 1991 and 2001. The actuarial 6-year resection-free tumor control rate was 98.6%. The 6-year actuarial rates for preserved facial nerve function, trigeminal nerve function, and hearing were 100%, 95.6 ± 1.8%, 78.6 ± 5.1%. Pollock et al. [15] were the first to prospectively demonstrate the advantage (in terms of functional outcome) of SRS over microsurgery in the management of VSs.

The Marseille Experience

In 1992, SRS was incorporated into VS management in Marseille. A strong otoneurosurgical team already present, provided for a comprehensive and successful program in the management of VSs. Between 1973 and 2004, a total of 2,577 VSs have been surgically resected or treated with SRS in Marseille. Surgical resections include translabyrinthine, middle fossa, retrosigmoid/suboccipital approaches. Approximately 1,500 patients have been treated with SRS using the Gamma Knife. All patients have been evaluated prospectively.

All VS patients treated with SRS in Marseille receive a 12-Gy tumor marginal dose. Three major technical advances have clearly influenced our practice. The availability of high-resolution stereotactic MRI [5], workstations to select the dose and treatment plan (GammaPlan) [17], and the installation of the robotic APS system have allowed our group to achieve more conformal and selective dose planning. The average number of isocenters used in 1992 was less than 5 and more than 15 in 2003 with the APS system [18]. Consequently, if we consider the first 100 patients of our experience representing our learning curve, 4 treatment periods can be defined. The rate of transient facial palsy and hemifacial spasm for VS patients treated by our group was: 3 and 3% during the first phase (June 1992 to December 1994; 100 patients), 1.4 and 2.8% during the second period (December 1994 to July 1997; 212 patients), 0.55 and 0.83% during the third period (July 1997 to May 2000; 360 patients), and 0 and 0% during the last period (May 2000 to January 2002, 258 patients), respectively.

Only patients with greater than 2 years of follow-up were included in our series [16].

Comparison with Microsurgery

In a comparison of 110 surgically resected VSs and 97 treated with SRS, a lower rate of facial palsy and a higher probability of functional hearing preservation were both achieved after SRS [19]. All patients had Koos stage 2-2 tumors with a minimum follow-up of 4 years.

Efficacy of Radiosurgery

In order to better define the accuracy and efficacy of SRS, we have systematically evaluated the morphologic imaging changes of tumors treated between July 1992 and January 2002 [2] by the otoneurosurgical group of the Timone Hospital in Marseille. Evaluation of MRI performed before and after SRS (intervals of 6 months, 1, 2, 3, 5, 7, and 10 years) have been reviewed. Systematic measurements have been performed on all tumors treated. Preoperatively, 129 patients presented with progressive tumors. At the time of SRS, the median tumor volume was 732 mm^3 (mean 1,346; range 20–14,405). According to the Koos topographical classification, there were 80 stage 1, 538 stage 2, 322 stage 3, and 56 stage 4 cases. Loss of central enhancement was visible on postoperative MRI at 6 months and/or 1 year in 45.5% patients. In 64% of these patients, loss of the central contrast enhancement occurred. A significant increase in tumor size was recorded in 15% of the patients. In 3% of the patients, progression led to a second procedure, either resection or a second SRS procedure. We have defined failure as continuous tumor progression after 3 years from treatment (SRS). Tumor control was achieved in 97% of cases. Since the natural history of the VSs include growth of 2 mm/year, our results confirm the efficacy of SRS.

Hearing Preservation

In spite of the technical advances in microsurgery, the majority of VS patients who undergo surgical resection lose functional hearing. In our SRS experience, 175 patients, with a VS and functional preoperative hearing (Gardner-Robertson 1 or 2), were initially treated with SRS. These patients all had follow-up longer than 3 years [6]. Hearing preservation after SRS was 60%

for all patients. Univariate and multivariate analysis have revealed parameters which influence the probability of functional hearing preservation at 3 years. These parameters include: a limited hearing loss (Gardner-Robertson stage 1), the presence of a tinnitus, younger age of the patient, and small lesion size. Functional hearing preservation at 3 years is 77.8% in patients with stage 1 hearing, 80% in patients with tinnitus as a first symptom, and 95% when the patient has both stage 1 hearing and tinnitus. In these patients, the probability of functional hearing preservation at 5 years is 84% [6].

Facial Nerve Preservation

Facial palsy is very rare (<1%) in our SRS management of VSs. Our results coincide with the Pittsburgh and Rhode Island experiences [16]. Schwannomas originating from the facial nerve itself are more prone to interfere with facial motor function. Surgical resection of 7th nerve schwannomas implies a higher risk of facial palsy after surgery. Due to the paucity of facial palsy after SRS of VSs, the use of SRS may be rational in this difficult group of patients [10]. Among the 1,000 schwannomas of the cerebellopontine angle treated with SRS in Marseille between July 1992 and March 2003, 9 have been diagnosed as originating from the 7th nerve. Criterion for diagnosis was the involvement of the second or third portion of the 7th nerve (7 patients) and/or intraoperative demonstration during a previous surgical resection (2 patients). Facial palsy occurring within 18 months of VS radiosurgery was determined in patients with more than 2 years of follow-up (8 patients). Four patients had previous facial paresis. Normal motor facial function was observed in 2 patients prior to SRS (House-Brackmann grade 2 in 6 patients; grade 3 in 1 patient). Follow-up ranged from 2 to 7 years in all patients. No patient developed worsening facial palsy, while 2 patients had improvement in their preoperative facial palsy. Our results confirm the leading role of SRS in the management of VSs in combination with facial nerve preservation.

Nervus Intermedius Dysfunction

The impact of radiosurgery on the facial nerve and nervus intermedius has recently been reported [26]. Due to the dual role of the facial nerve and the nervus intermedius in the mechanical protection of the eye, VS management can interfere with visual function. We have sought to evaluate and compare the impact of microsurgery or SRS on eye function. A functional questionnaire evaluating patient complaints related to the eye was sent to 100 patients who underwent SRS 3 years before. Another questionnaire was sent to a group of 100 patients who underwent surgical resection. A Shirmer test was performed before radiosurgery and 2 years after SRS in 46 patients. The incidence of a dry and burning eye was much higher in patients who underwent surgical resection of their VSs (57/99 patients), while no patients reported a dry and burning eye in the SRS group. The presence of a permanent facial deficit was reported by the majority of patients who underwent surgical resection (57/99 patients). In patients from both groups with no facial palsy, a dry eye was reported in 8/63 after SRS and 7/42 after surgical resection. Patients reported a burning eye in 9/63 after SRS and 9/42 after surgical resection. As a result, 15% of patients with no facial palsy present with possible injury of the intermedius nerve. When no permanent facial palsy is observed, a crocodile tear syndrome occurs predominantly after surgical resection (4/42 vs. 1/63; $p = 0.07$). This could suggest an early lesion of the 7th cranial nerve and nervus intermedius and subsequent abnormal regrowth. The only patient reporting a crocodile tear syndrome after SRS presented transiently with a slight deficit of the orbicularis muscle. In the absence of facial palsy, a weeping eye was reported more frequently after surgical resection (16/42 vs. 9/63, $p = 0.01$). This leads us to suspect a subclinical injury of the 7th nerve. Of patients with a Shirmer test prior to SRS and 2 years after, 28.3% had improvement, 56.5% had a stable test, and 15.2% worsened. This study was the first to demonstrate that radiosurgery can induce nervus intermedius injury in a small percentage of cases (15%). Symptoms related to the eye either due to the injury of the nervus intermedius and/or the 7th nerve are much more frequent after surgical resection than after SRS. We believe evaluation of the lacrimal function must be part of the systematic evaluation of radiosurgery studies involving VSs [26].

Vestibular Symptoms

The influence of radiosurgery on vestibular symptoms is poorly understood. Our comparative study of the functional outcome of patients treated with SRS vs. surgical resection have globally shown no superiority of one technique over the other for imbalance and vertigo [19]. The probability to observe a worsening at 3 years was 22% for microsurgery and 26% for radiosurgery [19]. However, the systematic study of imbalance in our patients has revealed the improvement in postural orientation and stability after SRS.

We have recently reported the study of postural, vestibular dependent performances in 218 patients before and after SRS [13]. Subjects were asked to stand at ease on a static dynamometric foot-plate, gazing at a fixed point (EO condition) or stand with their eyes closed (EC condition). Statokinesigrams were registered during two consecutive sessions of 51.2 s, under EO and EC conditions. These sessions were performed before (J − 1), and after (J + 1) irradiation; others were performed later (J + 1–5 years; n = 37). The center of pressure, mediolateral (X), and sagittal (Y) positions were quantified every 100 ms. Mean Xm session value (with SD) was defined as a personal parameter for left or right body inclination. Area S for 90% of the XY successive placements of the C of P observed during a session was defined as an index for 2D postural sway. Before irradiation grand average the 218 personal Xm mean values has evidenced a statistically significant body inclination toward the affected side, however under EC condition only. The day after irradiation, a significant reduction in the grand mean value of body inclination was observed. Statistics of paired Xm confirmed this trend toward usual symmetry. The day after stereo-irradiation averaging areas S of ellipses has indicated a shift of instability toward normality. For the two parameters, the pseudo-Romberg ratios (performance EC/performance EO) have indicated that a special visual contribution to balance control is present under vestibula nerve tumor (here 1 and 2 grades). The relative importance of this visual support diminished shortly after ionizing treatment. Because the radiation is neither noxious nor excitatory, we think such a rapid recovery is due to some recovery of vestibular nerve afferent conduction, and a rapid neural reprogramming of the balance control. These attractive results call for deeper vestibular investigations.

Hydrocephalus

Obstructive hydrocephalus (HCP) in association with a VS is a well-known phenomenon. In order to investigate whether SRS contributes to HCP, we studied our own series of patients [22]. Among the 1,000 patients treated using SRS at the Timone hospital between July 1992 and January 2002, 43 patients displayed HCP. Thirty-two patients displayed HCP prior to treatment (group A) and 11 after treatment (group B). Age at the time of treatment (median age of 70 years in A and B) and tumor volume were higher than for the entire treated population. Following radiosurgery, 75% of the patients from group A did not require a shunting device whereas all the patients from group B required a shunt. Three patients had tumor progression requiring surgery. Occurrence of de novo HCP was a rare event (1%) that required a shunt early after radiosurgery, at a mean interval of 14.8 (range 4–31) months. Results from this study suggest that radiosurgery is not responsible for a significant increase in the risk of developing HCP. We can postulate that SRS might have a protective effect on HCP progression since the number of preexisting patients with HCP which required a shunt was small [22].

Microsurgery after Radiosurgery

One of the primary criticisms of VS radiosurgery is the increased risk of microsurgery morbidity in those patients with tumor progression after SRS. We have recently reviewed our experience with patients who have undergone surgical resection after failed SRS [21]. From July 1992 to December 2000, 25 out of 1,000 patients underwent a second procedure after SRS failure. Excluding NF2 patients, 21 patients underwent surgical resection. In order to analyze the potential difficulties encountered during surgical resection, a questionnaire was sent to the primary surgeon.

The mean interval between radiosurgery and surgical resection was 36 months, ranging from 10 to 83 months. The mean increase in volume was 559% (range 37–3,036%, median 160%). Evaluation by the Koos staging system revealed 8 stage 2, 10 stage 3, 2 stage 4 tumors. Patients underwent surgical resection for radiographic tumor progression in 7 cases and for clinicoradiological progression in 13 cases. In 9 cases, the surgeon reported unusual difficulty related to adhesion of the tumor to neurovascular structures. Tumor removal was complete in 14 cases, near total in 4 cases, and subtotal in 2 cases. One case of venous infarction occurred following surgical resection associated with hemiparesis and aphasia which gradually recovered. At last follow-up, facial nerve function was near normal (House-Brackmann grade 1 and 2) in 10 cases while 7 cases had grade 3, and 3 cases had grade 4 and 5 function. We recommend that surgical resection of a progressive VS after SRS be performed after a sufficient follow-up period. Our results conclude that surgical resection may be more problematic and facial nerve preservation might be impaired by radiosurgery in half of our cases. However, these results do not support a change in our decision making of radiosurgical treatment of small to medium-size VSs [21].

Long-Term Complications

The use of SRS for many benign tumors has increased significantly over the last 2 decades. The long-term potential carcinogenic risk of SRS was not evaluated until recently. The definition of radio-induced tumors is based on the criteria by Cahan: the tumor must occur in a previously irradiated field, after a long time interval from irradiation, and must be pathologically different from the primary tumor and not present at the time of irradiation. In addition, the patient must not have a genetic predisposition for the tumor. A low dose of radiation, such as 1 Gy, has been associated with second tumor formation and a relative risk between 1.57 and 8.75. This relative risk increases to 18.4 for an interval time between 20 and 25 years. Radiation-associated tumor incidence is linked to different factors such as age and individual genetic susceptibility. At this time, three radiation-associated gliomas and five malignant VSs have been reported in the literature. Moreover, these second tumors do not meet all the Cahan criteria. We have reported two cases from our radiosurgical experience to discuss these points [11]. Long-term follow-up, ranging from 5 to 30 years, is needed to observe the crude incidence of radiation-induced tumors. The relative risk is estimated less than 1 per 1,000 and must be reported to each patient prior to any radiosurgical procedure.

Type 2 Neurofibromatosis

NF2 was present in 37 patients (50 VSs treated with SRS) among the VS patients treated in Marseille between July 1992 and January 2002 [25]. Prior to SRS treatment, surgical resection was performed on 16 patients. Tumor volumes ranged from 120 to 14,405 mm^3 (mean 3,468 mm^3) at the time of treatment. Twelve tumors were categorized as Koos stage 4. Median clinical and radiological follow-up was 62 months and ranged from 27 to 123 months. The 5- and 10-year actuarial survival rates were 90 and 85%, respectively. The 5-year actuarial survival rate without hearing decrement was 36% in patients with useful hearing (Gardner 1 and 2) at the time of treatment. Severe phenotype of the disease ($p = 0.05$) and dose (>12 Gy) delivered to the tumor margin ($p = 0.032$) correlated with hearing deterioration in a univariate analysis. Permanent facial nerve palsy occurred in 2%. These results confirm SRS is a valuable alternative treatment for NF2 patients with VSs. However, SRS does not provide the same level of tumor control and hearing preservation in comparison to treatment of patients with sporadic VSs. These results may improve with early treatment of NF2 VSs with SRS.

SRS Indications

Young patients with small and medium-sized VSs and few symptoms are the best candidates for radiosurgery. Patients with Koos stage 2 and 3 tumors are good candidates as well. Intracanalicular, cystic, previously resected, and Koos stage 4 tumors may be candidates as well.

Intracanalicular Schwannomas

Until 1999, Koos class 1 tumors were considered for radiosurgery only in cases of tumor progression at our institution. Our retrospective analysis of tumor growth rate, functional hearing preservation, and patients requesting radiosurgery have led us to modify our practice. Patients treated with SRS have a higher probability of functional hearing preservation [20]. Consequently, patients presenting with a stage 1 lesion and functional hearing are now considered for radiosurgery at our institution in the absence of tumor progression.

Large VSs

Surgical resection and facial nerve preservation is reserved for large tumors. In a small number of patients, microsurgery is not warranted because of contralateral deafness or the presence of comorbidities. We have analyzed our results of SRS treatment of large VSs [24]. Between July 1992 and December 2000, we treated 50 patients harboring large VSs, defined as Koos stage 4. Follow-up data were available for 44 patients, including 12 NF2 patients. Mean age at the time of treatment was 43.5 years (range 14–84 years), mean diameter of the tumor was 18 (range 12–30) mm, and the mean volume was 4,301 (range 1,340–11,405) mm^3. Gamma Knife treatment was undertaken utilizing an average of 13.4 (range 4–48) isocenters and a dose of 10.2 (range 8–14) Gy at the tumor margin. Median follow-up of patients was 45.5 months (range 24–108 months). Tumor control was 69% (confidence interval: 52–83%) and 3 patients had surgical resection because of tumor progression. Statistical analysis revealed the tumor volume correlated with SRS failure in a uni- and multivariate model ($p = 0.027$). No brain stem complication was observed in any patient. No facial nerve deterioration was found and useful hearing preservation was obtained in 12 out of 20 cases (60%). These results suggest that in a highly selected subgroup of large VSs, radiosurgery can be a potential alternative to open surgery, particularly if hearing preservation is pursued. Patients need to understand the risk of SRS failure is much greater when large VSs are treated [24].

Cystic VSs

Patients with cystic VSs are a well-defined subgroup of patients that historically have a poor outcome after microsurgical resection. These patients are considered poor candidates for radiosurgery based on Pendl's report of a high SRS failure rate [14]. Among the 1,000 consecutive patients treated with SRS in Marseille between July 1992 and January 2002, 54 patients had cystic tumors at the time of treatment [1]. The median follow-up for this group of patients was 26 months (mean 33 months; range 6–90 months). A failure rate of 6.4% resulted in microsurgical tumor removal in 2 patients and repeat SRS in 1 patient. No patients developed a facial palsy. Two patients developed transient facial hypesthesia. Among the 32 patients with functional hearing at the time of SRS, 53% had preserved hearing at 3 years follow-up. In summary, SRS treatment failure was higher in patients harboring cystic tumors in comparison to patients with solid tumors (93.6 vs. 98%).

Residual or Recurrent VSs after Microsurgical Resection

Significant morbidity is expected after a second microsurgical procedure for recurrent or growing residual VSs. Among the first 1,000 VSs treated with SRS in Marseille, 60 patients (including 12 NF2 patients) underwent radiosurgical treatment after one or more surgical resection attempts. There were 27 residual and 19 recurrent VSs. The mean time interval between surgical removal and radiosurgery was 71.5 months (range 1.8–127.8 months). Difficulty with radiosurgery planning occurred with 12 patients due to problematic target identification. Median follow-up for these patients was 51.6 months. Four out of 58 patients (7%, confidence interval: 1.9–16.7) were considered treatment failures. Statistical evaluation failed to identify significant parameters influencing failure. Facial and trigeminal nerve function was not impaired in any patient. One patient developed a radiation-induced pontine injury responsible for lower cranial nerve deficits. Our results confirm SRS is an acceptable treatment alternative for patients that have undergone prior surgical resection [23].

Conclusion

We have evaluated the outcome results of our prospective series of patients with vestibular schwannomas treated with Gamma Knife SRS. Between July 1992 and March 2001, 1,000 patients with VSs were treated consecutively in Marseille Timone University Hospital. Patients without NF2 and tumors originating from the facial nerve represented a total of 927 patients (414 males and 513 females). According to the Koos classification, 77 patients had stage 1, 520 stage 2, 287 stage 3, and 42 stage 4 tumors. Average tumor volume was 12.7 mm^3. Hearing prior to radiosurgery was useful, according to the Gardner-Robertson classification, in 47% of the patients. Tumor control at last follow-up was 97%. Trigeminal nerve injury was reported in 0.6% of the patients while 1.3% developed facial palsy. Among the last 258 patients treated with SRS, no patient has developed facial palsy. The rate of functional hearing preservation for patients with class 1 hearing was 77.8% at 3 years and 47.6% for class 2 hearing. In patients initially presenting with tinnitus, this rate of functional hearing preservation increased to 95%.

Based on our results and those of others, SRS may be superior to VS surgical resection in terms of cranial nerve preservation while equal in efficacy. Radiosurgery should be the preferred treatment modality for young patients with few symptoms presenting with small to medium-sized VSs (Koos stage 1–3). Determination of the potential long-term complications and mechanisms of action of radiosurgery should be future goals as the paradigm of SRS evolves.

References

1 Delsanti C, Regis J: Cystic vestibular schwannomas. Neurochirurgie 2004;50:401–406 (in French).
2 Delsanti C, Tamura M, Galanaud D, Regis J: Changing radiological results, pitfalls and criteria of failure. Neurochirurgie 2004;50:312–319 (in French).
3 Flickinger JC, Kondziolka D, Lunsford LD: Dose and diameter relationships for facial, trigeminal and acoustic neuropathies following acoustic neuroma radiosurgery. Radiother Oncol 1996;41: 215–219.
4 Flickinger JC, Kondziolka D, Niranjan A, Voynov G, Maitz A, Lunsford LD: Acoustic neuroma radiosurgery with marginal tumor doses of 12 to 13 Gy. Int J Radiat Oncol Biol Phys 2004;60: 225–230.
5 Flickinger JC, Kondziolka D, Pollock BE, Lunsford LD: Evolution in technique for vestibular schwannoma radiosurgery and effect on outcome. Int J Radiat Oncol Biol Phys 1996;36:275–280.
6 Gabert K, Regis J, Delsanti C, Roche PH, Facon F, Tamura M, Pellet W, Thomassin JM: Preserving hearing function after Gamma Knife radiosurgery for unilateral vestibular schwannoma. Neurochirurgie 2004;50(pt 2):350–357.
7 Henschen F: Zur histolgie und pathogenese der kleinhirnbruckenwinkel tumoren. Arch Psychiatry 1915;56:21–122.
8 Leksell L: A note on the treatment of acoustic tumors. Acta Chir Scand 1969;137:763–765.
9 Leksell L: A note on the treatment of acoustic tumours. Acta Chir Scand 1971;137:763–765.
10 Mdarhri D, Touzani A, Tamura M, Regis J: Gamma Knife surgery for VII nerve schwannomas. Neurochirurgie 2004;50(pt 2):407–413.
11 Muracciole X, Cowen D, Regis J: Radiosurgery and brain radio-induced carcinogenesis: update. Neurochirurgie 2004;50(pt 2):414–420.
12 Noren G: Gamma knife radiosurgery of acoustic neurinomas. A historic perspective. Neurochirurgie 2004;50:253–256.
13 Ouaknine M, Hugon M, Roman S, Thomassin JM, Sarabian N, Regis J: Improvement in postural orientation and stability after stereotactic gamma irradiation of acoustic neurinomas. Neurochirurgie 2004;50(pt 2):358–366.
14 Pendl G, Ganz J, Kitz K, Eustacchio S: Acoustic neurinomas with macrocysts treated with Gamma Knife radiosurgery. Stereotact Funct Neurosurg 1996;66(suppl 1):103–111.
15 Pollock B, Lunsford L, Kondziolka D, Flickinger J, Bissonette D, Kelsey S, Jannetta P: Outcome analysis of acoustic neuroma management: a comparison of microsurgery and stereotactic radiosurgery [published erratum appears in Neurosurgery 1995;36:427]. Neurosurgery 1995;36: 215–224; discussion 224–219.
16 Regis J, Delsanti C, Roche PH, Thomassin JM, Pellet W: Functional outcomes of radiosurgical treatment of vestibular schwannomas: 1,000 successive cases and review of the literature. Neurochirurgie 2004;50:301–311.
17 Regis J, Hayashi M, Porcheron D, Delsanti C, Muracciole X, Peragut JC: Impact of the model C and Automatic Positioning System on gamma knife radiosurgery: an evaluation in vestibular schwannomas. J Neurosurg 2002;97(suppl):588–591.

18 Regis J, Levivier M, Wikler D, Porcheron D: Dosimetric planning for radiosurgical treatment of vestibular schwannomas. Neurochirurgie 2004;50(pt 2):289–300.
19 Regis J, Pellet W, Delsanti C, Dufour H, Roche PH, Thomassin JM, Zanaret M, Peragut JC: Functional outcome after gamma knife surgery or microsurgery for vestibular schwannomas. J Neurosurg 2002;97:1091–1100.
20 Regis J, Roche PH, Delsenti C, Soumare O, Thomassin JM, Pellet W: Stereotactic radiosurgery for vestibular schwannoma; in Pollock BE (ed): Contemporary Stereotactic Radiosurgery: Thechnique and Evaluation. Armonk, New York, Futura Publishing Company, 2002, pp 181–212.
21 Roche PH, Regis J, Deveze A, Delsanti C, Thomassin JM, Pellet W: Surgical removal of unilateral vestibular schwannomas after failed Gamma Knife radiosurgery. Neurochirurgie 2004;50(pt 2): 383–393.
22 Roche PH, Ribeiro T, Soumare O, Robitail S, Pellet W, Regis J: Hydrocephalus and vestibular schwannomas treated by Gamma Knife radiosurgery. Neurochirurgie 2004;50(pt 2):345–349.
23 Roche PH, Robitail S, Delsanti C, Marouf R, Pellet W, Regis J: Radiosurgery of vestibular schwannomas after microsurgery and combined radio-microsurgery. Neurochirurgie 2004;50(pt 2): 394–400.
24 Roche PH, Robitail S, Pellet W, Deveze A, Thomassin JM, Regis J: Results and indications of gamma knife radiosurgery for large vestibular schwannomas. Neurochirurgie 2004;50(pt 2): 377–382.
25 Roche PH, Robitail S, Thomassin JM, Pellet W, Regis J: Surgical management of vestibular schwannomas secondary to type 2 neurofibromatosis. Neurochirurgie 2004;50(pt 2):367–376.
26 Tamura M, Murata N, Hayashi M, Regis J: Injury of the lacrimal component of the nervus intermedius function after radiosurgery versus microsurgery. Neurochirurgie 2004;50(pt 2):338–344.

Prof. Jean Régis
Service de Neurochirurgie Fonctionnelle et Stéréotaxique
264 Bvd St Pierre
FR-13385 Marseille Cedex 05 (France)
Tel. + 33 4 91 38 70 58, Fax + 33 4 91 38 70 56, E-Mail jregis@ap-hm.fr

Szeifert GT, Kondziolka D, Levivier M, Lunsford LD (eds): Radiosurgery and Pathological Fundamentals. Prog Neurol Surg. Basel, Karger, 2007, vol 20, pp 142–149

9.3. Radiosurgery for Intracranial Meningiomas

John Y.K. Lee[a,d], *Douglas Kondziolka*[a,b,d], *John C. Flickinger*[a,b,d], *L. Dade Lunsford*[a–d]

Departments of [a]Neurological Surgery, [b]Radiation Oncology, [c]Radiology, and [d]Center for Image-Guided Neurosurgery, University of Pittsburgh School of Medicine and University of Pittsburgh Medical Center, Pittsburgh, Pa., USA

Abstract

Introduction: Meningiomas are common intracranial benign tumors that can be surgically excised. However, their intimate involvement with critical neurovascular structures often prevent their complete resection. Gamma Knife radiosurgery is a minimally invasive option which provides excellent tumor control as both an adjunct and primary therapy. **Materials and Methods:** Between September 1987 and December 2004, 964 patients underwent Gamma Knife radiosurgery at the University of Pittsburgh for the diagnosis of meningioma. The majority of patients had tumors located at the skull base. All imaging and clinical follow-up was reviewed. **Results:** Overall, Gamma Knife radiosurgery provides 5- and 10-year actuarial tumor control rates of 93% for benign meningiomas. The 5-year actuarial control rate for patients with atypical and malignant meningiomas was 83 ± 7 and 72 ± 10%, respectively. The incidence of adverse radiation effect ranged from 5.7 to 16%; however, the incidence was gradually reduced with the advent of magnetic resonance imaging and lower dosing since 1991. **Conclusion:** Gamma Knife radiosurgery is an attractive option for patients with intracranial meningiomas. It can be used as both primary treatment based on imaging diagnosis alone, or as an adjunct treatment after craniotomy. It provides long-term tumor control with minimal adverse sequelae.

Meningiomas represent 15% of adult intracranial neoplasms, and surgical resection is the preferred method of treatment whenever surgical morbidity is within reasonable limits [1–3]. Considering the known benefit of total resection of an intracranial meningioma and its dural attachments, surgeons have traditionally opted to use Gamma Knife stereotactic radiosurgery (SRS) as an adjunctive treatment modality after surgical resection or for patients who are at high risk for operative morbidity or mortality. Multiple studies have demonstrated the efficacy and safety of this treatment with actuarial tumor control rates ranging from 60 to 100% depending on the proportion of atypical or malignant meningiomas [4–10]. Given the benefit of radiosurgery as an adjunct in treatment, Gamma Knife radiosurgery has been increasingly used to treat patients as a primary therapy based on imaging criteria only [11]. Here, we review the indications, technique, results, and complications of Gamma Knife radiosurgery for intracranial meningiomas.

Methods

Patient Selection

The first step in performing radiosurgery is proper patient selection. Patients referred to our Center for radiosurgery are reviewed by neurosurgeons with experience in both microsurgery and radiosurgery. Younger patients with larger tumors associated with regional mass effect are counseled to undergo tumor resection in order to quickly relieve mass effect. In contrast, elderly patients with an incidentally discovered tumor may be advised to undergo a period of observation. Between these two extremes lie the bulk of patients who present to the University of Pittsburgh for radiosurgery.

Preoperative considerations in the management of intracranial meningiomas include the involvement of critical neurovascular structures which limit the ultimate ability of any surgeon to resect the entire tumor and its meningeal attachment. Cavernous sinus location, attachment to the middle or posterior third of the superior sagittal sinus, direct compression of the brainstem and obstructive hydrocephalus are all anatomic concerns that may influence the decision to perform open craniotomy or radiosurgery. Another preoperative consideration is the overall size of the tumor. In general, larger tumors with average diameters >3 cm are referred for either complete surgical resection or surgical debulking. Patient age is another important consideration as younger patients are generally given the option for open craniotomy and older patients are given the option of radiosurgery. Another important factor during the preoperative period is the decision whether to treat the meningioma based on imaging criteria alone. Since Gamma Knife radiosurgery is a noninvasive treatment option, primary radiosurgery requires that the imaging diagnosis of meningioma be accurate. Given our experience of 'misdiagnosis' based on imaging in only 2% of cases, most of whom would have underwent radiosurgery anyway, we do not hesitate to treat patients with radiosurgery based on MR criteria alone.

Radiosurgery Procedure

Patients are admitted to the hospital on the day of surgery, and most patients are given supplemental anxiolytics such as 1.0 mg lorazepam and/or 50 μg of fentanyl prior to frame placement. After the patient's head has been cleaned with alcohol, the Leksell Model G stereotactic frame (Elekta Instruments, Atlanta, Ga., USA) is placed. In patients who are undergoing adjunct radiosurgery, it is important to palpate the patient's skull to avoid placing the pins through prior craniotomy defects. Patients are given 1% lidocaine and 0.5% bupivacaine at the four pin sites. Measurements of the patient's skull dimensions are recorded and used by the computer dose-planning software to calculate the attenuation of the photon beams prior to reaching the target. The patient is then taken to the MRI unit for stereotactic imaging. On rare occasions, patients are unable to undergo MRI due to metallic implants or the patient's weight. In these cases we utilize contrast-enhanced, stereotactic CT scanning for dose planning.

Upon arrival in the MRI suite, patients are given a paramagnetic contrast agent. An initial sagittal imaging sequence is obtained to define regions of interest for subsequent sequences. The primary imaging sequence we use is a volume acquisition, spoiled GRASS gradient recovery technique performed in the axial plane. Between 28 and 60 images can be obtained with images spaced from 1 to 2 mm apart. The time of this sequence using a 512×256 matrix with two excitations is from 5 to 10 min. Fat suppression images are important for tumors near the orbit or in patients with fat grafts after transsphenoidal procedures. After the fiducial measurements on the images are checked for stereotactic accuracy at the MR console, the patient is returned to the gamma unit. The images are transferred to our computer workstation via Ethernet. Our current dose-planning software (GammaPlan version 5.33, Elekta Instruments, Atlanta, Ga., USA) rapidly creates stereotactic coronal and sagittal reformatted images from the axial images, significantly decreasing our scanning time by eliminating the need to perform multiplanar imaging at the MR unit.

Dose planning is performed at the computer workstation in the radiosurgical unit. The goal of dose planning is to create a conformal isodose configuration that completely covers the tumor with a minimum amount of radiation being delivered to the surrounding structures. This is particularly important in the treatment of cavernous sinus lesions which contain cranial nerves and which lie adjacent to the brainstem. Using a combination of multiple irradiation isocenters of different sizes (4, 8, 14, and 18 mm), differential weighting of the individual isocenters and selective blocking of the collimated beams of radiation, it is possible to produce dose plans that closely conform to the irregular shape of all tumors. With regard to meningiomas, it is important to target the dural tail, and although the precise edge of the dural tail can be difficult to determine, we make a concerted effort to treat the tail carefully [12].

Three factors have been critical in our ability to design more complex and highly conformal dose plans. First, the use of MRI instead of CT as our primary stereotactic imaging modality provides superior resolution of the tumor margins. Second, high-speed computer workstations and advanced dose-planning software have reduced the calculation time for dose plans from several minutes to seconds. This real-time feedback facilitates the design of more sophisticated dose plans as well as the ability to view the images in multiple planes simultaneously, allowing a three-dimensional assessment of the dose plan at all times. Third, the new Model C Gamma Knife, with automated patient positioning system, facilitates the use of more isocenters to improve the conformality of the delivered radiosurgical treatment.

After the plan is completed, the neurosurgeon, in conjunction with the radiation oncologist and medical physicist, decide the appropriate radiation dose to be given for each case. Dose prescription is based on clinical experience and the integrated logistic formula for predicting radiation-related complications after radiosurgery. The goal is to provide the lowest radiation dose possible that will give long-term tumor growth control, thereby minimizing the likelihood of adverse radiation effects on nearby structures. Although it appears that some cranial nerves may tolerate high doses of radiation (60–70 Gy) when it is delivered in multiple fractions, cranial nerves may be more susceptible to injury after single-fraction, high-dose radiation. For example, we observed trigeminal and facial neuropathy rates of approximately

30% after acoustic neuroma radiosurgery when the maximum radiation dose was 36–40 Gy. Such high doses were used in the 1980s and have not been used for over 12 years. Different classes of cranial nerves appear to have distinct tolerances for radiation. Special sensory nerves such as the optic nerve may not tolerate single fraction doses >10 Gy [13], whereas general somatic nerves such as the oculomotor nerve are not adversely affected by much higher doses. We try to restrict the dose to the optic apparatus to less than 8 Gy. Within the cavernous sinus, we noted that when exposed to the same high, single-fraction dose, the trigeminal nerve was more susceptible to adverse radiation effects than the oculomotor nerves [10].

After the radiosurgical procedure is completed (which usually takes between 30–60 min), the stereotactic frame is removed and a gauze headwrap is applied to the pin sites. A single dose of methylprednisolone (40 mg) is given to the patient prior to his/her leaving the surgical suite. The patient is then returned to the general neurosurgical ward and is given a normal diet. Patients are instructed to resume their normal activities the day after surgery.

Results

We reviewed our consecutive experience of 964 patients with meningiomas managed at the University of Pittsburgh. We have performed radiosurgery on 646 females and 317 males with meningiomas located in various locations. The mean age at time of treatment was 57 years. Approximately half of the patients (46%) had prior craniotomies, whereas another half of the patients (54%) had primary radiosurgery. Only 6.3% had prior fractionated radiation therapy. Eighty-three percent of patients had Karnofsky scores of 90 or greater at the time of radiosurgery. The mean number of isocenters used in this series was 7.8. The average tumor margin dose was 13.9 Gy and the mean central dose was 27.9 Gy.

We have previously published the excellent actuarial tumor control rate that can be achieved after radiosurgical treatment of meningiomas. For example, in patients with cavernous sinus meningiomas, the single-center University of Pittsburgh study demonstrated a 10-year actuarial tumor control rate of 93% [10]. Lee et al. [10] studied 159 patients who had meningiomas centered within the cavernous sinus. Seventy-six patients (48%) underwent adjuvant radiosurgery after one or more attempts at surgical resection. Eighty-three patients (52%) underwent primary radiosurgery. Conformal multiple isocenter Gamma Knife radiosurgery with a median marginal tumor dose of 13 Gy was performed. Tumor volumes decreased in 54 (34%) patients, remained stable in 96 (60%), and increased in 9 (6%). The actuarial tumor control rate at 5 years for patients who underwent primary radiosurgery was 96.9 ± 3.0%. The tumor control rate at 5 years for patients who underwent adjuvant radiosurgery was 79.6 ± 7.1%. If the patients with known atypical or malignant meningiomas are excluded from the analysis, the actuarial tumor control rate for patients undergoing adjuvant radiosurgery was 90.4 ± 5.1%. Adverse radiation effects occurred after 11 procedures (6.7%). For patients who had radiosurgery as their only treatment (n = 83), the actuarial tumor control rate at 5 years was 96.9 ± 3.0%.

In a multicenter study of Gamma Knife radiosurgery for parasagittal meningiomas, a 5-year actuarial tumor control rate of 93% was achieved. Kondziolka's group studied 203 patients with histologically benign meningiomas. The tumors were located in the anterior superior sagittal sinus in 52 patients, at the middle of the sinus in 91, and at the posterior portion of the sinus in 60. The mean tumor volume at the time of radiosurgery was 10 cm^3. In patients who underwent radiosurgery as the primary therapy (n = 66), the 5-year actuarial tumor control rate was 93 ± 4%. No clinical failure (need for additional therapy or worsened neurological function) occurred in patients who had smaller tumors ($<7.5\,cm^3$) and who had never undergone resection (n = 410). The 5-year control rate for patients with previous surgery was only 60 ± 10%; the control rate for the radiosurgery-treated volume was 85%. Most failures resulted from remote tumor growth. Multivariate analyses identified significantly decreased tumor control with increasing tumor volume ($p = 0.002$) and previous neurological deficits ($p = 0.002$). The rate of transient, symptomatic edema after radiosurgery was 16%, was more common with larger tumors, and occurred within 2 years.

Gamma Knife radiosurgery of meningiomas as a primary treatment modality is associated with better actuarial tumor control rates as compared to treatment as an adjunct. Flickinger et al. [11] studied a single-center University of Pittsburgh series of 219 patients with meningiomas diagnosed by imaging criteria only. Patients were treated with a median marginal tumor dose of 14 Gy, and a median treatment volume of 5.0 cm^3. The median follow-up period was 29 months. Tumor progression developed in 7 cases, 2 of which turned out to be different tumors (metastatic nasopharyngeal adenoid cystic carcinoma and chondrosarcoma). One tumor was controlled, but the development of other brain metastases suggested a different diagnosis. The actuarial tumor control rate was 93.2 ± 2.7% at 5 and 10 years. The actuarial rate of identifying a diagnosis other than meningioma was 2.3 ± 1.4% at 5 and 10 years. The actuarial rate of developing any postradiosurgical injury reaction was 8.8 ± 3.0% at 5 and 10 years. No pretreatment variables correlated with tumor control in univariate or multivariate analysis. The risk of postradiosurgery sequelae was lower (5.3 ± 2.3%) in patients treated after 1991 (with stereotactic MRI and lower doses; $p = 0.0104$) and tended to increase with treatment volume ($p = 0.0537$).

The role of Gamma Knife radiosurgery in the treatment of malignant meningioma remains unclear. Harris et al. [14] studied 30 patients who had SRS for treatment of malignant (n = 12) or atypical (n = 18) meningiomas. The median imaging follow-up was 2.3 years. The 5-year actuarial tumor control rate was 59% for both atypical and malignant meningiomas. Atypical meningiomas had a 5-year progression-free survival (PFS) of 83 ± 7%, while malignant meningiomas had a 5-year PFS of 72 ± 10% ($p = 0.018$). On multivariate analysis, early SRS and smaller tumor volumes were associated with better PFS, while younger age was associated with better survival. One patient had an adverse radiation effect after SRS.

Discussion

Simpson [15] provided data on meningioma recurrence after surgical resection. He reported a 9% recurrence rate for tumors completely resected along with their dural attachment, a 19% recurrence rate if the tumor was completely resected and the adjacent dura cauterized, and a 40% recurrence rate in patients with partial resection. We have provided evidence that the actuarial tumor control rate at 5 years and even up to 10 years is 93% for meningiomas treated with primary radiosurgery. This is equivalent and possibly marginally better than the 9% recurrence rate by Simpson. In patients where a complete resection is impossible or a complete cauterization is impossible, radiosurgery offers a better chance for tumor control rate. Hence, meningiomas located along the convexity, lateral sphenoid ridge and anterior fossa floor should be treated with a craniotomy and surgical resection. However, in patients with deeply seated tumors which are adjacent to neurovascular structures, radiosurgery can be offered as primary treatment or as an adjunct after surgical debulking.

The tumor control rate of atypical and malignant meningiomas treated with radiosurgery is not as well established. Radiosurgery provides only a 59% tumor control rate at 5 years. However, surgical resection combined with radiosurgery and fractionated radiation therapy provide three different treatment modalities that can be used in conjunction to treat these types of difficult tumors [14, 16].

Radiosurgery of meningiomas at the skull base poses particular concern to the vascular and neural structures that are often embedded within or around the meningioma tumor. We have not found the motor cranial nerves within the cavernous sinus to be particularly sensitive to the radiosurgery doses used in meningioma radiosurgery. In our series of 159 patients with cavernous sinus meningiomas, no patient developed oculomotor, abducens, or trochlear nerve complication [10]. In this same series, however, 5 patients developed trigeminal nerve dysfunction including facial pain, keratitis and paresthesias. The sensory nerves appear to be more sensitive. Hence, for skull base meningiomas that arise near the optic nerve we keep the radiation dose to the optic nerve to 8–10 Gy [13].

In addition to risk of damage to neural structures, radiosurgery of skull base meningiomas poses particular susceptibility to major vascular structures.

In our experience of radiosurgery for parasagittal meningiomas, we have not observed any increased risk to bridging veins or the sinus. Although it is possible that radiosurgery may cause progressive sinus occlusion, this occlusion may be so slow as to be asymptomatic in most patients. Increased time for follow-up will allow us to observe this late complication.

Conclusion

We have performed radiosurgery in almost 1,000 patients with meningiomas at the University of Pittsburgh. This treatment modality can be performed both as an adjunct to surgical resection or as a primary procedure. The 5- and 10-year actuarial tumor control rate is above 90%, as demonstrated in multiple studies. The complication rate remains low, and thus Gamma Knife radiosurgery is an effective treatment strategy for meningiomas.

References

1 Mahmood A, Qureshi NH, Malik GM: Intracranial meningiomas: analysis of recurrence after surgical treatment. Acta Neurochir 1994;126:53–58.
2 Mirimanoff RO, Dosoretz DE, Linggood RM, Ojemann RG, Martuza RL: Meningioma: analysis of recurrence and progression following neurosurgical resection. J Neurosurg 1985;62:18–24.
3 Borovich B, Doron Y: Recurrence of intracranial meningiomas: the role played by regional multicentricity. J Neurosurg 1986;64:58–63.
4 Kondziolka D, Levy EI, Niranjan A, Flickinger JC, Lunsford LD: Long-term outcomes after meningioma radiosurgery: physicians and patients perspective. J Neurosurg 1999;91:44–50.
5 Muthukumar N, Kondziolka D, Lunsford LD, Flickinger JC: Stereotactic radiosurgery for anterior foramen magnum meningiomas. Surg Neurol 1999;51:268–273.
6 Liscak R, Simonova G, Vymazal J, Janouskova L, Vladyka V: Gamma knife radiosurgery of meningiomas in the cavernous sinus region. Acta Neurochir 1999;141:473–480.
7 Hakim R, Alexander E, Loeffler JS, Shrieve DC, Wen P, Fallon MP, Stieg PE, Black PM: Results of linear accelerator-based radiosurgery for intracranial meningiomas. Neurosurgery 1998;42: 446–453.
8 Tanaka T, Kobayashi T, Kida Y: Growth control of cranial base meningiomas by stereotactic radiosurgery with a gamma knife unit. Neurol Med Chir 1996;36:7–10.
9 Pendl G, Schrottner O, Eustacchio S, Feichtinger K, Ganz J: Stereotactic radiosurgery of skull base meningiomas. Minim Invasive Neurosurg 1997;40:87–90.
10 Lee JY, Niranjan A, McInerney J, Kondziolka D, Flickinger JC, Lunsford LD: Stereotactic radiosurgery providing long-term tumor control of cavernous sinus meningiomas. J Neurosurg 2002;97: 65–72.
11 Flickinger JC, Kondziolka D, Maitz AH, Lunsford LD: Gamma knife radiosurgery of imaging-diagnosed intracranial meningioma. Int J Radiat Oncol Biol Phys 2003;56:801–806.
12 DiBiase SJ, Kwok Y, Yovino S, Arena C, Naqvi S, Temple R, Regine WF, Amin P, Guo C, Chin LS: Factors predicting local tumor control after gamma knife stereotactic radiosurgery for benign intracranial meningiomas. Int J Radiat Oncol Biol Phys 2004;60:1515–1519.
13 Leber KA, Bergloff J, Pendl G: Dose-response tolerance of the visual pathways and cranial nerves of the cavernous sinus to stereotactic radiosurgery. J Neurosurg 1998;88:43–50.

14 Harris AE, Lee JY, Omalu B, Flickinger JC, Kondziolka D, Lunsford LD: The effect of radiosurgery during management of aggressive meningiomas. Surg Neurol 2003;60:298–305; discussion 305.
15 Simpson D: The recurrence of intracranial meningiomas after surgical treatment. J Neurochem 1957;20:22–39.
16 Ojemann SG, Sneed PK, Larson DA, Gutin PH, Berger MS, Verhey L, Smith V, Petti P, Wara W, Park E, McDermott MW: Radiosurgery for malignant meningioma: results in 22 patients. J Neurosurg 2000;93(suppl 3):62–67.

John Y.K. Lee, MD
Department of Neurological Surgery
University of Pennsylvania School of Medicine
Penn Gamma Knife at Pennsylvania Hospital
Philadelphia, PA 19107 (USA)
Tel. +1 215 829 7144, Fax +1 215 829 6645, E-Mail John.Lee3@uphs.upenn.edu

Szeifert GT, Kondziolka D, Levivier M, Lunsford LD (eds): Radiosurgery and Pathological Fundamentals. Prog Neurol Surg. Basel, Karger, 2007, vol 20, pp 150–163

9.4. The Role of the Gamma Knife in the Management of Cerebral Astrocytomas

György T. Szeifert[a], *Dheerendra Prasad*[b], *Toshifumi Kamyrio*[b], *Melita Steiner*[b], *Ladislau E. Steiner*[b]

[a]National Institute of Neurosurgery and Department of Neurological Surgery, Semmelweis University, Budapest, Hungary; [b]Lars Leksell Center for Gamma Knife Surgery, Department of Neurological Surgery, University of Virgina, Charlottesville, Va., USA

Abstract

The aim of this study was to assess the role of Gamma Knife radiosurgery in the complex management of cerebral astrocytomas. Out of a series with more than 1,000 brain tumor cases treated at the Lars Leksell Center for Gamma Knife Surgery, UVA, 74 astrocytomas were selected for the present review. The tumor either disappeared or decreased in 60% of grade 1 astrocytomas (n = 15), and 71% tumor control was achieved in grade 2 astrocytomas (n = 17) following radiosurgery. In the high-grade glioma group (grades 3 and 4; n = 42) median survival time was 14 (range 2–58) months, and 25% of the patients were alive at 5 years after the treatment. The best results were presented by the subgroup wherein previous craniotomy and debulking of the tumor were followed by radiosurgery (n = 7) with a median survival period of 24 (range 2–53) months. Results of the present analysis suggest that stereotactic radiosurgery represents an alternative or supplementary treatment modality to conventional surgery in small-volume low-grade astrocytomas especially in deep-seated critical locations. There is also evidence for the beneficial effect of radiosurgery on the survival of patients with high-grade gliomas; however, the limitations of a focused irradiation technique on a malignant infiltrative process are obvious.

The quest for ideal management of astrocytomas is one of the most challenging tasks for neurosurgeons and neurooncologists. Forty to 50% of the brain tumors arise from the astrocytic series, and malignant gliomas constitute the most common primary, supratentorial cerebral neoplasm in adulthood [1]. The conventional treatment protocols usually consist of surgical resection, followed by radiotherapy or chemotherapy according to histopathological grading.

More recently, brachytherapy [2], interstitial chemotherapy [3], monoclonal antibodies [4] and gene therapy [5] have enriched the therapeutic arsenal. Nevertheless, the outcome in glioblastoma is one of the poorest in the oncological practice and the results remain depressing. The median survival time in glioblastoma is around 1 year following diagnosis, and survival of more than 2 years is less than 20% [6, 7]. The expected survival benefit following surgery improves with the enhanced dose of external radiotherapy [8, 9], but the possibility to use high dosage is limited by the risk for radiation-induced injuries to the surrounding normal brain tissue. This is increasing with fractionated doses exceeding 60 Gy. Significant improvement in survival was achieved in selected patients with small, unifocal, localized lesions using interstitial brachytherapy boost to enhance local disease control [10, 11]. Nowadays more and more units have the chance to use one of the single high-dose radiosurgery modalities as a boost technique to conventional radiotherapy.

The aim of the present study was to assess the role of the Gamma Knife (GK) in the complex management of cerebral astrocytomas.

Materials and Methods

At the Lars Leksell Center for Gamma Knife Surgery, Department of Neurological Surgery, University of Virginia, more than 1,000 brain tumors have been treated using the GK between 1989 and 1997; of those, 81 were astrocytomas. Follow-up data were available in 74 cases, included in the present study. The complete patient population consisted of 40 males and 34 females. The mean age of the cases was 34.4 (range 4–84) years. Karnofsky performance status of the patients varied between 60 and 100%.

There were 15 patients (4 males and 11 females) harboring astrocytoma grade 1. The mean age was 24.1 (range 4–53) years. Surgical resection was performed in 7 (twice in 3) cases and 1 patient had radiotherapy prior to GK treatment. Histologically, 13 were diagnosed as pilocytic astrocytomas and 2 subependymal giant cell astrocytomas. Ten of the 15 tumors were deep seated in the pons, midbrain, hypothalamus, thalamus, basal ganglia and optic chiasm. The mean volume of the neoplasm was 3.5 (0.7–11.3) cm^3 before radiosurgery.

The astrocytoma grade 2 group included 17 patients (9 males and 8 females). The mean age was 29.4 (9–56) years. One or repeated surgical resection was carried out in 6 cases before GK treatment, and 2 patients underwent a second radiosurgery intervention. Out of the 17 lesions, 10 were located in deep-seated structures. The mean volume of the tumor was 3.4 (0.7–9.7) cm^3 at the time of GK surgery.

The astrocytoma grade 3 and 4 population consisted of 42 patients (27 males and 15 females). Their mean age was 49.6 (range 7–93) years. Histological diagnoses were high-grade astrocytoma (grade 3) in 27, and glioblastoma multiforme or gliosarcoma (grade 4) 15 cases. Eighteen of these tumors were situated in, or extended to involve deeper critical elements of the brain. The mean volume of the neoplasms was 11.85 (range 0.1–93.0) cm^3.

Treatment planning was performed on CT and MR images using the KULA system between 1989 and 1993, and following that with the GammaPlan (Elekta Instruments AB,

Stockholm, Sweden). Prescribed doses were calculated on the basis of tumor volume, location, previous fractionated radiotherapy and the prescription isodose line. Radiosurgery treatments were carried out using the Leksell Gamma Knife Model U (Elekta). Astrocytoma grade 1 cases were treated with a 12.8 Gy mean dose at the periphery, which usually corresponded to the 40% isodose (30–50%) line and a maximum dose of mean 33.3 Gy (25.6–42.6). The mean number of the isocenters was 4 (range 1–8). In the grade 2 group, the margin of the tumors at the 40% isodose (30–50%) received a mean dose of 13.4 Gy, and 36.3 Gy as a maximum dose. A mean of 5 (range 2–11) isocenters was used. In high-grade gliomas, a mean dose of 7.6 Gy was administered to the margin of the lesion using generally the 30–50% isodose curve, with the corresponding mean maximum dose of 24.3 Gy.

GK surgery was carried out as a primary treatment for tumors in critical locations: in the brainstem, thalamus, hypothalamus and the basal ganglia. Radiosurgery was used either as a secondary treatment following partial surgical resection, or to escalate the dose already delivered by radiotherapy, with or without previous surgical intervention. In the latter case, tumor size, location, patient age and condition had not been the selecting criteria. However, lesions with multifocal appearance or spreading to the opposite side have not been treated.

The mean follow-up period was 28.8 (range 8–96) months for grade 1 cases, 33.4 (range 6–81) months for grade 2 tumors, and 17.7 (range 2–58) months for grade 3 and 4 astrocytomas. Follow-up imaging studies were regularly carried out at 3- to 6-month intervals depending on histology. Tumor margin delineated at the time of the treatment and the follow-up image was used for volume assessment by the NETRA, a computer-assisted image-analyzing software developed at the UVA. The clinical, histological and treatment variables as well as the length of follow-up were correlated to the imaging outcome which was classified on the basis of volume changes as tumor disappeared, decreased, did not change or increased.

Results

Astrocytoma Grade 1

The tumor disappeared in 1 (6.7%), decreased in 8 (53.3%), and increased in 6 (40%) cases following GK treatment (fig. 1). Hence, the tumor either disappeared or decreased in 9 (60.0%) cases out of 15. A 15–25% shrinkage occurred in 1, 26–50% in 2, 51–90% in 3, and 91–100% in 2 cases. In 2 cases, a cystic component which was present prior to GK treatment increased, in 1 case despite of decrease in the irradiated solid component. Best results occurred when the pretreatment volume was less than 3 cm^3. The mean volume of tumors with response to the treatment was 2.7 cm^3. All but 1 patient of 15 remained neurologically unchanged. This one patient developed hemiparesis and ptosis related to the increase of the cystic component of a tumor. Three patients had surgery because of tumor increase in 2, and bleeding in 1 case. Five patients had seizures prior to GK surgery, 2 of them became seizure free on medication, 2 had decreased frequency of seizures, and 1 had shown no change.

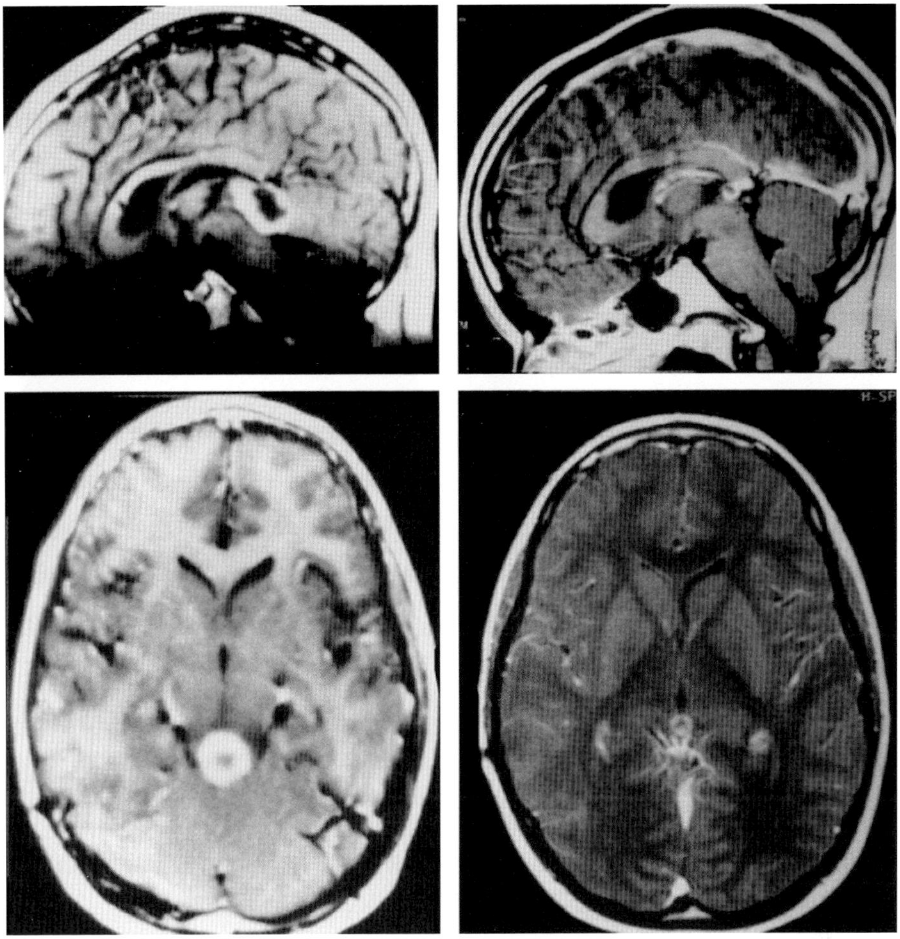

a b c d

Fig. 1. GK surgery for astrocytoma grade 1. Sagittal and axial contrast-enhanced MR images before GK treatment (***a***, ***c***) and 96 months following radiosurgery (***b***, ***d***). The small residual enhancement which has remained unchanged over the last several years is presumed to be gliosis secondary to radiation.

Astrocytoma Grade 2

The tumor disappeared in 3 (17.6%), shrunk in 7 (41.1%), remained unchanged in 2 (12.5%) and increased in 5 (31.3%) cases (fig. 2). Hence, the tumor either disappeared or decreased in 10 cases (58.8%) out of 17. A 25% shrinkage occurred in 1, 51–90% in 5, and 91–100% in 4 tumors. Out of the 17 cases in this group 3 patients developed transient neurological deficits, while the

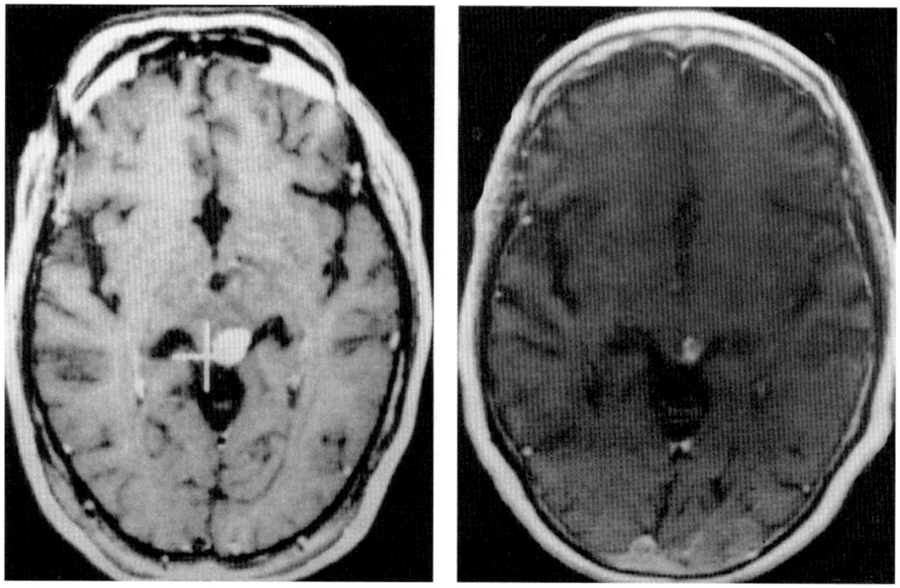

Fig. 2. GK surgery for astrocytoma grade 2. Axial postcontrast MR, T_1SE images before (*a*) and 12 months after (*b*) radiosurgery demonstrating a small residual gliosis. Subsequent MRIs revealed the gliotic changes to be stable over the last 3 years.

others remained neurologically unchanged following GK treatment. Craniotomy was necessary in 1 case. Increase in the size of the tumor led to death in 1 case 46 months following irradiation. In 3 patients with history of seizures, a decrease in the frequency of seizures was registered after the treatment.

Astrocytoma Grades 3 and 4

Out of the 42 cases, a decrease in the tumor size was observed in 11 (22%) cases with complete disappearance in 2 (fig. 3). There was no change in the tumor volume of 12 (28.5%) cases, and increase in size was noticed in 19 (45%) of the cases. The mean survival time interval was 26 (range 2–58) months with a median of 14 months, and 27 patients died during the observation period (fig. 4). At 5 years, 25% of patients were alive. Survival was better in patients with tumors that revealed radiological stabilization or decrease and/or disappearance (mean 33 months), as compared to patients with tumors that continued to increase (19 months) by the Kaplan-Meier method ($p = 0.003$).

Patients were divided on the basis of therapeutic modalities into those that underwent surgical resection + radiotherapy + GK; surgery + GK; radiotherapy + GK, and GK alone. When comparing these different treatment modalities

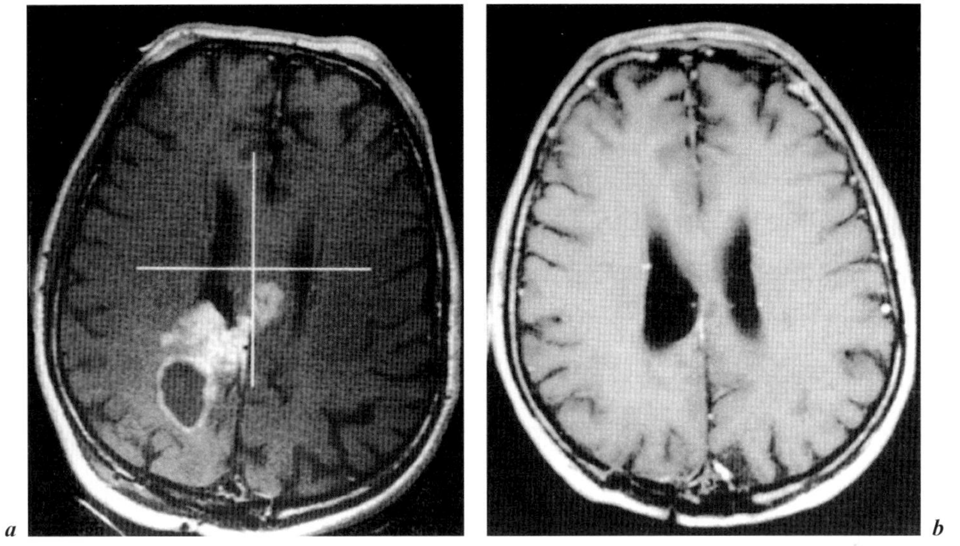

Fig. 3. GK surgery for astrocytoma grade 4. Stereotactic postcontrast axial T_1SE MR images at the time of treatment (***a***) and 6 months following radiosurgery (***b***) showing almost complete resolution of enhancing abnormality. Subsequent MRI 18 months after the first follow-up disclosed recurrent tumor, but the patient was asymptomatic. (This scan was not available at the time of publication.)

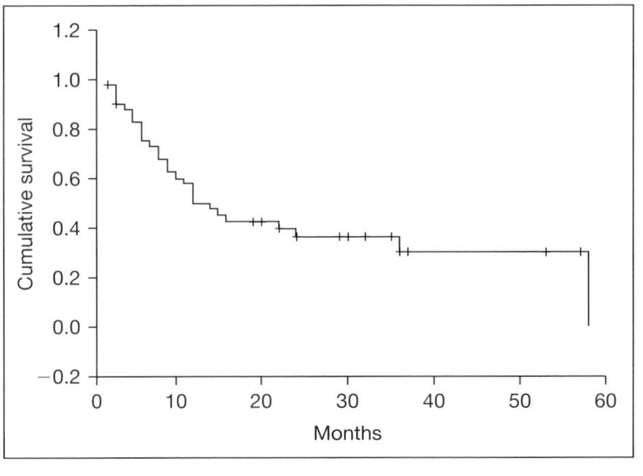

Fig. 4. Overall survival of patients with grades 3 and 4 astrocytomas.

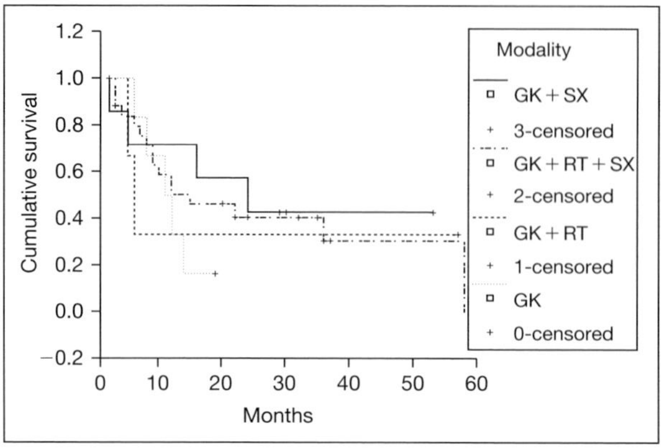

Fig. 5. Survival functions related to modalities of therapy.

(fig. 5), the poorest results were seen in the subgroup where the conventional radiotherapy was followed by radiosurgery without previous surgical debulking of the tumor (3 cases). However, percentile plots revealed that these data were biased by the preponderance of tumors with larger volume at treatment as compared to the other therapeutic groups. In these cases, the mean tumor volume was 20.7 (range 4.8–43.0) cm^3 and the median survival was 6 months. Results in patients who underwent GK surgery as the initial and only treatment following biopsy (n = 6) were better, with a median survival of 11.5 months for mean tumor volume 7.1 (range 1.9–12.0) cm^3. In the subgroup treated with surgical resection followed by full dose (60 Gy) conventional radiotherapy and finally an escalation of the dose to the more restricted area of the tumor with the GK, the median survival was 15 (range 2–58) months. The mean volume of tumors in this group was 12.6 (range 0.125–93.0) cm^3. Finally, in the subgroup of 7 cases where previous craniotomy and debulking of the tumor was followed by GK radiosurgery the median survival period was 24 (range 2–53) months. The mean tumor volume was 6.45 (range 1.5–12.5) cm^3 in this population.

Survival figures were not statistically different in the above four categories by either the log-rank or the Breslow method of comparison. But the series are small and even so there is a tendency for the patients that undergo resection rather than biopsy to do better. No statistical difference was seen in survival when correlated to age, sex, initial tumor volume or to parameters of radiosurgical treatment, on univariate and multivariate analysis. Patients with grade 3 histological subtype did better than those with grade 4. We analyzed our patients based on the recursive analysis Radiation Therapy Oncology Group

Table 1. Definition of prognostic class from the RTOG recursive analysis

RTOG prognostic class	Definition
1	AA, Age < 50, normal mental status
2	AA, Age ≥ 50, KPS ≥ 70, duration of symptoms > 3 months
3	AA, Age < 50, abnormal mental status
	GBM, Age < 50, KPS = 90
4	AA, Age ≥ 50, KPS ≥ 70, duration of symptoms ≤ 3 months
	GBM, Age < 50, KPS < 90
	GBM, Age > 50, KPS ≥ 70, partial or total resection, NFS = working
5	GBM, Age ≥ 50, KPS ≥ 70, partial or total resection, NFS < working
	GBM, Age ≥ 50, KPS ≥ 70, biopsy only
	GBM/AA, Age ≥ 50, KPS < 70, normal mental status
6	GBM/AA, Age ≥ 50, KPS < 70, normal mental status

AA = Anaplastic astrocytoma, WHO grade 3; GBS = glioblastoma multiforme, WHO grade 4; KPS = Karnofsky performance score; NFS = neurological functional status.

Table 2. Outcomes in the present series based on prognostic classes described by recursive analysis of RTOG data

RTOG class	Median survival time, months	2-year survival, %	n
1	58	80	6
2			
3	15	12	58
4	19	50	17
5	7	0	11
6			

(RTOG) prognostic categories (table 1) as well [12], and our results are demonstrated in table 2. The RTOG prognostic class criterion was significantly correlated to survival in both the Kaplan-Meier method (fig. 6) and multivariate analysis ($p = 0.005$). A summary of the statistical results of the multivariate analysis is presented in table 3.

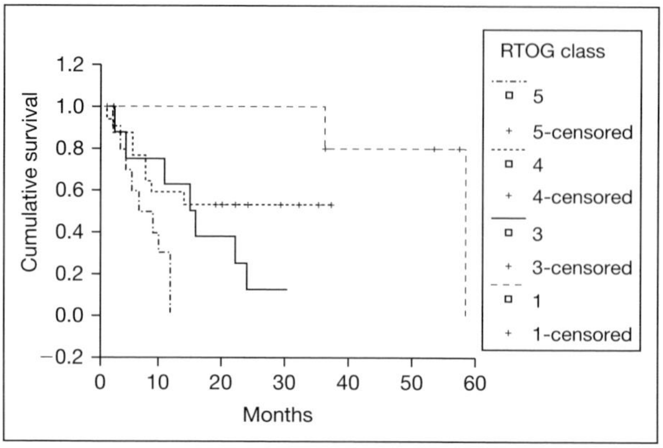

Fig. 6. Survival functions related to RTOG prognostic classes.

Table 3. Summary of multivariate analysis grade 3 and 4 tumors in the present series

Variable	p value
Age	0.173
Radiosurgery dose (Maximum)	0.726
Radiosurgery dose (Minimum)	0.503
Histological grade	0.366
Conventional radiotherapy	0.168
Surgical resection	0.140
RTOG prognostic class	0.005
Radiological reduction in tumor	0.003

Discussion

Options in Current Therapy of Gliomas

Surgery

The goals of surgical resection in the complex management of gliomas usually are debulking of the volume, relief of intracranial pressure, histological diagnosis and removal of obstruction to CSF circulation. While in low-grade tumors reduction of tumor burden may facilitate survival, delay recurrence and increase the efficacy of adjuvant therapy, there is no conclusive evidence that these issues are relevant to infiltrative high-grade gliomas. However, there are several series, including the present material, that present improved survival when at least a partial resection has been performed. The RTOG protocol [13] has demonstrated that the extent of resection is the third most important factor after age and Karnofsky performance scores (KPS).

Conventional Radiotherapy

The role of conventional radiotherapy for low-grade glioma is controversial [14], and has been used only in limited numbers for astrocytoma grade 2, and rarely for astrocytoma grade 1 except for tumors in special locations, such as optic pathways or brain stem. This is due to the fact that the long-term side effects of radiation on the white matter, and endocrinological or neuropsychological untoward effects can outweigh the otherwise benign course of these tumors [15]. This is particularly true of the pediatric patient population. Shaw et al. [16] concluded that postoperative radiation therapy had no effect on astrocytoma grade 1, but it improved survival particularly in adults with grade 2 tumors. Lunsford et al. [17] reported the usefulness of fractionated radiation therapy for nonpilocytic low-grade astrocytoma as initial treatment after histological diagnosis by biopsy.

Concerning high-grade astrocytomas, evidence exists for the role of radiation therapy in prolonging survival and perhaps improving quality of life [18]. However, no additional benefits are derived over the dose of 60 Gy. Increasing doses beyond this limit are associated with an increased risk for radiation necrosis. The main problem with XRT or surgery + XRT series is local recurrence. Attempts have been made to increase the biological efficacy of the treatment by hyperfractionation and with neutron therapy. However, the role of local dose escalation has led to the use of brachytherapy and radiosurgery in these cases.

Brachytherapy

Mundinger et al. [19] reported a retrospective study on interstitial radiation therapy for low-grade gliomas of the brain stem ^{125}I and ^{192}Ir. The treatment with ^{125}I produced favorable outcome and the 5-year survival rate was 54.8% compared to 26.9% by ^{192}Ir treatment and 14.7% without radiation therapy. Voges et al. [20] published good results with interstitial radiation therapy for inoperable or partially resected grade 1 and 2 gliomas with stereotactically implanted ^{125}I seeds. In the case of high-grade astrocytomas, candidates for brachytherapy are patients with smaller localized lesions and good KPS. Improvement in survival has been demonstrated by randomized and phase 1/2 trials [21]. However, selection criteria differ and results therefore vary from center to center [22].

Radiosurgery

Connected to brachytherapy, the role of radiosurgery has been proposed in the local escalation of radiation dose to visible (enhancing) tumor tissue in malignant gliomas and to deliver therapeutic doses in low-grade astrocytomas without the concomitant long-term effects of radiation in low-grade tumors. However, despite the similarities of selection criteria for brachytherapy and radiotherapy, the similarity is superficial. The dose rates with the GK usually exceed 1 Gy/min, and the biology of cell destruction at these rates are different from dose rates typical for brachytherapy (0.006 Gy/min).

Colombo [23] was the first to publish results of radiosurgery in low-grade gliomas, but grade 1 and 2 astrocytomas were not separated and fractionation was used in the treatments. Barcia et al. [24] in 16 cases of low-grade astrocytomas found disappearance of tumor in 50% and decrease or static tumor size in 31% of cases. However, 6 patients received conventional radiotherapy in addition to radiosurgery, and histology was available only in 7 cases. Grabb et al. [25] used the GK in 8 cases of pilocytic astrocytoma and 5 cases of low-grade astrocytoma in children. In pilocytic astrocytoma, the tumor either disappeared or decreased in 7 cases with median follow-up of 21 months. In nonpilocytic low-grade astrocytoma, the tumor either disappeared or decreased in 2 cases with a median follow-up of 19 months.

There are several papers summarizing the experience of radiosurgical treatment in high-grade astrocytomas. Masciopinto et al. [26] presented 32 patients with glioblastoma multiforme who underwent tumor debulking or biopsy, stereotactic radiosurgery with a 6 Mev modified LINAC, and standard radiation therapy. Radiosurgery delivered a central dose of 15–35 Gy, the peripheral isodose line varied from 40 to 90% with a median of 72.5% and a mode of 80%. The mean follow-up period was 12.84 months with a median of 9.5 months. Actuarial 12-month survival was 37% with a median of 9.5 months. They concluded that the curative value of radiosurgery is significantly limited by peripheral recurrences. Sarkaria et al. [27] evaluated the impact of stereotactic radiosurgery on the survival of patients treated with malignant gliomas and found that the actuarial 2-year and median survival for all patients was 45% and 96 weeks, respectively. In comparison with the results from a previously published analysis of 1,578 patients entered in three RTOG external beam radiotherapy protocols from 1974 to 1989 [12], patients treated with radiosurgery had a significantly improved 2-year and median survival (p = 0.01). This improvement in survival was seen predominantly for the worse prognostic classes (classes 3–6). Although Karnofsky performance status and prognostic class were significant on univariate analysis, only the KPS was a significant predictor of outcome on multivariate analysis. To determine factors associated with survival differences, Larson et al. [28] analyzed 189 patients treated with GK radiosurgery for primary or recurrent glioma grades 1–4. Multivariate analysis showed that increased survival was associated with 5 variables: lower pathologic grade, younger age, increased KPS, smaller tumor volume, and unifocal tumor. Survival was not found to be significantly related to radiosurgical technical parameters. Kondziolka et al. [29]

reported their 8-year experience of the survival benefit of stereotactic radiosurgery performed on 43 patients with grade 3, and 64 patients with grade 4 astrocytomas. The median survival time was 21 (range 3–93) months with a 2-year survival rate of 67% in grade 3 cases after GK radiosurgery. In grade 4 tumors, the median survival time after GK radiosurgery was 16 months (1–74) and the 2-year survival rate was 51%. No survival benefit was identified for patients who underwent chemotherapy in addition to radiosurgery ($p = 0.97$).

Current Series

Selection Bias

Most of the patients in this series were symptomatic due to the tumor growth. Following resection or only biopsy, they underwent GK surgery for residual tumors. The tumors were preselected by referring doctors and tended to be small, located in the deep part of the brain, and close to the eloquent areas in the low-grade cases. The high-grade group was a similarly selected patient material where the referring physician or the family requested treatment and therefore included tumors of various sizes. Three cases were excluded from statistics due to incorrect initial histological classification or incomplete histology.

Treatment Outcomes

No acute morbidity was observed in any case among all histological groups after GK surgery. In astrocytoma grade 1 category, enlargement of the cystic component or progress of the tumor volume occurred in 6 cases (40%), radiation-induced edema and hemorrhage presented in 1 case. There were 5 cases (31.3%) in astrocytoma grade 2 population with continuous growing of the tumor mass following GK treatment. Failure of tumor control was seen overall in 45% of the high-grade cases, and in the subgroup of grade 4 astrocytomas in 42%. Masciopinto et al. [26] reported a higher failure rate, 64.5% in a series of 31 cases, but the median volume of tumors treated by them was higher ($16.4\,cm^3$) than in our series ($7.0\,cm^3$). It is noteworthy that their cases were treated with 1–2 isocenters, and the impact of dose inhomogeneity with multiple isocenter treatment should not be discounted. Barker et al. [30] reported a 35% failure rate with conventional radiation, without alluding to the size of the tumor. Kondziolka et al. [29] reported that 12 patients (19%) needed craniotomies and tumor resection at a mean of 8 months following initial GK treatment, and 4 cases (6%) underwent subsequent radiosurgery for local or distant tumor recurrence.

Our material confirms the observations of Barker et al. [30] that there is a significant correlation of radiologically assessed response and clinical survival and the probability of death ($p < 0.002$). Systematic MR follow-up and meticulous image analysis of treated patients is therefore a good predictor of clinical behavior. The issue of tumor enhancement versus radiation necrosis of tumor tissue remains a challenging question in follow-up management. This requires the integration of recently developed functional imaging techniques, like PET, to obtain additional metabolic data for more precise targeting to sophisticated treatment planning, and to promote decision making in glioma radiosurgery [31].

Whereas the limitations of a focused irradiation technique on a malignant infiltrative disease are obvious, the psychological impact of the offered therapy on the patients and their families should not be neglected. Although the expected relief is restricted only to a short period, it might be meaningful to the patients and their families; therefore, we believe that it is worthwhile.

Conclusion

Stereotactic radiosurgery represents an alternative or supplementary treatment modality to conventional surgery in small-volume well-circumscribed low-grade astrocytomas, especially in deep-seated critical locations. There is also evidence for the beneficial impact of radiosurgery on the survival of patients with high-grade gliomas; however, the limitations of a focused irradiation technique on a malignant infiltrative process are obvious.

References

1 Levin VA, Gutin PH, Leibel S: Neoplasms of the central nervous system; in De Vita VT Jr, Hellman S, Rosenberg SA (eds): Cancer: Principles and Practice of Oncology. Philadelphia, Lippincott Williams & Wilkins, 1993, pp 1679–1737.

2 Shrieve DC, Gutin PH, Larson DA: Brachytherapy; in Mauch P, Loeffler JS (eds): Radiation Oncology, Technology and Biology. Philadelphia, WB Saunders, 1994, pp 216–236.

3 Brem H, Piantadosi S, Burger PC, et al: Placebo-controlled trial of safety and efficacy of intraoperative controlled delivery by biodegradable polymers of chemotherapy for recurrent gliomas. The Polymer Brain Tumor Treatment Group. Lancet 1995;345:1008–1012.

4 Sipos L, Wakabayashi T, Szeifert GT, et al: Characterization of human gliomas by a monoclonal antibody both on tissue culture and paraffin-embedded sections. Neurol Res 1992;14:263–266.

5 Kramm CM, Sena-Esteves M, Barnett FH, et al: Gene therapy for brain tumors. Brain Pathol 1995;5:345–381.

6 Salcman M: Survival in glioblastoma: historical perspective. Neurosurgery 1980;7:435–439.

7 Salford LG, Brun A, Nirfalk S: Ten-year survival among patients with supratentorial astrocytomas grade III and IV. J Neurosurg 1988;69:506–509.

8 Walker MD, Strike TA, Sheline GE: An analysis of dose-effect relationship in the radiotherapy of malignant gliomas. Int J Radiat Oncol Biol Phys 1979;5:1725–1731.

9 Bleehen NM, Stenning SP: A Medical Research Council trial of two radiotherapy doses in the treatment of grades 3 and 4 astrocytoma. The Medical Research Council Brain Tumor Working Party. Br J Cancer 1991;64:769–774.

10 Scharfen CO, Sneed PK, Wara WM, et al: High activity iodine-125 interstitial implant for gliomas. Int J Radiat Oncol Biol Phys 1992;24:583–591.

11 Wen PY, Alexander E 3rd, Black PM, et al: Long term results of stereotactic brachytherapy used in the initial treatment of patients with glioblastomas. Cancer 1994;73:3029–3036.
12 Curran W, Scott C, Weinstein A, et al: Survival comparision of radiosurgery-eligible and -ineligible malignant glioma patients treated with hyperfractionated radiation therapy and Carmustine; A report of Radiation Therapy Oncology Group 83–02. J Clin Oncol 1993;11:857–862.
13 Simpson JR, Horton J, Scott C, et al: Influence of location and extent of surgical resection on survival of patients with glioblastoma multiforme: results of three consecutive Radiation Therapy Oncology Group (RTOG) clinical trials. Int J Radiat Oncol Biol Phys 1993;26:239–244.
14 Philippon JH, Clemenceau SH, Fauchon FH, et al: Supratentorial low-grade astrocytomas in adults. Neurosurgery 1993;32:554–559.
15 North CA, North RB, Epstein JA, et al: Low-grade cerebral astrocytomas. Survival and quality of life after radiation therapy. Cancer 1990;66:6–14.
16 Shaw EG, Scheithauer BW, O'Fallon JR: Management of supratentorial low-grade gliomas. Oncology 1993;7:97–111.
17 Lunsford LD, Somaza S, Kondziolka D, et al: Survival after stereotactic biopsy and irradiation of cerebral nonanaplastic, nonpilocytic astrocytoma. J Neurosurg 1995;82:523–529.
18 Walker MD, Green SB, Byar DP, et al: Randomized comparison of radiotherapy and nitrosoureas for the treatment of malignant glioma after surgery. N Engl J Med 1980;303:1323–1329.
19 Mundinger F, Braus DF, Krauss JK, et al: Long-term outcome of 89 low-grade brain-stem gliomas after interstitial radiation therapy. J Neurosurg 1991;75:740–746.
20 Voges J, Treuer H, Schlegel W, et al: Interstitial irradiation of cerebral gliomas with stereotactically implanted iodine-125 seeds. Acta Neurochir 1993;58(suppl):108–111.
21 Scharfen CO, Sneed PK, Wara WM, et al: High activity iodine-125 interstitial implant for gliomas. Int J Radiat Oncol Biol Phys 1992;24:583–591.
22 Viola A, Major T, Julow J: The importance of postoperative CT image fusion verification of stereotactic interstitial irradiation for brain tumors. Int J Radiat Oncol Biol Phys 2004;60:322–328.
23 Colombo F: Linear accelerator radiosurgery. A clinical experience. J Neurosurg Sci 1989;33: 123–125.
24 Barcia JA, Barcia-Salorio JL, Ferrer C, et al: Stereotactic radiosurgery of deeply seated low grade gliomas. Acta Neurochir 1994;62(suppl):58–61.
25 Grabb PA, Lunsford LD, Albright AL, et al: Stereotactic radiosurgery for glial neoplasms of childhood. Neurosurgery 1996;38:696–701.
26 Masciopinto JE, Levin AB, Mehta MP, et al: Stereotactic radiosurgery for glioblastoma: a final report of 31 patients. J Neurosurg 1995;82:530–535.
27 Sarkaria JN, Mehta MP, Loeffler JS, et al: Radiosurgery in the initial management of malignant gliomas: survival comparison with the RTOG recursive partitioning analysis. Radiation Therapy Oncology Group. Int J Radiat Oncol Biol Phys 1995;32:931–941.
28 Larson DA, Gutin PH, McDermott M, et al: Gamma Knife for glioma: selection factors and survival. Int J Radiat Oncol Biol Phys 1996;36:1045–1053.
29 Kondziolka D, Flickinger JC, Bissonette DJ, et al: Survival benefit of stereotactic radiosurgery for patients with malignant glial neoplasms. Neurosurgery 1997;41:776–783.
30 Barker FG 2nd, Prados MD, Chang SM, et al: Radiation response and survival time in patients with glioblastoma multiforme. J Neurosurg 1996;84:442–448.
31 Levivier M, Wikler d, Goldman S, et al: Integration of metabolic data of positron emission tomography in the dosimetry planning of radiosurgery with the gamma knife: early experience with brain tumors. J Neurosurg 2000;93(suppl 3):233–238.

György T. Szeifert, MD, PhD
National Institute of Neurosurgery and Department of Neurological Surgery
Semmelweis University
Amerikai út 57
HU–1145 Budapest (Hungary)
Tel. +36 1 2512 999, Fax +36 1 2515 678, E-Mail gyorgyszeifert@yahoo.com

Szeifert GT, Kondziolka D, Levivier M, Lunsford LD (eds): Radiosurgery and Pathological Fundamentals. Prog Neurol Surg. Basel, Karger, 2007, vol 20, pp 164–171

9.5.1. Radiosurgery for Pituitary Adenomas

Bruce E. Pollock

Department of Neurological Surgery and the Division of Radiation Oncology, Mayo Clinic College of Medicine, Rochester, Minn., USA

Abstract

Stereotactic radiosurgery has been used to manage patients with pituitary adenomas for over 30 years. Numerous studies have documented that more than 95% of pituitary adenoma patients have either tumor shrinkage or stabilization after radiosurgery. Biochemical remission is possible in approximately 80% of properly selected patients with hormone-producing pituitary adenomas. The time to endocrine normalization typically ranges from 1 to 5 years. Factors associated with endocrine cure include the absence of pituitary suppressive medications at the time of radiosurgery and higher radiation doses. Delayed anterior pituitary deficits occur in 20–50% of patients depending on the length and quality of the endocrine follow-up. Visual loss after radiosurgery is rare if the maximum radiation dose to the optic apparatus is kept below 12 Gy. Since the effects of radiosurgery are gradual compared to surgical removal of pituitary adenomas, surgical resection remains the primary therapy for the majority of patients with large tumors causing visual loss or for patients with symptomatic acromegaly or Cushing's disease. However, radiosurgery is effective for pituitary adenoma patients with persistent or recurrent tumors after prior surgery, or for patients considered high risk for open surgical procedures due to coexisting medical conditions.

Pituitary adenomas are benign tumors that are generally diagnosed due to symptoms from hormonal overproduction, visual loss, pituitary insufficiency, or pituitary apoplexy. Although medical therapy and surgical resection are the primary treatments for the majority of patients with pituitary adenomas, some patients do not respond to medical therapy and complete tumor resection is not possible in every patient. Fractionated radiation therapy has been employed for patients who fail medical and surgical treatment of their pituitary adenoma. However, radiotherapy frequently causes hypothalamic-pituitary dysfunction, typically requires several years to correct hormonal overproduction, and is associated with the risk of radiation-induced neoplasms. In recent years, stereotactic

Table 1. Pituitary adenoma patients (n = 176) having radiosurgery

Type	Patients (%)
Hormone producing	
GH producing	59 (34)
ACTH producing	17 (10)
PRL producing	20 (11)
FSH producing	2 (1)
Nelson's syndrome	14 (8)
Nonfunctional	64 (36)

radiosurgery has been increasingly used as an alternative to surgery or radiation therapy to manage patients with pituitary adenomas [1–14]. This paper will review the results of radiosurgery for hormone-producing pituitary adenomas, including patients with Nelson's syndrome, and for patients with nonfunctional pituitary adenomas.

Patients and Methods

Proper patient selection is the most important factor associated with good outcomes after radiosurgery. As a general rule, pituitary adenomas with significant suprasellar extension are typically not considered good candidates for radiosurgery. This is because patients with larger lesions often have visual loss related to mass effect. So although radiosurgery does result in growth control and size reduction in the majority of pituitary adenomas, this is generally a gradual process requiring several years [14]. Therefore, surgical resection is the preferred approach for patients with large pituitary adenomas. However, for many patients it is recognized in advance that complete tumor removal is not possible because the tumor extends into the cavernous sinus. In this setting, radiosurgery can be part of staged approach with microsurgery. Initially, the tumor is debulked to create a separation between the top surface of the tumor and the optic apparatus without an attempt at resection of the tumor involving the cranial nerves, major arteries, or dural venous sinuses. Radiosurgery can then be performed for the remaining tumor volume with little risk of cranial nerve deficits. Such multimodality treatment should result in reduced patient morbidity, with long-term tumor control.

From January 1990 until December 2004, 176 patients with pituitary adenomas (from a total experience of 2,945 patients) have undergone stereotactic radiosurgery at the Mayo Clinic (table 1). Over 90% of patients have undergone prior surgery and approximately 75% had tumors with extension into the cavernous sinus. At our Center, radiosurgery is performed using the Leksell Gamma Knife (Elekta Instruments, Norcross, Ga., USA). Unless contraindicated, dose planning is based on volumetric MRI to allow clear delineation of the sellar contents and the adjacent optic nerves and chiasm. Dose prescription is based on several factors including histology, tumor size, the distance from the optic apparatus, and the history of prior radiation therapy. For patients with hormone-producing tumors, every effort is made to provide a minimum tumor margin dose exceeding 20 Gy (fig. 1). For nonfunctional

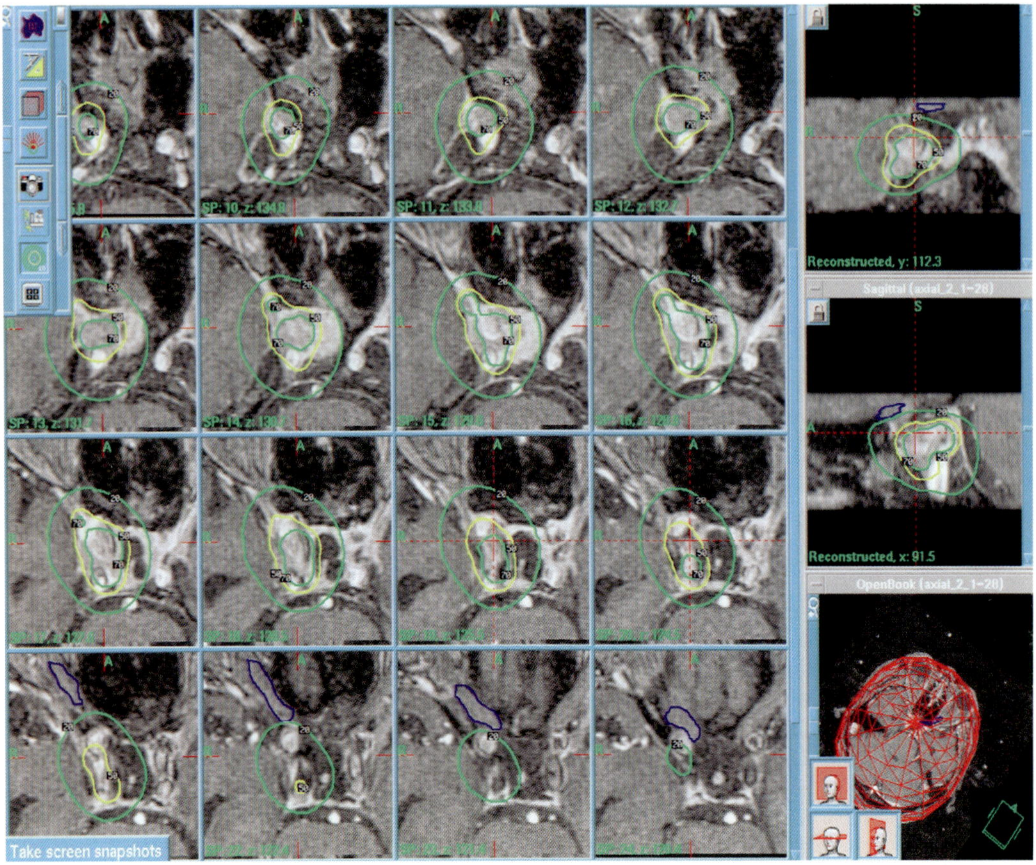

Fig. 1. Dose plan of a patient with persistent acromegaly after prior transsphenoidal surgery. The tumor margin received 25 Gy; the maximum dose to the adjacent optic nerve was 9.8 Gy.

tumors, the tumor margin dose generally ranges from 14 to 16 Gy. The incidence of postradiosurgical visual deficits is less than 2% if the maximum radiation dose received by the optic apparatus is less than 12 Gy [15, 16].

Results

Hormone-Producing Pituitary Adenomas

Hormonal oversecretion from pituitary adenomas can result in significant morbidity and reduced life expectancies for affected patients. Whereas tumor control and preservation of pituitary function is adequate for non-hormone-producing

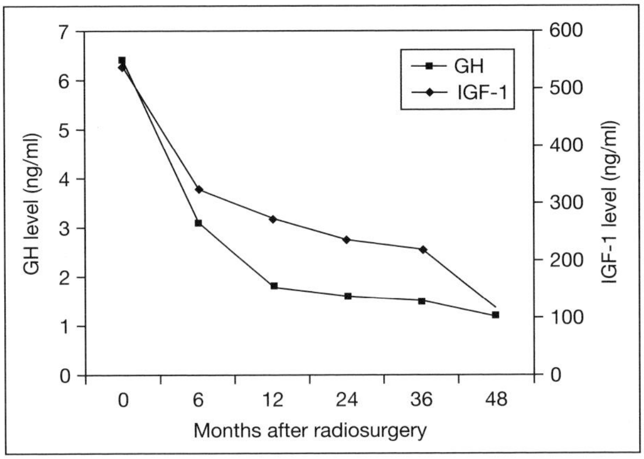

Fig. 2. Graph showing the serum values of GH and IGF-1 for a patient with acromegaly having radiosurgery. The age- and sex-adjusted normal range of IGF-1 for this patient was 290 ng/ml.

tumors, correction of endocrinopathies is critical to good outcomes for patients with hormone-producing pituitary adenomas. Surgical resection of pituitary adenomas as a primary treatment is able to rapidly normalize hormone levels in the majority of patients. However, patients with persistent or recurrent endocrinopathies after surgical resection less frequently achieve biochemical remission after repeat surgery.

Endocrine normalization (cure) was defined as normal or below normal hormonal levels off all pituitary suppressive or cortisol-lowering medications. Specifically, acromegalic patients were required to have fasting growth hormone (GH) level less than 2 ng/ml and normal age and sex-adjusted insulin-like growth factor-1 (IGF-1) levels; patients with Cushing's disease needed a 24-hour UFC $<$90 μg, and patients with prolactinomas needed PRL levels $<$23 ng/ml. By actuarial statistics, we have found that approximately 80% of patients not on pituitary suppressive medications receiving a maximum tumor dose greater than 40 Gy have correction of their hormonal overproduction 3 years after radiosurgery (fig. 2). No correlation was found between tumor type and endocrine cure. This supports the results of other radiosurgical centers [1–5, 7]. We have found by multivariate analysis that the absence of suppressive medications (dopamine agonists, octreotide) at the time of radiosurgery correlates with hormonal cure [8], similar to the studies of Landolt et al. [4] and Landolt and Lomax [5]. Higher radiation doses (maximum radiation doses greater than 40 Gy) have also been associated with hormone normalization in our experience [8]. New anterior pituitary deficits have occurred in approximately 20% of our patients. Other complications have included temporal lobe necrosis, asymptomatic internal carotid artery stenosis, and unilateral blindness in a patient who had failed prior surgery and fractionated radiation therapy.

To date, we have used radiosurgery in 14 patients with ACTH-producing tumors after bilateral adrenalectomy. In 12 patients, tumor growth was documented prior to radiosurgery. Two patients underwent radiosurgery prophylactically to prevent future tumor enlargement. Tumor growth control has been documented in 12 patients (86%). So although our experience is limited, it appears that radiosurgery provides tumor control for the majority of patients with ACTH-producing pituitary adenomas who have undergone bilateral adrenalectomy.

Nonfunctional Pituitary Adenomas

Nonfunctioning pituitary adenomas comprise approximately 30% of diagnosed pituitary tumors. Patients with nonfunctional tumors generally experience anterior pituitary deficits, visual loss, headaches, or less frequently apoplexy. However, because the symptoms typically develop slowly and may be rather nonspecific, many years may pass before patients with nonfunctioning pituitary adenomas are correctly diagnosed. Consequently, most patients present with macroadenomas and the primary treatment is surgical resection to decompress adjacent structures. Still, many tumors extend into the cavernous sinuses, and complete resection is not possible with acceptable morbidity. Stereotactic radiosurgery has become increasingly utilized to manage patients with progressive or recurrent nonfunctional pituitary adenomas [10, 12, 14].

The management of patients with nonfunctioning pituitary adenomas is relatively straightforward compared to patients with hormone-producing tumors. The goals for these patients are freedom from tumor mass effect with low treatment-associated morbidity (fig. 3). Adenoma progression after radiosurgery is rare: the risk of documented tumor progression has ranged from 0 to 7% [10, 12, 14]. However, the average follow-up in these series has been less than 5 years. Therefore, long-term data are still required to ensure that late tumor progression does not occur. In our experience, the primary risk of radiosurgery for patients with nonfunctioning pituitary adenomas has been the development of new anterior pituitary deficits. We have found that more than 40% of patients develop deficits in one or more pituitary axes after radiosurgery. Although some authors have found an incidence of new anterior pituitary deficits from 0 to 14% after radiosurgery of nonfunctioning pituitary adenomas [12, 14], other centers have documented an incidence closer to our estimate [17]. Vladyka et al. [17] found that the mean radiation dose to the hypophysis was associated with hormonal insufficiency. By 90 months after

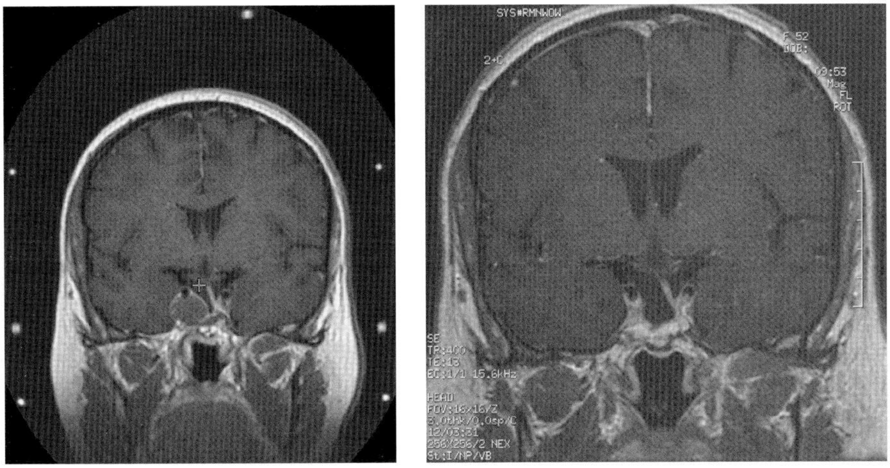

a *b*

Fig. 3. MRIs of a patient with a recurrent nonfunctional pituitary adenoma after prior transsphenoidal surgery. ***a*** MRI at the time of radiosurgery. ***b*** MRI performed 6 years later showing the tumor significantly smaller.

radiosurgery, the risk of new deficits was 85% if the mean dose to the hypophysis was greater than 17 Gy. Conversely, if the mean dose was 17 Gy or less, only 15% of patients developed new anterior pituitary insufficiency. In the hope of balancing the goals of tumor control and reduced risk of hormonal insufficiency, dose prescription for nonfunctioning pituitary adenomas is generally limited to 16 Gy of less.

Discussion

Radiosurgery for patients with pituitary adenomas has been performed for over 30 years. Yet, patients having pituitary adenoma radiosurgery before the mid-1990s underwent a rather crude procedure compared to our modern techniques. The early cases relied upon skull radiographs or computed tomography as the imaging database for dose planning. Also, the radiation dosimetry was frequently calculated manually without the aid of sophisticated computerized dose-planning software. Despite these shortcomings, early reports found this procedure to be effective. However, the information available from these studies had numerous flaws making direct comparisons with the published results of best medical and surgical treatments difficult. First, the definition of hormonal cure has continued to evolve, especially for acromegalic patients. Second, in some studies, the number of patients reported as cured continued to require either pituitary suppressive or cortisol-lowering medicines at last follow-up. Third, another problem for most of these papers were the small number of patients and the relative short follow-up presented. The importance of longer follow-up has become increasingly recognized because late complications after radiosurgery of the sellar region such as anterior pituitary deficiency or vascular injury typically occur only after a number of years have passed since the procedure. Nonetheless, this initial information provided the impetus for better and more accurate reporting of pituitary adenoma radiosurgery.

Our center has found radiosurgery to be an important tool in the management of patients with pituitary adenomas. Our overall tumor control rate exceeds 95% with follow-up that now extends up to 15 years. Patients with persistent or recurrent hormonal overproduction syndromes now typically undergo radiosurgery rather than either reoperation or fractionated radiation therapy. Patients are taken off all pituitary suppressive medications for 4–6 weeks before radiosurgery. At radiosurgery, every attempt is made to provide a maximum tumor margin dose that exceeds 20 Gy while still limiting the maximum radiation dose to the optic apparatus to less than 12 Gy. In this manner, biochemical remission is possible for approximately 80% of patients. The majority of patients achieve normalization 12–24 months after radiosurgery. Likewise, radiosurgery has essentially replaced radiation therapy for patients with recurrent or progressive nonfunctioning pituitary adenomas. For these patients, the tumors can extend up to the optic nerves or chiasm over a short segment because the necessary tumor margin dose is lower compared to hormone-producing tumors. Following radiosurgery, our patients are generally seen in follow-up at 6-month intervals for the first 2 years, then yearly thereafter. Close endocrinological observation is needed to detect the onset of pituitary deficits that may require replacement therapy. Follow-up imaging becomes less critical after several years because of the very low chance of tumor growth and delayed radiation-related complications. However, additional follow-up is still needed to establish the long-term success of pituitary adenoma radiosurgery, and more accurately determine the chance of rare complications such as radiation injury to the internal carotid artery [18].

References

1 Höybye C, Grenbäck E, Rähn T, Degerblad M, Thoren M, Hulting AL: Adrenocorticotrophic hormone-producing pituitary tumors: 12- to 22-year follow-up after treatment with stereotactic radiosurgery. Neurosurgery 2001;49:284–292.

2 Ikeda H, Jokura H, Yoshimoto T: Transsphenoidal surgery and adjuvant gamma knife treatment for growth hormone-secreting pituitary adenoma. J Neurosurg 2001;95:285–291.

3 Landolt AM, Dieter H, Lomax N, Scheib S, Schubiger O, Siegfried J, Wellis G: Stereotactic radiosurgery for recurrent surgically treated acromegaly: comparison with fractionated radiotherapy. J Neurosurg 1998;88:1002–1008.

4 Landolt AM, Haller D, Lomax N, Scheib S, Schubiger O, Siegfried J, Wellis G: Octreotide may act as a radioprotective agent in acromegaly. J Clin Endocrinol Metab 2000;85:1287–1289.
5 Landolt AM, Lomax N: Gamma knife radiosurgery for prolactinomas. J Neurosurg 2000;93(suppl 3): 14–18.
6 Mitsumori M, Shrieve DC, Alexander E III, Kaiser UB, Richardson GE, Black PM, Loeffler JS: Initial clinical results of LINAC-based radiosurgery and stereotactic radiotherapy for pituitary adenomas. Int J Radiat Oncol Biol Phys 1998;42:573–580.
7 Morange-Ramos I, Régis J, Dufour H, Andrieu JM, Grisoli F, Jaquet P, Peragut JC: Gamma knife surgery for secreting pituitary adenomas. Acta Neurochir 1998;140:437–443.
8 Pollock BE, Nippoldt TB, Stafford SL, Foote RL, Abboud CF: Results of stereotactic radiosurgery for patients with hormone producing pituitary adenomas: factors associated with endocrine normalization. J Neurosurg 2002;97:525–530.
9 Pollock BE, Young WF Jr: Stereotactic radiosurgery for patients with ACTH-producing pituitary adenomas after prior adrenalectomy. Int J Radiat Oncol Biol Phys 2002;54:839–841.
10 Pollock BE, Carpenter PC: Stereotactic radiosurgery as an alternative to fractionated radiation therapy for patients with recurrent or residual nonfunctioning pituitary adenomas. Neurosurgery 2003;53:1086–1094.
11 Sheehan JM, Vance ML, Sheehan JP, Ellegala DB, Laws ER Jr: Radiosurgery for Cushing's disease after failed transsphenoidal surgery. J Neurosurg 2000;93:738–742.
12 Sheehan JP, Kondziolka D, Flickinger JC, Lunsford LD: Radiosurgery for residual or recurrent nonfunctioning pituitary adenoma. J Neurosurg 2002;97(suppl 5):408–414.
13 Thoren M, Rähn T, Guo WY, Werner S: Stereotactic radiosurgery with cobalt-60 gamma unit in the treatment of growth hormone-producing tumors. Neurosurgery 1991;29:663–668.
14 Wowra B, Stummer W: Efficacy of gamma knife radiosurgery for nonfunctioning pituitary adenomas: a quantitative follow up with magnetic resonance imaging-based volumetric analysis. J Neurosurg 2002;97(suppl 5):429–432.
15 Leber KA, Berglöff J, Pendl G: Dose-response of the visual pathways and cranial nerves of the cavernous sinus to stereotactic radiosurgery. J Neurosurg 1998;88:43–50.
16 Stafford SL, Pollock BE, Leavitt JA, Foote RL, Brown PD, Gorman DA, Schomberg PJ: A study on the radiation tolerance of the optic nerves and chiasm after stereotactic radiosurgery. Int J Radiat Oncol Biol Phys 2003;55:1177–1181.
17 Vladyka V, Liscak R, Novotny J Jr, Marek J, Jezkova J: Radiation tolerance of functioning pituitary tissue in gamma knife surgery for pituitary adenomas. Neurosurgery 2003;52:309–317.
18 Lim YJ, Leem W, Park JT, Kim TS, Rhee BA, Kim GK: Cerebral infarction with ICA occlusion after gamma knife radiosurgery for pituitary adenoma: a case report. Stereotact Funct Neurosurg 1999;72(suppl 1):132–139.

Bruce E. Pollock, MD
Department of Neurological Surgery, Mayo Clinic
200 First Street SW
Rochester, MN 55905 (USA)
Tel. +1 507 284 5317, Fax +1 507 294 5206, E-Mail pollock.bruce@mayo.edu

Szeifert GT, Kondziolka D, Levivier M, Lunsford LD (eds): Radiosurgery and Pathological Fundamentals. Prog Neurol Surg. Basel, Karger, 2007, vol 20, pp 172–179

9.5.2. Pathological Findings following Radiosurgery of Pituitary Adenomas

Jason Sheehan[a], *M. Beatriz Lopes*[b], *Edward Laws*[a]

[a]Department of Neurological Surgery and [b]Division of Neuropathology, University of Virginia, Charlottesville, Va., USA

Abstract

Pituitary adenomas represent approximately 10–20% of all primary brain tumors. Surgical resection is the mainstay of treatment for most pituitary adenomas. At times, complete surgical resection may be impossible or the adenoma may recur. The Gamma Knife has become an important neurosurgical tool for the treatment of recurrent or residual pituitary adenomas. Gamma surgery typically affords a high rate of tumor volume control but a more variable rate of endocrinological remission. When radiosurgery fails to provide a good outcome, surgical resection often needs to be repeated. At the University of Virginia during a 15-year time period, 434 patients have been treated for recurrent or residual pituitary adenomas with the Gamma Knife. Upon review of their follow-up neuroimaging studies, we have not observed a case of a radiation-induced neoplasm. The incidence of Gamma Knife-induced neoplasia is likely low and will require longer follow-up to ascertain the true incidence. Pre- and post-Gamma Knife histological specimens were available in 4 patients (0.92% of patients). A comparison of these specimens was significant for necrosis but not vessel wall hyaline thickening, fibrinoid necrosis, vascular occlusions, or teleangectatic dilatations. Further study must be performed to determine the histological changes that accompany the frequently beneficial effects of radiosurgery in recurrent or residual pituitary adenomas.

Pituitary adenomas represent between 10–20% of all primary brain tumors [1–3]. Epidemiological studies have demonstrated that nearly 20% of the general population has a pituitary adenoma [1, 2, 4, 5]. Pituitary adenomas are broadly classified into two groups – secretory and nonsecretory adenomas. The first category of tumors is those that secrete excess amounts of pituitary hormones and, consequently, present with a variety of clinical syndromes depending upon hormones secreted. The most common of these is the prolactinoma which causes amenorrhea and galactorrhea in women and impotence and infertility in men.

Prolactinomas can usually be managed medically with dopamine agonists. The second most common functioning pituitary adenoma is the growth hormone-secreting variant in which patients present with acromegaly in adults and gigantism before closure of the epiphyseal plates [6]. Corticotrophin-secreting tumors produce Cushing's disease or, if bilateral adrenalectomies have been performed, Nelson's syndrome [7].

The second category of pituitary adenomas is composed of tumors that do not secrete any known biologically active pituitary hormones, and these represent approximately 30% of all pituitary tumors [8]. These so-called nonsecretory pituitary adenomas progressively enlarge in the pituitary fossa and may even extend outside of the confines of the sella turcica. These tumors may cause symptoms related to mass effect, whereby the optic nerves and chiasm are compressed, and a bitemporal visual field loss characteristically results. Those with nonfunctioning adenomas can also have hypopituitarism as a result of compression of the normal-functioning pituitary gland.

Other than for prolactinomas, surgical resection is typically the initial treatment of choice. Extirpation permits immediate decompression of the optic apparatus and the chance for hormonal normalization. Unfortunately, for both secretory and nonsecretory pituitary adenomas, recurrence as a result of tumor invasion into surrounding structures or incomplete tumor resection is all too common. Long-term tumor control rates after microsurgery alone vary from 50 to 80% [2, 3, 9–11]. Radiation therapy or radiosurgery can be administered postoperatively as prophylaxis to inhibit recurrent growth or, later, when clinical symptoms or radiographic signs indicate recurrence. They may also be utilized postoperatively to treat known residual tumor following incomplete resection. The presence of residual tumor is not uncommon in adenomas with either a suprasellar component or cavernous sinus involvement, and the incidence of recurrence has been shown to correlate with dural invasion by a pituitary adenoma [12, 13].

In 1951, stereotactic radiosurgery was described by Lars Leksell as the 'closed skull destruction of an intracranial target using ionizing radiation' [14]. In 1968, Leksell treated the first pituitary adenoma patient with the Gamma Knife. Since that time, stereotactic radiosurgery has been utilized in more than 20,000 patients to control tumor growth and normalize hormonal production. Tumor control rates after stereotactic radiosurgery vary from 68 to 100% but are generally around 90% [15–27]. Hormonal normalization rates vary substantially. The wide range of remission rates following radiosurgery is likely due to differences in the endocrinological criteria employed to define a 'cure', length and rigorousness of follow-up, and targeting methodology. Generally, Cushing's disease and acromegaly are more responsive to radiosurgery whereas prolactinomas and Nelson's syndrome are less so.

When radiosurgery fails to effectuate tumor control and/or hormonal normalization, surgical resection is generally warranted. To date, little has been written about the pathological considerations of pituitary adenomas following stereotactic radiosurgery. This speaks to the fact that extirpation followed by radiosurgery for recurrent or residual adenomas typically affords effective treatment. This paper details our findings when microsurgical tumor resection is employed after radiosurgery.

Materials and Methods

This study encompasses all those patients with pituitary adenomas who underwent radiosurgery at the University of Virginia. In total, from 1989 to 2004, 434 patients with pituitary adenomas have undergone Gamma Knife surgery at Virginia. The radiosurgery was performed by Dr. Ladislau Steiner. Whenever possible, patients were followed up with postoperative neuroimaging at 6-month intervals. All neuroimaging was evaluated both by Dr. Steiner and one of the attending neuroradiologists at the University of Virginia.

In order to evaluate the neuropathological findings, attention was also focused upon those patients who underwent surgical resection following radiosurgery. The surgical resections were all performed by the senior author (E.L.). These patients represent 0.92% of the 434 patients with pituitary adenomas who have been treated with Gamma Knife surgery at Virginia. All tumor histology was evaluated by Dr. M. Beatriz Lopes.

Results

Radiation-Induced Neoplasia

At the University of Virginia, more than 400 patients with recurrent or residual pituitary adenomas have been treated with Gamma Knife surgery and followed for more than 12 months. None of these patients have had demonstrable radiation-induced neoplasia on follow-up neuroimaging. Moreover, in the fraction of those who underwent surgical resection following radiosurgery, no cases of a different tumor pathology (e.g. malignant degeneration following radiosurgery) have been observed.

Neuropathological Findings

Comparison of the histopathological findings from specimens obtained before and after Gamma Knife radiosurgery was performed in 4 patients (table 1, fig. 1). Three of the patients had a corticotroph (ACTH-immunoreactive) adenoma and 1 had a null-cell (immunonegative) adenoma.

In two of the corticotroph adenomas, surgical specimens obtained after radiosurgery showed increased cellular pleomorphism, prominent mitotic activity

Table 1. Summary of 4 pituitary adenoma patients with histological results after gamma surgery

Patient	Tumor type	Gamma Knife maximal dose, Gy	Gamma Knife margin dose, Gy	Pathological findings following gamma surgery
1	Nonsecretory	30	9	increased cellular pleomorphism, mitotic activity and high Ki-67; tumor necrosis
2	ACTH secreting	40	20	increased cellular pleomorphism, prominent mitotic activity, and moderate Ki-67; tumor necrosis
3	ACTH secreting	10	3	increased cellular pleomorphism, prominent mitotic activity, and moderate Ki-67
4	ACTH secreting	50	25	no tumor seen; specimen contained normal dura and anterior pituitary gland

and moderate to high proliferative index as measured by the Ki-67 antigen (MIB-1 monoclonal antibody) in comparison to the surgical specimen obtained before radiosurgery. In one of these two corticotroph adenomas, tumor necrosis was evident. In the third corticotroph adenoma, the surgical specimen obtained by transsphenoidal microsurgery after radiosurgery failed to show neoplastic tissues. The patient was not cured from Cushing's disease at that point and subsequently underwent a second radiosurgery treatment and, ultimately, an adrenalectomy.

The patient with a null-cell adenoma had progressive disease despite radiosurgery and several tumor resections (a total of 7 surgical procedures). The patient underwent radiosurgery after the second surgical resection. The specimen obtained before radiosurgery (i.e. at the time of the first recurrence) was histologically different from the original tumor as it showed increased cellular pleomorphism, mitotic activity and high Ki-67. The surgical specimens obtained after radiosurgery (total of five) continue to show similar histological appearance, increased mitotic activity and high Ki-67 labeling index. There was no significant histological anaplastic progression on the surgical specimens other than the presence of necrosis.

Overall, in all 4 cases analyzed, there was no evidence of radiation-induced changes other than necrosis. Vascular radiation-induced alteration including vessel wall hyaline thickening, fibrinoid necrosis, vascular occlusions, and teleangectatic dilatations were not seen. Changes unrelated to radiation include

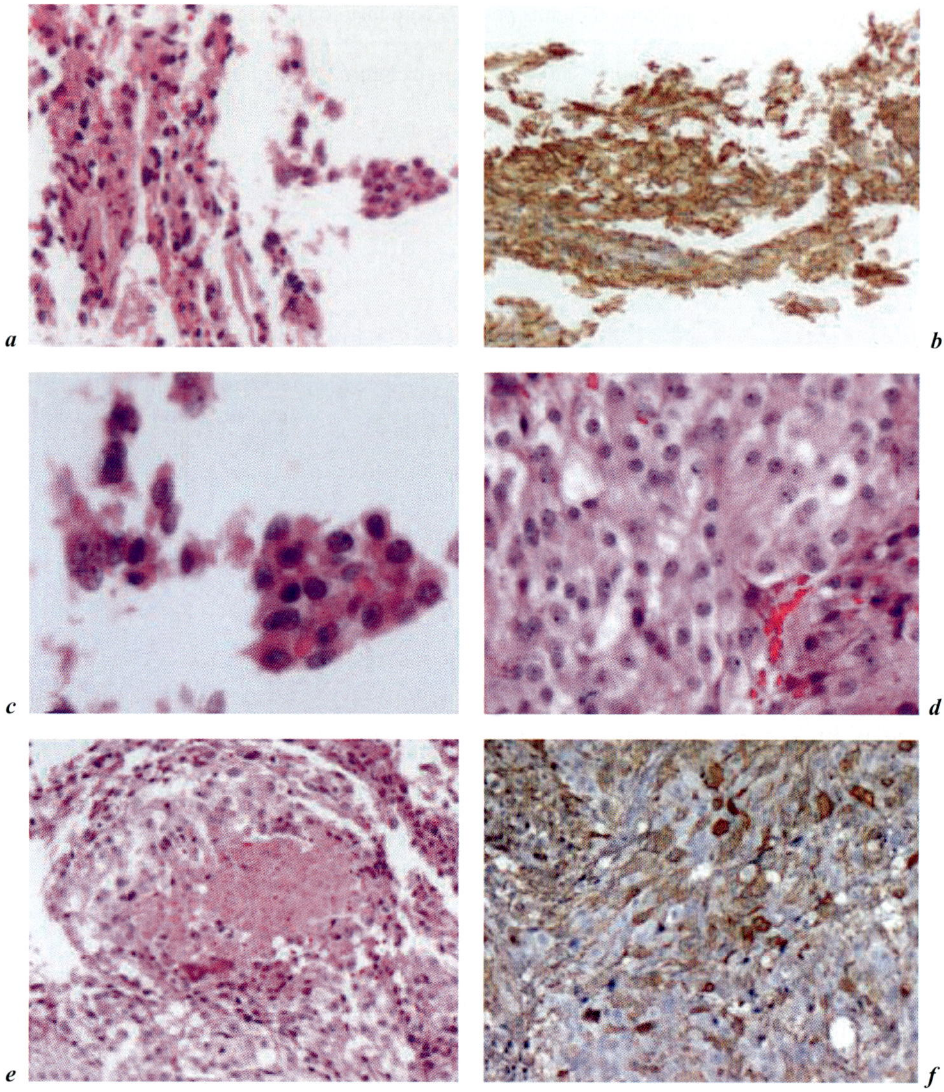

Fig. 1. ***a–c*** Biopsy of a patient with Cushing's and a corticotroph adenoma which underwent Gamma Knife surgery 1 year before showing regular-sized cells with nuclei displaying prominent nucleoli (***c***), and intense immunoreactivity for ACTH (***b***). ***d–f*** Subsequent transsphenoidal tumor resection in the same patient 18 months after Gamma Knife surgery showed cellular pleomorphism, increased mitotic activity (***d***) and focal tumor necrosis (***e***). ***f*** The adenoma still displayed intense immunoreactivity for ACTH.

progressive invasion of the adenomas into adjacent fibrous tissues including the dura mater and sinus mucosa.

Discussion

Stereotactic radiosurgery has been shown to induce a high rate of volume control in pituitary adenomas. Its effectiveness in terms of inducing hormonal remission is more variable.

Despite radiosurgery having been performed in over 250,000 patients for more than 30 years, the precise incidence of radiosurgery-induced neoplasms is difficult to estimate because of the delayed fashion in which such lesions may develop and the apparently low rate of occurrence. Based upon the literature, the incidence of stereotactic radiosurgery-induced neoplasia has been reported to range between 0–3 per 200,000 patients [28]. The true incidence of radiosurgery-induced neoplasms following Gamma Knife surgery is difficult to ascertain. It is conceivable that the true incidence may be greater than that estimated by Dr. Ganz. Longer-term studies will help to ascertain the overall incidence of radiation-induced tumors following gamma surgery. We have not observed a case of a radiation-induced tumor in our patients treated for recurrent or residual pituitary adenomas, but we mention this as a possible risk during preoperative discussion. We continue to follow these patients with serial neuroimaging studies.

The relatively scarce data on pathology after gamma surgery point to the large degree of success following treatment of recurrent or residual pituitary adenomas. Many of the patients who underwent surgical resection following gamma surgery had tumors which demonstrated refractoriness to prior therapies (e.g. medical management, surgical resection, and radiation therapy). Thus, the findings reported here are derived from a patient population not representative of the vast majority of pituitary adenoma patients. Our neuropathological findings must be viewed in that context.

Sutter et al. [29] reported on the histological findings of 3 patients who failed radiosurgery. In 1 case, atypical features (e.g. cellular and nuclear pleomorphism and multinucleated cells) were observed. These features were thought to be a result of previous fractionated radiation therapy. The other 2 cases did not show histological changes attributable to radiation. Moreover, no histological alterations as a result of radiosurgery were evident. The lack of definitive histological changes may have been a result of the low radiosurgical dose delivered in these 3 cases and the relatively short interval of follow-up. The present neuropathological analysis of 4 cases was similar in that we observed no evidence of radiosurgery-induced changes other than necrosis. Most notably, we did not observe vessel wall hyaline thickening, fibrinoid necrosis, vascular occlusions, and teleangectatic dilatations in any of the 4 cases.

Histological changes in the anterior pituitary have been reported after radiosurgery [30]. The dose delivered to regions of necrosis was approximately 185 Gy. In 1 patient from that same radiosurgical series, changes seen on postmortem examination were consistent with pyknosis and nuclear alterations, but no necrosis was present. Backlund and Ganz [30] postulated that the normal human anterior pituitary lobe is relatively resistant to radiation and that 185 Gy or more is needed to induce necrosis.

Conclusions

Gamma Knife surgery is quite effective for the treatment of recurrent or residual pituitary adenomas. The incidence of a radiation-induced neuropathological lesion following gamma surgery is likely quite low. The histological changes following Gamma Knife surgery may include necrosis. It remains to be determined to what extent gamma surgery induces vessel wall hyaline thickening, fibrinoid necrosis, vascular occlusions, and teleangectatic dilatations in recurrent or residual pituitary adenomas. Further study of the neuropathological changes in pituitary adenomas following radiosurgery must be performed to answer these questions.

References

1 Sanno N, Teramoto A, Osamura RY, Horvath E, Kovacs K, Lloyd RV, Scheithauer BW: Pathology of pituitary tumors. Neurosurg Clin N Am 2003;14:25–39.

2 Laws ER, Ebersold MJ, Piepgras DG, et al: The results of transsphenoidal surgery in specific clinical entities; in Laws ER, Randall RV, Kern EB, et al. (eds): Management of Pituitary Adenomas and Related Lesions with Emphasis on Transsphenoidal Microsurgery. New York, Appleton-Century-Crofts, 1982, pp 277–305.

3 Laws ER, Vance ML: Radiosurgery for Pituitary Tumors and Craniopharyngiomas. Neurosurg Clin N Am 1999;10:327–336.

4 Radhakrishnan K, Mokri B, Parisi JE, O'Fallon WM, Sunku J, Kurland LT: The trends in incidence of primary brain tumors in the population of Rochester, Minnesota. Ann Neurol 1995;37:67–73.

5 Annegers JF, Schoenberg BS, Okazaki H, Kurland LT: Epidemiologic study of primary intracranial neoplasms. Arch Neurol 1981;38:217–219.

6 Laws ER Jr, Fode NC, Redmond MJ: Transsphenoidal surgery following unsuccessful prior therapy. An assessment of benefits and risks in 158 patients. J Neurosurg 1985;63:823–829.

7 Sheehan JM, Vance ML, Sheehan JP, Ellegala DB, Laws ER Jr: Radiosurgery for Cushing's Disease after failed transsphenoidal surgery. J Neurosurg 2000;93:738–742.

8 Milker-Zabel S, Debus J, Thilmann C, Schlegel W, Wannenmacher M: Fractionated stereotactically guided radiotherapy and radiosurgery in the treatment of functional and nonfunctional adenomas of the pituitary gland. Int J Radiat Oncol Biol Phys 2001;50:1279–1286.

9 Chandler WF, Schteingard DE, Lloyd RV, McKeever PE, Ibarra-Perez G: Surgical treatment of Cushing's disease. J Neurosurg 1987;66:204–212.

10 Friedman RB, Oldfield EH, Nieman LK, Chrousos GP, Doppman JL, Cutler GB Jr, Loriaux DL: Repeat transsphenoidal surgery for Cushing's disease. J Neurosurg 1989;71:520–527.
11 Mampalam TJ, Tyrrell JB, Wilson CB: Transsphenoidal microsurgery for Cushing disease. Ann Intern Med 1988;109:487–493.
12 Shaffi OM, Wrightson P: Dural invasion by pituitary tumours. N Z Med J 1975;81:386–390.
13 Meij BP, Lopes MB, Ellegala DB, Alden TD, Laws ER Jr: The long-term significance of microscopic dural invasion in 354 patients with pituitary adenomas treated with transsphenoidal surgery. J Neurosurg 2002;96:195–208.
14 Leksell L: The stereotaxic method and radiosurgery of the brain. Acta Chir Scand 1951;102:316–319.
15 Feigl GC, Bonelli CM, Berghold A, Mokry M: Effects of gamma knife radiosurgery of pituitary adenomas on pituitary function. J Neurosurg 2002;97(suppl 5):415–421.
16 Inoue HK, Kohga H, Hirato M, Sasaki T, Ishihara J, Shibazaki T, Ohye C, Andou Y: Pituitary adenomas treated by microsurgery with or without gamma knife surgery: experience in 122 cases. Stereotact Funct Neurosurg 1999;72(suppl 1):125–131.
17 Hayashi M, Izawa M, Hiyama H, Nakamura S, Atsuchi S, Sato H, Nakaya K, Sasaki K, Ochiai T, Kubo O, Hori T, Takakura K: Gamma knife radiosurgery for pituitary adenomas. Stereotact Funct Neurosurg 1999;72(suppl 1):111–118.
18 Izawa M, Hayashi M, Nakaya K, Satoh H, Ochiai T, Hori T, Takakura K: Gamma knife radiosurgery for pituitary adenomas. J Neurosurg 2000;93(suppl 3):19–22.
19 Lim YL, Leem W, Kim TS, Rhee BA, Kim GK: Four years' experiences in the treatment of pituitary adenomas with gamma knife radiosurgery. Stereotact Funct Neurosurg 1998;70(suppl 1):95–109.
20 Martinez R, Bravo G, Burzaco J, Rey G: Pituitary tumors and gamma knife surgery. Clinical experience with more than two years of follow-up. Stereotact Funct Neurosurg 1998;70(suppl 1):110–118.
21 Mitsumori M, Chrieve DC, Alexander E 3rd, Kaiser UB, Richardson GE, Black PM, Loeffler JS: Initial clinical results of LINAC-based stereotactic radiosurgery and stereotactic radiotherapy for pituitary adenomas. Int J Radiat Oncol Biol Phys 1998;42:573–580.
22 Mokry M, Ramschak-Schwarzer S, Simbrunner J, Ganz JC, Pendl G: A six year experience with the postoperative radiosurgical management of pituitary adenomas. Stereotact Funct Neurosurg 1999;72(suppl 1):88–100.
23 Muramatsu J, Yoshida M, Shioura H, Kawamura Y, Ito H, Takeuchi H, Kubota T, Maruyama I: Clinical results of LINAC-based stereotactic radiosurgery for pituitary adenoma. Nippon Igaku Hoshasen Gakkai Zasshi 2003;63:225–230.
24 Petrovich Z, Yu C, Giannotta SL, Zee CS, Apuzzo ML: Gamma knife radiosurgery for pituitary adenoma: early results. Neurosurgery 2003;53:51–59.
25 Pollock BE, Carpenter PC: Stereotactic radiosurgery as an alternative to fractionated radiotherapy for patients with recurrent or residual nonfunctioning pituitary adenomas. Neurosurgery 2003;53: 1086–1094.
26 Sheehan JP, Kondziolka D, Flickinger J, Lunsford LD: Radiosurgery for residual or recurrent nonfunctioning pituitary adenoma. J Neurosurg 2002;97(suppl 5):408–414.
27 Wowra B, Stummer W: Efficacy of gamma knife radiosurgery for nonfunctioning pituitary adenomas: a quantitative follow-up with magnetic resonance imaging-based volumetric analysis. J Neurosurg 2002;97(suppl 5):429–432.
28 Ganz JC: Gamma knife radiosurgery and its possible relationship to malignancy: a review. J Neurosurg 2002;97(suppl 5):644–652.
29 Sutter B, Steiner M, Lopes MBS, Prasad D, Steiner L: Failure in management of pituitary tumors: discussion of 3 cases. Acta Neurochir (Wien) 1995;134:159–166.
30 Backlund EO, Ganz J: Pituitary adenomas: gamma knife; in Alexander E, et al. (eds): Stereotactic radiosurgery. New York, McGraw-Hill, 1993, pp 167–173.

Jason Sheehan
Department of Neurological Surgery
Box 800-212, Health Sciences Center
Charlottesville, VA 22908 (USA)
Tel. +1 434 924 8129, Fax +1 434 243 6726, E-Mail jps2f@virginia.edu

Szeifert GT, Kondziolka D, Levivier M, Lunsford LD (eds): Radiosurgery and Pathological Fundamentals. Prog Neurol Surg. Basel, Karger, 2007, vol 20, pp 180–191

9.6. Treatment Strategy and Pathological Background of Radiosurgery for Craniopharyngiomas

Tatsuya Kobayashi

Nagoya Radiosurgery Center, Nagoya Kyoritsu Hospital, Nagoya, Japan

Abstract

In this paper, pathological aspects of diagnosis, classification, treatment strategy and interstitial radiotherapy for craniopharyngiomas have been discussed and reviewed. The classification based on the location of squamous cell nests is useful for clinical evaluations and/or surgical approaches. Two pathological patterns, adamantinomatous and squamous cell types, are well correlated to the age of the patient, nature and response of tumor to radiation therapy. The originating portion of tumor (so called 'R site') at the retrochiasmal and anterior part of the stalk showed close contact of tumor with hypothalamic neurons without arachnoid membrane or glial cleavage. This means that the total removal of the tumor is difficult without damage to the stalk and optic pathway. A new concept of strategy can be proposed that a small tumor at this portion is intentionally left behind and is treated by gamma radiosurgery. The treatment strategy for large cystic tumor has been important and two methods can be recommended. The use of an Ommaya draining system has been useful not only for internal irradiation but also for collapse of the cyst prior to gamma radiosurgery. The effectiveness of interstitial radiation therapy has been evaluated by the surgical specimen using various immunohistochemical studies.

Various tumors are known to arise in the sellar-parasellar region, and each type shows characteristic biological behaviors depending upon its pathological nature.

In order of frequency, these tumors are pituitary adenomas, craniopharyngiomas, parasellar meningiomas, optic nerve gliomas, suprasellar germ cell tumors. Other far more rare primary tumors include the choristoma or infundibuloma (pituitocytoma), colloid cysts in the third ventricle, Rathke's cleft cyst and so on. The different responses of these benign tumors to Gamma Knife radiosurgery have been studied and pilocytic astrocytomas of optic nerves, suprasellar germinomas and craniopharyngiomas were found to be

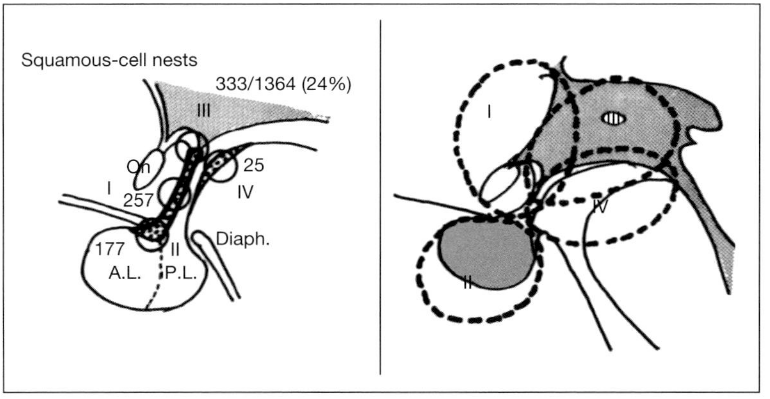

Fig. 1. Origins and classification of craniopharyngiomas. The origins are squamous cell nests [21] and four tumor locations are classifiable according to the origins [13]. I = Type 1, anterior; II = type 2, intrasellar; III = type 3, intraventricular; IV = type 4, posterior.

radiosensitive, with a complete response (CR) being obtained even with marginal doses as low as approximately 10 Gy. However, pituitary adenomas and meningiomas are less sensitive, and the so-called 3D strategy (detachment and decompression of optic nerves, and debulking of the tumor) is necessary prior to Gamma Knife radiosurgery [17]. The pathological background and basis of interstitial radiotherapies for craniopharyngiomas are discussed.

Characteristics and Classification Based on Pathology

Craniopharyngiomas are benign congenital tumors thought to be derived from squamous cell nests at the pars tuberalis, believed to be a remnant of the embryonic craniopharyngeal duct [21]. There are two age-peak incidences around 10 (children) and 40 (adults) years of age. Craniopharyngiomas account for 5.8% of all brain tumors and 12.5% of pediatric tumors, according to the Japan Brain Tumor Registry [3].

The frequency of these tumors has also been recognized as higher in Asian than in western countries, although this tumor is not uncommon (incidence: 3%) in the USA with no difference according to gender or race [2]. The location of these tumors correlates with the sites of squamous cell nests [21] from which such tumors originate and develop. There are four types based on the location of the main mass [13]: anterior type (1; 30%), intrasellar type (2; 20%), intraventricular type (3; 40%) and posterior type (4; 10%). This classification is important and useful for understanding biological behavior, clinical signs and symptoms, and surgical approaches to craniopharyngiomas [13] (fig. 1).

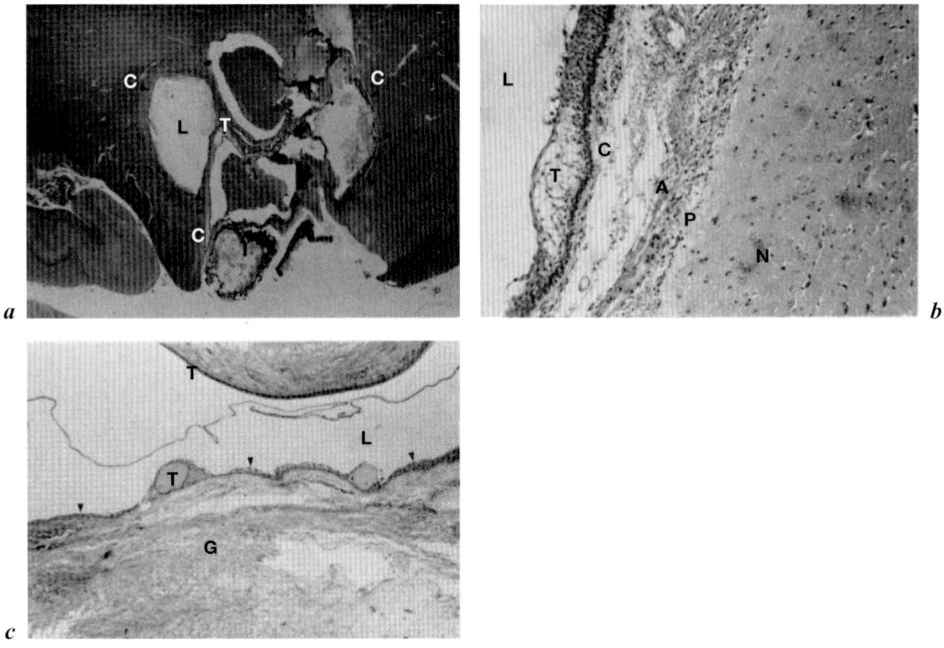

Fig. 2. Pathological findings of adamantinomatous type. ***a*** Multiple cysts are located in the third ventricle and hypothalamus. Each cyst has a thin tumor layer (T) and cavity (L) with an external connective tissue capsule (C). HE stain, ×1.5. ***b*** The cyst wall is composed of several layers of tumor cells (T) on the luminal side (L) and an external connective tissue layer (C). Arachnoid (A) and pial (P) membranes exist between the capsule and brain (N). Masson-Trichrome stain, ×200. ***c*** The sheet of tumor cells (T) is attached to brain tissue without a connective tissue layer. Abundant gliosis (G) is found between the tumor layer and neurons. PTAH stain, ×100.

Pathological Types

Macroscopic findings are mainly those of cystic, mixed and solid tumors. Clinicopathological features were extensively studied in surgically treated tumors [1, 28]. Cystic and mixed types involve a single large cyst or multiple small cysts in the tumors of both children and adults, and account for 70% of total tumors. In this type, the recurrence rate after surgery was as high as 13% in adults and 9% in pediatric patients. The solid tumors were found in one third of the adult patients but did not occur in children. Outcomes were good, without recurrence. The microscopic characteristics of the former tumors are consistent with the adamantinomatous type, in which the cyst contains motor oil-like fluid with cholesterine crystals, and sand-like or nodular calcifications in the tumor are another landmark of this pathological type (fig. 2). The tumor cells are

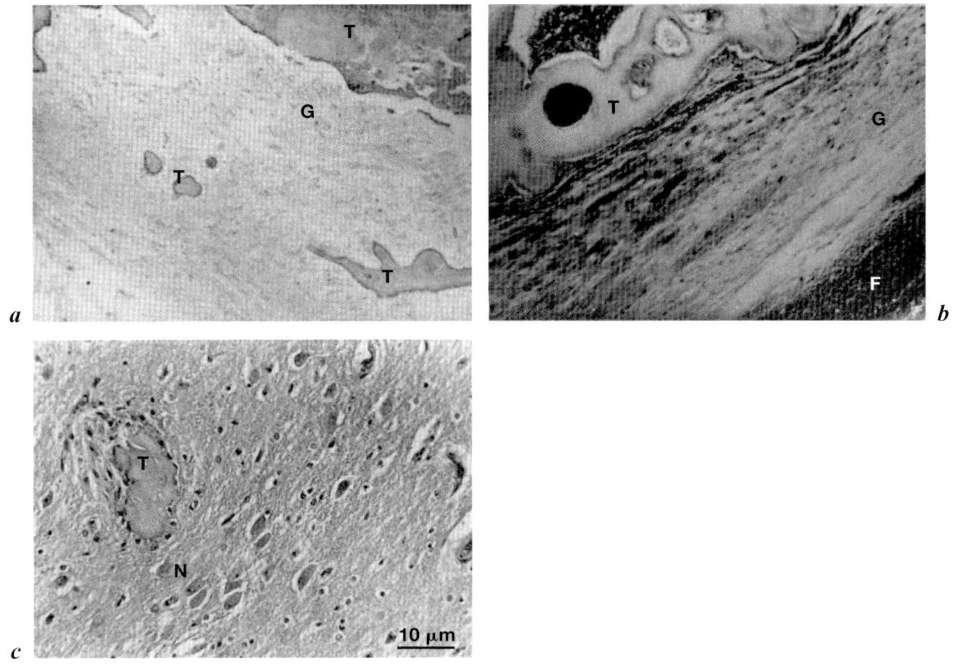

Fig. 3. Pathological findings of squamous cell type. ***a*** Finger-shaped or island-like protrusions of tumor cells (T) are seen in the adjacent brain tissue. Surrounding gliosis (G) is rich in Rosenthal fibers and fibrillary astrocytes. HE stain, ×100. ***b*** A tumor sheet (T) shows invasion of the hypothalamus. A thick layer of demyelinated fibers and gliosis (G) is present between the tumor and normal axons (F). Kluver-Barrera stain, ×200. ***c*** A tumor island (T) is close to neurons (N) of the hypothalamus without glial cleavage or arachnoid membrane. HE stain, ×400.

basically epithelial in origin, for example stratified epithelial cells of the epidermis, and show a three-layer arrangement. The most external layer is composed of single cuboidal or cylindrical cells, an intermediate thick layer of stratified polygonal or spindle-shaped cells, and an inner layer of stellate cells in a loose or island arrangement. Lamellar structures derived from keratinization and calcification are found in the centers of the islands. In contrast, solid tumors show neither cysts nor calcification and are found mostly in adults (fig. 3). The pathological characteristics are those of squamous cell type tumors. The tumor is composed of polygonal prickle cells which have distinctive intercellular bridges and show a stratified, sheet or island-like arrangement. The stroma is rich in vessels and connective tissue but there is no cyst formation, keratinization or calcification.

Important Pathological Findings for the Treatments

Pathological findings have been examined in numerous studies of surgical specimens, and many reported autopsy findings [9, 11]. Autopsy findings are extremely valuable as they can serve as controls for the evaluation of radiation or surgical effects, and are especially useful for determining relationships between the tumor and surrounding brain tissues. We have previously reported on 8 untreated autopsy cases in which craniopharyngioma tumor cells invaded the hypothalamus in some areas and were within a few microns of nerve cell contact with neither arachnoidal membrane involvement nor glial cleavage (fig. 3c), although most of the tumor was covered by arachnoid membrane [11]. This finding has been the basis of our philosophy that total removal of craniopharyngioma is difficult to achieve without damaging hypothalamic structures such as optic nerves and the pituitary stalk.

Craniopharyngioma treatments have long been controversial. Although total removal is ideal [29], it has been difficult to achieve complete resection without loss of neuroendocrinological functions because of tumor proximity to the hypothalamus, pituitary gland and optic pathway. Another method involves combining partial removal of the tumor with subsequent fractionated focal irradiation, and good, long-term control has been obtained [24, 25]. However, late-onset radiation-induced injury of the surrounding organs can produce long-term sequelae such as hypopituitarism, optic neuropathy or cognitive disturbance, especially in children [25, 26].

Recently, stereotactic radiosurgery (Gamma Knife) has been shown to be effective and safe for craniopharyngiomas not only as an adjuvant but also as an initial treatment [4, 14–16]. We have reported long-term results of 100 craniopharyngioma cases treated by gamma radiosurgery [16]. The results were evaluated in terms of MRI changes after treatment. The overall tumor response was complete (diminished) in 19, partial (decreased >25%) in 47, no change (unchanged or <25% decrease) in 12 and progression (increased) in 20 cases. Thus, a CR rate of 19.4%, response rate of 67.3%, tumor control rate of 79.5% and progression rate of 20.4% were obtained during a mean follow-up of 65 months. It was also found that the main cause of tumor progression was cyst enlargement, which accounted for half of the cyst-mixed tumors.

A New Treatment Strategy

A strategy for the treatment of craniopharyngiomas based on pathological and radiological features has been proposed and is summarized in table 1. Cure can be achieved by total removal without severe neuroendocrine deficits in

Table 1. A treatment strategy for craniopharyngioma

Tumor type	Approaches	Goal of treatment
1 Anterior	Subfrontal Pterional	
1 + 2	Combined Intracranial and transsphenoidal	Radical surgery (total removal)
2 Intrasellar (includes Rathke's)	Transsphenoidal	
3 Intraventricular	Transcallosal Transventricular Trans-lamina terminalis	Subtotal or partial removal + Radiation therapy (interstitial)
4 Posterior	Subtemporal Posterior fossae	1. Cystic … intracavitary 2. Solid … radiosurgery

type 1 and 2 tumors, while total removal is often difficult in type 3 and 4 tumors. It has been found that solid residual or recurrent tumors after surgery can be effectively and safely treated with stereotactic radiosurgery [16]. Large cystic tumors, in contrast, can be cured with intracavitary irradiation using radioisotopes [6, 12]. However, two important issues must be emphasized in these two combined-treatment protocols. The small amount of tumor remaining after extensive removal is usually in the retro-chiasm and anterior part of the pituitary stalk where the tumor originated, and marked invasion into both organs may be present. This point is the so-called 'R site' where residual or recurrent tumor is often encountered, and complete removal is difficult without risking severe visual disturbances and diabetes insipidus (fig. 4). It has been emphasized that these small tumors can be cured by Gamma Knife radiosurgery without side effects [16] (fig. 5).

The second issue is that the cystic part of the tumor has been known to be less responsive to radiosurgery, such that a different surgical strategy is necessary for cystic tumors. After open biopsy to make the diagnosis, cyst drainage through an Ommaya system is recommended for large cystic tumors; the cyst can be collapsed at the time of dose planning for Gamma Knife and good results have been obtained (fig. 6). The other goal is the introduction or retrieval of the radioisotopes used for intracavitary irradiation [12]. We treated 10 cysts in 8 patients using P-32 and Au-198 by this method and complete collapse of the cyst was obtained in 8 cysts during a mean follow-up of 64 months. The effective and safe wall dose was calculated to be between 80 and 200 Gy with

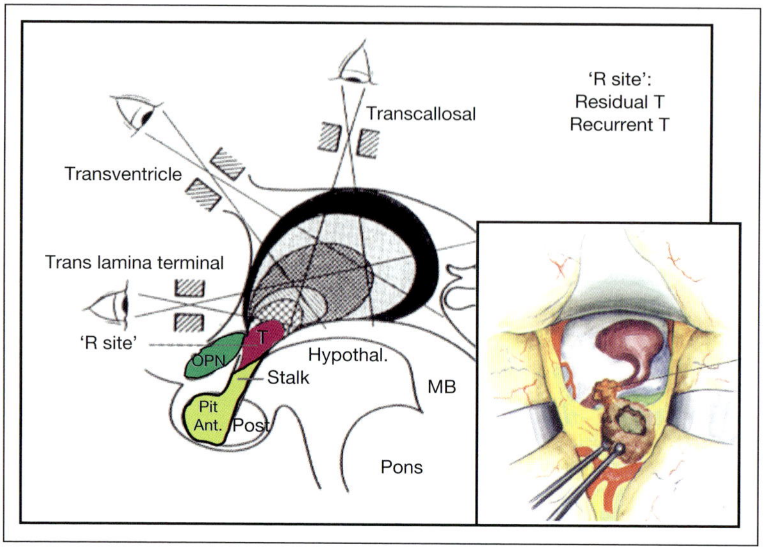

Fig. 4. Residual tumor at 'R site' and surgical view of the region. Schematic drawing of residual or recurrent tumor (T) between the optic nerve and anterior part of the stalk where surgical removal is difficult to achieve without producing neuroendocrinological deficits. The surgical view shows this region.

only 1 patient showing oculomotor palsy due to an excessive dosage. The effects were originally confirmed by positive-dye cystography, but more recently by MRI in which 3 of 8 patients were confirmed to be tumor free for more than 20 years. The effects were also confirmed by a pathological study of a surgical specimen 8 months after 170 Gy intracavitary irradiation using 2.3 mCi of P-32. The tumor in the cyst wall showed coagulation necrosis (fig. 7a) and a tumor-free state was verified by MRI 25 years after the treatment (fig. 7b). Pathological changes after intracavitary irradiation using yttrium-90 have also been reported: the epithelial cell layer was destroyed and an abundance of collagen fibers with focal hyaline degeneration was found, although the cyst wall dose was not specified in their report [26].

A pathological diagnosis and definition of the tumor type prior to treatment are essential for selecting optimal surgical approaches and radiation therapy strategies. This is because the squamous cell type is known to be more radiosensitive than the adamantinoma type [1, 10], and intracavitary irradiation is thought to be more effective than external irradiation for cystic craniopharyngioma [6, 12]. Recently, pathological diagnosis has become more

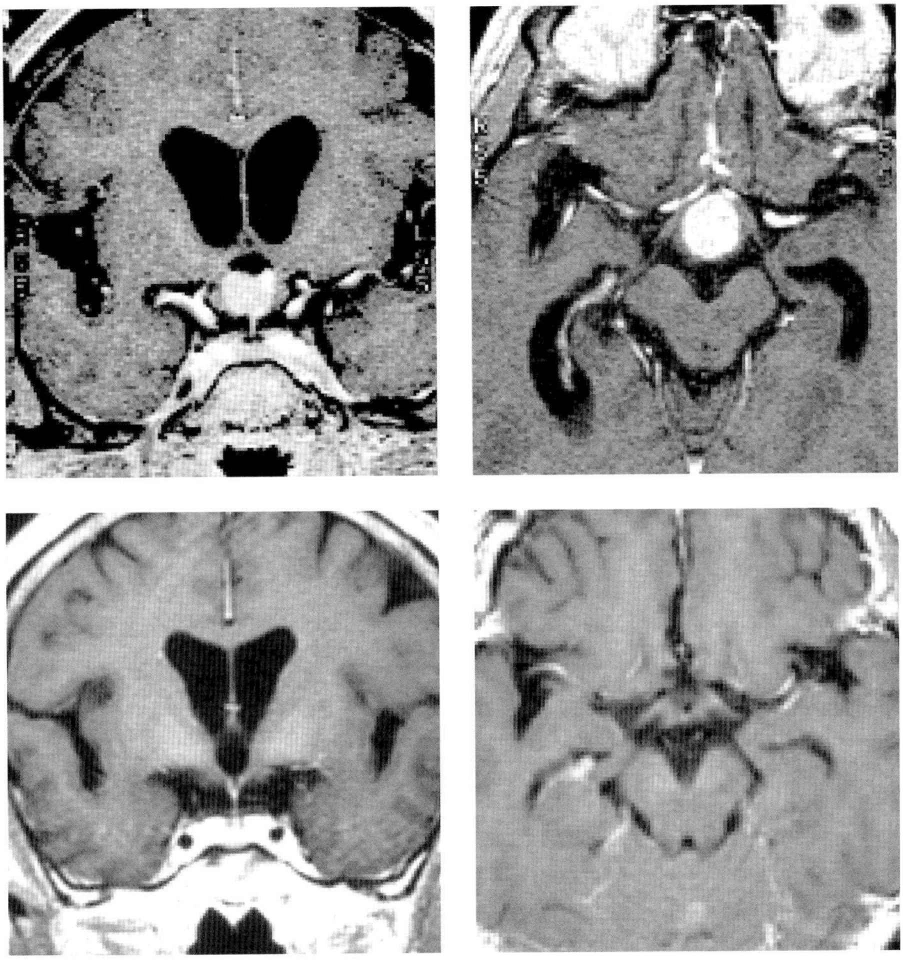

a

b

Fig. 5. Small tumor at 'R site' and follow-up MRI after Gamma Knife radiosurgery. ***a*** A 45-year-old man showed visual and memory disturbance; MRI revealed a small mass compressing the optic nerves and hydrocephalus. After open biopsy, the tumor was treated by Gamma Knife with a maximum dose of 15 Gy and a marginal dose of 9.8 Gy. ***b*** Follow-up MRI at 30 months showed disappearance of the tumor (CR) and improvement of hydrocephalus, as well as the symptoms. The optic nerves and stalk structures were restored.

specific, and the biological behaviors of tumors are better understood because the characteristics of tumors are demonstrated by immunohistochemical techniques using cytokeratins [18], PCNA [23], p53 [22], MIB-1 [5] and cathepsins B, D and K [20].

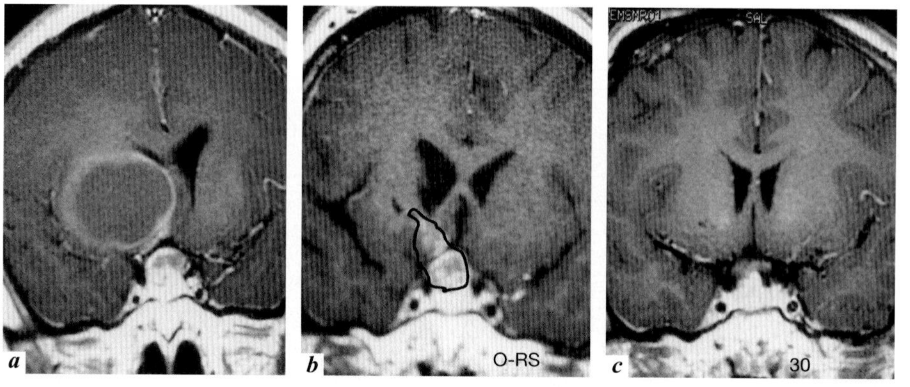

Fig. 6. Treatment strategy for large cystic craniopharyngioma. ***a*** An 18-year-old girl experienced sudden onset of severe headache with vomiting; MRI revealed a large cyst contiguous with a suprasellar tumor. ***b*** After biopsy and cyst drainage using an Ommaya system, the collapsed cyst and tumor were treated by Gamma Knife radiosurgery (26.6 mm) with a maximum dose of 16 Gy and a marginal dose of 10.4 Gy. ***c*** Follow-up MRI at 30 months showed complete disappearance of the cyst and a marked decrease in tumor size. This patient is now married and has recently become pregnant.

Pathological Changes after Radiation Therapy

After radiation therapy, changes in the tumor and surrounding tissues are evaluated using repeated CT or MRI [7], and more recently by SPECT or PET scan [19]. Recently, Szeifert et al. [27] reported that the tumor changes shown by PET imaging were due to vascular changes demonstrated by immunohistochemical study of marginal brain tissue using factor VIII and CD34 antigens. However, direct evaluation of the effects or side effects relies on pathological studies of surgical specimens taken after irradiation or autopsy materials. Hirato et al. [8] reported the proliferative capacity of two tumors to be increased after Gamma Knife radiosurgery. The specimens were surgically removed and examined using Ki-67, and showed a labeling index higher than average for craniopharyngiomas. These authors also reported that 5 of 10 craniopharyngioma cases treated by Gamma Knife showed cyst enlargement after 1–2 years, with the main pathological changes being fibrinoid necrosis and fibrous thickening of the vascular wall, along with partial necrosis and fibrosis of the tumor cells [8].

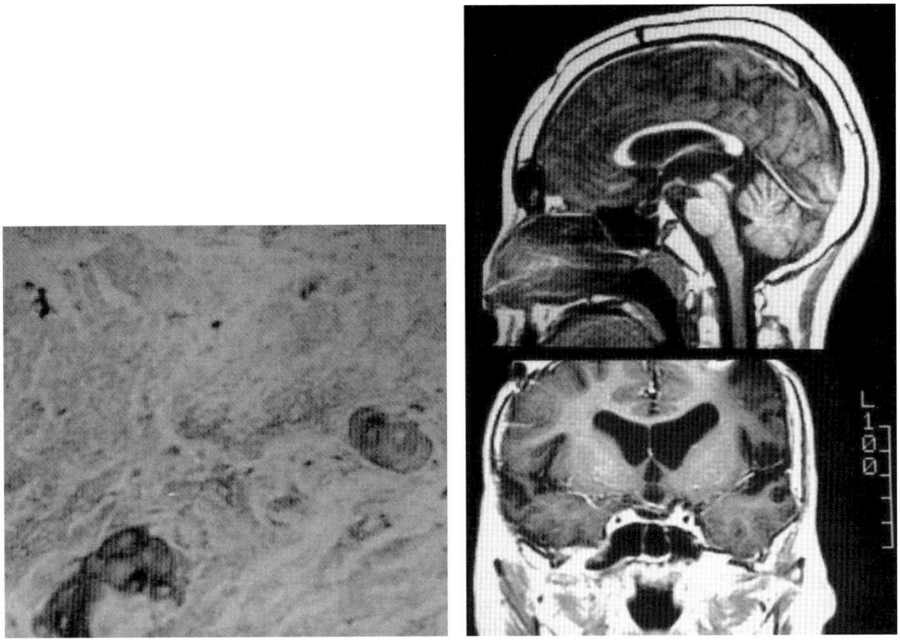

a *b*

Fig. 7. ***a*** Pathological findings of the cyst wall after intracavitary irradiation. A suprasellar cyst was treated by intracavitary irradiation using 2.3 mCi of P-32, with a calculated wall dose of 170 Gy. The cyst was collapsed at 6 months, but was surgically removed at 8 months when a new cyst appeared. The tumor cells in the wall showed coagulation necrosis with ghost-like structures containing keratinization and calcifications. HE stain, ×400. ***b*** MRI findings 25 years after intracavitary irradiation. Two large cysts were treated by intracavitary irradiation using 2.3 mCi of P-32 and 10 mCi of Au-198, separately, at the age of 4. The MRI 25 years after the treatments confirmed this 29-year-old man to be tumor free.

Conclusion

Pathological findings of tumors have greatly contributed to the understanding of the classification, nature, symptomatology and/or treatment strategy of craniopharyngiomas.

The responses and effects of interstitial radiotherapy, i.e. internal irradiation or stereotactic radiosurgery, can be evaluated clinically by repeated CT or MRI, and more recently by dynamic images obtained with SPECT or/and PET. However, definite changes can only be confirmed by pathological examination of surgical specimens or autopsy materials after treatment. Tumor cells show a variety of changes from minute alterations to complete necrosis, especially when using recent immunohistochemical techniques.

References

1 Adamson TE, Wiestler OD, Kleihues P, Yasargil MG: Correlation of clinical and pathological features in surgically treated craniopharyngiomas. J Neurosurg 1990;73:12–17.

2 Bunin GR, Surawicz TS, Witman PA, Preston-Martin S, Davis F, Bruner JM: The descriptive epidemiology of craniopharyngioma. J Neurosurg 1998;89:547–551.

3 The Committee of Brain Tumor Registry of Japan: The Report of Brain Tumor Registry of Japan.1990, vol 7 [Jpn].

4 Chung WY, Pan DHC, Shiau CY, Guo WY, Wang LW: Gamma knife radiosurgery for craniopharyngiomas. J Neurosurg 2000;93(suppl 3):45–56.

5 Duo D, Gasverde S, Benech F, Zenga F, Giordana MT: MIB-1 immunoreactivity in craniopharyngioma: a clinicopathological analysis. Clin Neuropathol 2003;22:229–234.

6 Hasegawa T, Kondziolka D, Hadjipanayis CG, Lunsford LD: Management of cystic craniopharyngioma with phosphorus-32 intracavitary irradiation. Neurosurgery 2004;54:813–820.

7 Hamamoto Y, Niino K, Adachi M, Hosoya T: MR and CT findings of craniopharyngioma during and after radiation therapy. Neuroradiology 2002;44:118–122.

8 Hirato M, Hirato J, Zama H, Inoue H, Ohye C, Shibasaki T, Andou Y: Radiobiological effects of Gamma Knife radiosurgery on brain tumors studied in autopsy and surgical specimens. Stereotact Funct Neurosurg 1996;66(suppl 1):4–16.

9 Inenaga C, Kakita A, Iwasaki Y, Yamatani K, Takahashi H: Autopsy findings of a craniopharyngioma with a natural course over 60 years. Surg Neurol 2004;61:536–540.

10 Inoue HK, Nakamura M, Ono N, Kohga H, Kakegawa T, Naitou I, Tamada J, Handa I: Radiosensitive squamous cell craniopharyngioma: clinical and pathological comparison with the adamantinomatous type. Noshuyou Byori 1993;10:27–31.

11 Kobayashi T, Kageyama N, Yoshida J, Shibuya N, Yonezawa T: Pathological and clinical basis of the indication for treatment of craniopharyngiomas. Neurol Med Chir 1981;21:39–47.

12 Kobayashi T, Kageyama N, Ohara K: Internal irradiation for cystic craniopharyngioma. J Neurosurg 1981;55:896–903.

13 Kobayashi T, Nakane T, Kageyama N: Combined transsphenoidal and intracranial surgery for craniopharyngioma. Prog Exp Tumor Res 1987;30:341–349.

14 Kobayashi T, Tanaka T, Kida Y: Stereotactic gamma radiosurgery of craniopharyngiomas. Pediatr Neurosurg 1994;21(suppl 1):69–74.

15 Kobayashi T, Kida Y, Mori Y: Effects and prognostic factors in the treatment of craniopharyngioma by Gamma Knife; in Kondziolka D (ed): Radiosurgery 1999. Basel, Karger, 2000, vol 3, pp 192–204.

16 Kobayashi T, Kida Y, Mori Y, Hasegawa T: Long-term results of gamma knife radiosurgery for the treatment of craniopharyngioma in 98 consecutive cases. J Neurosurg 2005;103(suppl pediatrics): 482–488.

17 Kobayashi T: A strategy for treating sellar-parasellar tumors based on long-term results of microsurgery and gamma knife radiosurgery; in Kondziolka D (ed): Radiosurgery. Basel, Karger, 2004, vol 5, pp 1–12.

18 Kurosaki M, Seager W, Luedecke DK: Immunohistochemical localization of cytokeratins in craniopharyngioma. Acta Neurochir (Wien) 2001;143:147–151.

19 Levivier M, Wikler D Jr, Massager N, David P, Devriendt D, Lorenzoni J, Pirotte B, Desmedt F, Simon S Jr, Goldman S, Van Houtte P, Brotchi J: The integration of metabolic imaging in stereotactic procedures including radiosurgery: a review. J Neurosurg 2002;97(suppl 5):542–550.

20 Lubansu A, Ruchoux MM, Brotchi J, Salmon I, Kiss R, Lefranc F: Catepsin B, D and K expression in adamantinomatous craniopharyngiomas related to their levels of differentiation as determined by patterns of retinoic acid receptor expression. Histopathology 2003;43:563–572.

21 Luse SA, Kernohan JW: Squamous cell nests of the pituitary gland. Cancer 1955;8:623–638.

22 Momota H, Ichiyama S, Ikeda T, Yamaki T, Kikuchi T, Houkin K, Sato N: Immuno-histochemical analysis of the P-53 family members in human craniopharyngiomas. Brain Tumor Pathol 2003;20: 73–77.

23 Pan J, Qi ST, Deng YJ, Ding YQ, Peng L, Li XQ: Expression of proliferating cell nuclear antigen in craniopharyngioma and tumor recurrence. Di Yi Jun Yi Da Xue Xue Bao 2002;22:363–365.

24 Rajan B, Ashley S, Gorman C, Jose CC, Horwich A, Bloom HJ, Marsh H, Brada M: Craniopharyngioma – a long-term results following limited surgery and radiotherapy. Radiother Oncol 1993;26:1–10.
25 Regine WF, Mohiuddin M, Kramer S: Long-term results of pediatric and adult craniopharyngiomas treated with combined surgery and radiation. Radiother Oncol 1993;27:13–21.
26 Szeifert GT, Julow J, Slowik F, Balint K, Lanyi F, Pasztor E: Pathological changes in cystic craniopharyngioma following intracavital 90 yttrium treatment. Acta Neurochir (Wien) 1990;102: 14–18.
27 Szeifert GT, Massager N, DeVriendt D, David P, De Smedt F, Rorive S, Salmon I, Brotchi J, Levivier M: Observation of intracranial neoplasms treated with gamma knife radiosurgery. J Neurosurg 2002;97(suppl 5):623–626.
28 Weiner HL, Wisoff JH, Rosenberg ME, Kupersmith MJ, Cohen H, Zagzag D, Shiminski-Maher T, Flamm ES, Epstein FJ, Miller DC: Craniopharyngiomas: a clinicopathological analysis of factors predictive of recurrence and functional outcome. Neurosurgery 1994;35:1001–1010.
29 Yasargil MG, Curcic M, Kis M, Siegenthaler G, Teddy PJ, Roth P: Total removal of craniopharyngiomas. Approaches and long-term results in 144 patients. J Neurosurg 1990;73:3–11.

Tatsuya Kobayashi, MD, PhD
Nagoya Radiosurgery Center, Nagoya Kyoritsu Hospital
1-172 Hokke, Nakagawa
Nagoya 454-0933 (Japan)
Tel. +81 52 362 5151, Fax +81 52 353 9126, E-Mail ttkobayashi@kaikou.or.jp

Szeifert GT, Kondziolka D, Levivier M, Lunsford LD (eds): Radiosurgery and Pathological Fundamentals. Prog Neurol Surg. Basel, Karger, 2007, vol 20, pp 192–205

9.7. Radiosurgery for Miscellaneous Skull Base Tumors

L. Dade Lunsford, Ajay Niranjan, Juan J. Martin, Sait Sirin, Amin Kassam, Douglas Kondziolka, John C. Flickinger

Department of Neurological Surgery and The Center for Image-Guided Neurosurgery, University of Pittsburgh Medical Center, Pittsburgh, Pa., USA

Abstract

Stereotactic radiosurgery has become an integral part of conventional and advanced skull base surgery. Despite the advances in skull base techniques, the goal of total resection of such tumors is often problematic and associated with significant risk to critical structures of the skull base, including those within the cavernous sinus, those in the petrous apex, and the jugular bulb. Aggressive resection of such tumors sometimes results in severe adverse neurological events, ranging from permanent extraocular movement deficits to hearing loss, facial weakness, and difficulties with vagal and glossopharyngeal function. Gamma Knife radiosurgery is a primary alternative option for these patients. It minimizes the risks of open surgical techniques and preserves existing cranial nerve function in most patients and achieves tumor growth arrest. Adjuvant radiosurgery is used for larger tumors after their initial partial resection. Gamma Knife radiosurgery becomes an adjuvant tool to provide long-term tumor growth control of a significantly reduced tumor volume.

Stereotactic radiosurgery over the last 25 years has become an integral part of conventional and advanced skull base surgery. Although the Gamma Knife was first created in order to be able to provide ablation of a normal intracranial target during functional neurosurgery for obsessive compulsive disorders and for trigeminal neuralgia, the first patient treated with the 179 Cobalt source prototype Gamma Knife in 1967 was a patient with a craniopharyngioma [Backlund, pers. commun.]. The patient was treated at the site of the construction of the Gamma Knife before it was moved to the Sophiahemmet in Stockholm, where Leksell initially pursued the further development of Gamma Knife radiosurgical techniques. The second generation unit, installed at the

Karolinska Hospital in 1975, had circular aperture collimator helmets more suitable for conformal volumetric stereotactic surgery of brain tumors and vascular malformations.

Over the last 15 years, major advances have characterized the phenomenal growth of radiosurgery: power of dose planning systems, more accurate photon beam algorithms, modern neurodiagnostic imaging tools performed to localize the tumor during the radiosurgical procedure itself, and the introduction of robotic technology in isocenter placement. During this same interval, longer-term outcome studies have caused a reevaluation of the goals of conventional skull base microsurgery. In the 1990s, previously unapproachable tumors became operable by using advanced skull base techniques derived from comprehensive understanding of the difficult skull base anatomy. Despite these advances, total resection of such tumors was often impossible. Patients sustained significant risks related to the critical nerve and vascular structures, in the cavernous sinus, the petrous apex, and the region of the jugular bulb. The role of Gamma Knife radiosurgery began to be evaluated during the decades of the 80s and 90s, eventually leading to publications of comprehensive outcome data. Currently, the Gamma Knife has a major primary role in the management of tumors without significant mass effect and as an adjuvant management after partial resection of large tumors. The pathological response after radiosurgery is defined in the chapter below, although to date limited pathologic material is available.

The Role of the Gamma Knife

Adjuvant radiosurgery is extremely important in larger tumors that have been partially resected. Such tumors are sometimes aggressively removed, only to have patients suffer adverse neurological events, ranging from permanent extraocular movement deficits to hearing loss, facial weakness, and difficulties with vagal and glossopharyngeal function. In many cases, because of the high tumor control rates achieved by radiosurgery, it is possible to stop short of complete resection, and thereby preserve adjacent cranial nerve function. Gamma Knife radiosurgery becomes an adjuvant tool to provide long-term tumor growth control of a significantly reduced volumetric tumor.

In other cases, newly diagnosed patients with relatively small volume tumors (e.g. those in the average diameter of ≤30 mm and not associated with significant brainstem mass effect or headache) may be suitable for primary management using the Gamma Knife. In such cases, the presumed pathological diagnosis is based on high resolution neurodiagnostic imaging, most commonly volumetric MRI scan. In almost all cases, we can differentiate the tumor type based on its contrast pattern, its long TR imaging appearance, the absence or presence of a dural tail, in conjunction with the neurological examination. For these patients, Gamma Knife radiosurgery may be a primary option, designed to minimize the risks of open surgical techniques and attempt to preserve existing cranial nerve function with a high success rate. For most patients, tumor controlling doses are similar for a wide spectrum of these benign tumors (discussion below will describe some exceptions such as chordoma). Standard three-dimensional volumetric radiosurgery provides equally effective control of schwannomas, meningiomas, hemangioblastomas, glomus tumors, and cavernous sinus hemangiomas.

Intraoperative Stereotactic Radiosurgical Imaging Techniques

Before intraoperative imaging, the standard Leksell Model G stereotactic head frame is attached to the head and usually placed as low as possible in the cranial base. The frame is shifted posteriorly for inferior skull base tumors. High-resolution neurodiagnostic intraoperative MRI scan is preferred. Occasionally, CT scan imaging is used with iodine contrast enhancement, using 1- to 2-mm slices, but only in those cases where intraoperative MRI scan is precluded by standard MRI concerns such as pacemakers or higher undefined metallic substances in the field of view. Pin artifacts are greatly reduced by MRI in comparison to CT.

Schwannomas, craniopharyngiomas and hemangioblastomas are best defined by high-resolution axial plane MRI with 1- to 2-mm volume acquisition slices (for GE scanners, an SPGR sequence). This volumetric slab can be reformatted in coronal and sagittal planes using current versions of GammaPlan®, for example version 5.34 or 4C. Other tumors may benefit from usage of long TR imaging sequences to define the tumor edge better. Certain cystic tumors may be enhanced by looking at long TR imaging sequences using a fast spin echo with long T_2 preference. Similarly, both chordomas and chondrosarcomas require high signal long TR imaging, especially in cases where there is distinct bone invasion. Normally, we obtain 2-mm serial stacking axial plane slices. In addition, cavernous sinus or orbital hemangiomas are characteristically defined by a dark T_2 signal surrounding the tumor volume of the cavernous sinus as well as by the absence of a dural tail, thereby distinctly defining the tumor volume, and eliminating the differential diagnosis of a cavernous sinus meningioma.

Glomus tumors must be looked at as special cases because the inferior extent of such patients at the time of presentation may preclude Gamma Knife as the sole radiosurgical technology unless the new Perfexion® model is used. Instead it may be combined with either primary surgery or linear accelerator-based extracranial

Table 1. Skull base tumors treated at the University of Pittsburgh (n = 238)

Diagnosis	Patients
Nonacoustic schwannoma	65
Trigeminal	35
Facial	4
9–10	26
Craniopharyngioma	43
Glomus tumor	16
Chordoma	26
Chondrosarcoma	17
Hemangioblastoma	36
Hemangioma	7
Invasive skull base tumors	28
Adenocarcinoma	14
Squamous cell carcinoma	13
Neuroendocrine carcinoma	1

radiosurgery as such CyberKnife® or Synergy®, which facilitates treatment of tumors that extend below the skull base into the neck. Most glomus tumors have significant extracranial extension.

Results and Experience

From September 1987 through December 2004, a total of 6,750 patients underwent Gamma Knife radiosurgery at the University of Pittsburgh Medical Center. During this interval, the 238 miscellaneous skull base tumors were treated. These tumors and their subsequent management are described below in more detail (table 1).

Nonacoustic Schwannomas

Thirty-five patients underwent radiosurgery for trigeminal nerve sheath tumors defined by clinical examination, high-resolution intraoperative imaging, and in selected cases prior surgery. Our results of trigeminal schwannoma have been recently published [1]. The records of 23 patients were reviewed with a median follow-up of 40 months. Twenty of 22 patients (91%) had tumor growth control, with regression noted in 15 and no further tumor growth in 5 (fig. 1). Patients who had subsequent tumor enlargement were re-treated effectively by a second radiosurgical procedure. Twelve of 23 trigeminal nerve sheath tumor patients (52%) reported systemic improvement. Nine (39%) had no change in

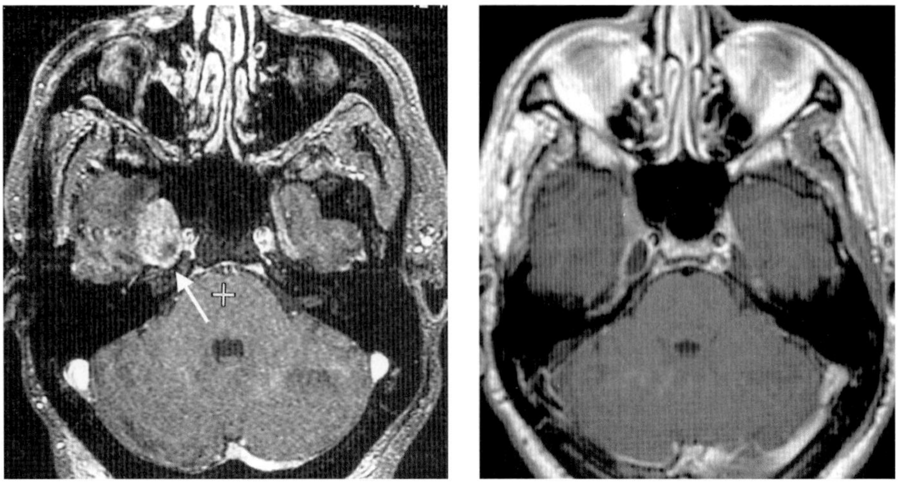

a b

Fig. 1. ***a*** Axial contrast-enhanced MRI showing a right-sided trigeminal schwannoma (arrow). ***b*** A follow-up MRI 31 months after radiosurgery shows significant regression of tumor.

their symptoms. Only 2 patients noted new neurological complaints such as facial weakness (1 patient) and worsening of the preradiosurgical facial numbness (1 additional patient).

Of interest, trigeminal nerve sheath tumors have a much higher likelihood of developing transient, but occasionally impressive short-term swelling in the 1st year after radiosurgery. This is quite distinct from those patients who have undergone acoustic tumor radiosurgery. In the majority of trigeminal neuroma patients, transient swelling is followed by delayed shrinkage, often of profound degree (fig. 2). Therefore, it is critical that patients and referring doctors do not despair during this transient tumor enlargement phase identified by imaging and sometimes associated with temporary concomitant neurological symptoms. Most such symptoms will resolve as the tumors regress during the next 3–6 months. Radiosurgery using the Gamma Knife proved to be an effective management strategy for those patients who had undergone both primary as well as adjuvant (postmicrosurgery) radiosurgery [2].

Tumors of the ninth and tenth cranial nerve also recognize special challenges. Currently, 26 patients underwent radiosurgery for jugular bulb schwannomas between August 1987 and September 2004. Most such patients present with symptoms related to imbalance, incoordination, dysphagia, or hearing loss. A total of 12 patients had previously undergone gross total resection with tumor recurrence, and four had undergone prior partial resection. Results to date show a high likelihood of long-term tumor growth control for such tumors. Three

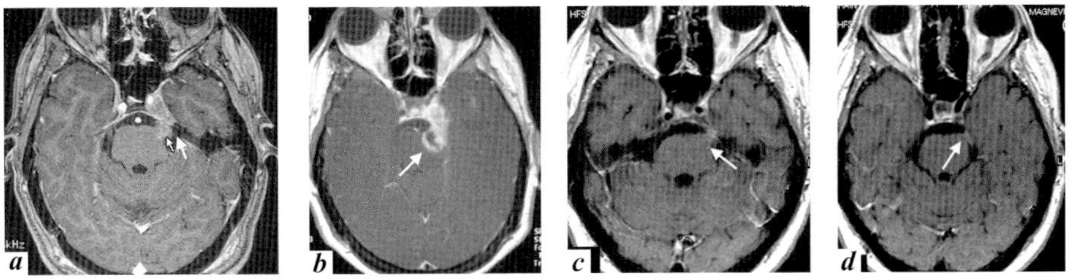

Fig. 2. ***a*** Axial contrast-enhanced MRI showing a left-sided trigeminal schwannoma (arrow). ***b*** A significant tumor swelling is noted on a 6-month follow-up MRI. ***c*** A 2-year follow-up MRI showing significant regression in tumor. ***d*** A 5-year follow-up MRI showing further tumor regression.

patients underwent Gamma Knife radiosurgery for facial schwannomas, all identified at the time of prior microsurgery and associated with recurrence or subtotal prior resection. In an earlier report including 17 patients, we reported a tumor control rate of 94% (8 decreased and 8 were stable in size) after jugular foramen schwannoma radiosurgery [3]. Zhang et al. [4] reported 96% (26/27) tumor growth control with a follow-up period of 38.7 months. In the series of nonvestibular schwannomas, Pollock et al. [5] reported 96% (22/23) tumor growth control after Gamma Knife radiosurgery. Mabanta et al. [6] reported 100% local control after LINAC-based radiosurgery for nonvestibular schwannomas with higher complication rate than Gamma Knife series.

Craniopharyngioma

Forty-three patients have undergone Gamma Knife radiosurgery as part of a primary or adjuvant management strategy for craniopharyngioma.

Radiosurgery is usually part of a multimodality management when prior therapies have failed. Earlier, we reported the outcomes in 10 consecutive patients (3 males and 7 females) who had radiosurgery for craniopharyngioma during a 10-year interval [7]. Twelve radiosurgical procedures were performed to treat 12 tumors in these 10 patients. Overall, 7 of 12 tumors became smaller or vanished with a median of 8.5 months. Prior visual defects improved subjectively in 6 patients. Multimodality therapy is often necessary for such patients because of the development of refractory cystic components of their tumors and occasionally new solid tumor growth. We found that stereotactic radiosurgery was a reasonable option in selected patients with small recurrent or residual craniopharyngiomas. Adverse radiation risks related to adjacent cranial nerve structures or the development of new extraocular movement deficits are rare, providing that the optic nerve and tract dose is kept lower than 8 Gy or less in a single procedure. In general, we prefer the use of multimodality management including microsurgery, radiosurgery, and intracavitary radiation rather than stereotactic or fractionated radiation therapy [8]. The goal has been to maintain endocrinological function whenever possible, reduce the risks of visual dysfunction, and subsequently control tumor growth. There are other reports that have similar results in the management of craniopharyngiomas using the Gamma Knife [9–12].

Glomus Tumors

Radiosurgery using the Gamma Knife has been performed in 16 patients in a 17-year interval. The sparse number of patients is accounted for by the tendency of such tumors to extend well below the skull base. When surgical resection is not feasible, we consider staged radiosurgery technologies such as LINAC-based radiosurgery for the extracranial component and the Gamma Knife for the intracranial portion. Some patients also have undergone elective embolization for shrinkage of their tumor or subtotal microsurgical resection. Only 1 patient in our series had a glomus tympanicum tumor.

Gamma Knife radiosurgery appears to have a long-term high rate of glomus tumor control, paralleling the benefit provided by fractionated radiation therapy (fig. 3). However, the Gamma Knife provides a superior biological effective tumor dose, with better dose sparing of the adjacent brainstem and cranial nerve structures. Pollock [13] in a series including 42 patients reported 98% tumor control after glomus jugulare radiosurgery at a mean follow-up of 44 months. Neurological improvement or stability was observed in the majority of patients in published series [14–19]. Centers using LINAC-based radiosurgery continue to support radiosurgery as an effective and safe method of treatment for glomus jugulare tumors that results in low rates of morbidity [20, 21].

Hemangiomas

Radiosurgery for hemangioma was performed in 7 patients. Hemangiomas of neurosurgical interest are histologically benign tumors of vascular epithelial cell origin that most often occur in the orbit or cavernous sinus or both. These patients tend to present with ocular symptoms or signs such as orbital pain, ophthalmoplegia, proptosis or impaired visual acuity. They can, in fact, be diagnosed by their characteristic imaging appearance by MRI. Since they may hemorrhage dramatically at the time of attempted removal, it is prudent for surgeons considering biopsy or resection of such tumors to get the appropriate imaging in

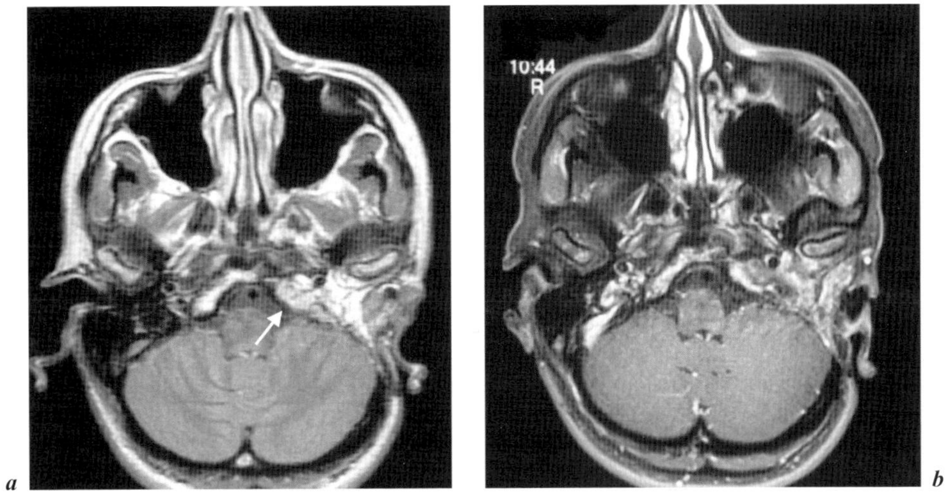

Fig. 3. ***a*** Axial contrast-enhanced MRI showing a left-sided glomus tumor (arrow) at Gamma Knife radiosurgery. This patient had undergone tumor resection and fractionated radiation therapy prior to radiosurgery. ***b*** A 22-month follow-up MRI showing significant regression of tumor.

advance. Asymptomatic lesions do not require intervention but are often approached surgically in pursuit of a diagnosis. Symptomatic lesions require treatment. Options include en bloc resection, embolization, or radiation. Radiosurgery is a better option. In our relatively limited experience, some patients have had incomplete resection because of excessive blood loss, and 1 patient had undergone unsuccessful embolization.

We recently reported the outcomes of 4 patients treated with radiosurgery with tumor doses ranging from 14 to 19 Gy at the margin [22]. All patients had symptomatic improvement, and all have shown a dramatic reduction in the overall volume of their tumor. One patient had persistent diplopia.

In our early experience, stereotactic radiosurgery proved to be a very effective management strategy which avoided potentially serious complications associated with skull base microsurgery or embolization [22]. The other reports including 3–5 cases in each, also achieved reduction in tumor volume after radiosurgery [23–25].

Hemangioblastoma

Thirty-six patients with intracranial hemangioblastomas, usually in conjunction with the syndrome of von Hippel-Lindau disease (VHL), have been treated by radiosurgery at our Center. Early experience from several centers indicated that radiosurgery could lead to tumor control or regression [26–32]. For the most part, we have treated tumors with documented tumor growth, which are usually solid, and almost exclusively located in the posterior fossa, cerebellum and brainstem [28, 33]. Such tumors are generally treated when they have shown evidence of objective growth and neurological symptoms develop. Prophylactic radiosurgery for hemangioblastomas in the case of VHL is not performed unless tumor growth or new symptoms are documented. Multifocality is often a characteristic of the 20% of hemangioblastomas that are associated with VHL. Radiosurgery is a potential therapeutic option for these patients where resection of multiple tumors might be precluded because of brain location. For those patients with cystic hemangioblastomas, we have less optimism related to the overall role of radiosurgery at least as a single option. Cyst-associated tumors with nonenhancing cyst cavities were controlled by including only the enhancing nodule in the target volume. However, surgical removal of a large cystic component of a tumor producing mass effect symptoms is usually appropriate followed by radiosurgery for any residual solid component. In selected cases, stereotactic aspiration of the cyst followed by subsequent radiosurgery is feasible. Repeat radiosurgery may be required over many years when other tumors show additional growth [33].

Chordoma and Chondrosarcoma

During our 17-year experience, 26 patients with chordomas and 17 patients with chondrosarcomas have undergone management with radiosurgery. We reported our experience in two prior publications [34, 35].

We continue to regard these tumors as difficult to manage. Almost invariably they require multimodality management over the course of many years. These invasive tumors provide a management challenge because of their critical location and their tendency to aggressively recur locally despite multimodality treatment [36]. Radiosurgery has been used both as a primary and adjuvant management strategy [37, 38]. Radiosurgery appears to be a safe and effective management for small volume tumors, but over the course of many years, especially from years 5–10 after initial surgery and radiosurgery, recurrence rates continue to increase. In such cases, repeat radiosurgery or perhaps fractionated radiation therapy and repeat radiosurgery should be considered [39–41]. Most such patients require one or more microsurgical approaches for tumor cytoreduction. More recently, we have embarked on the usage of endoscopic transsphenoidal resection followed by radiosurgery (fig. 4). In our 1998 report, with an average of 4 years of experience, 15 patients were evaluated. In 13 cases, it was used as an adjunctive treatment, and in 2 patients as an alternative

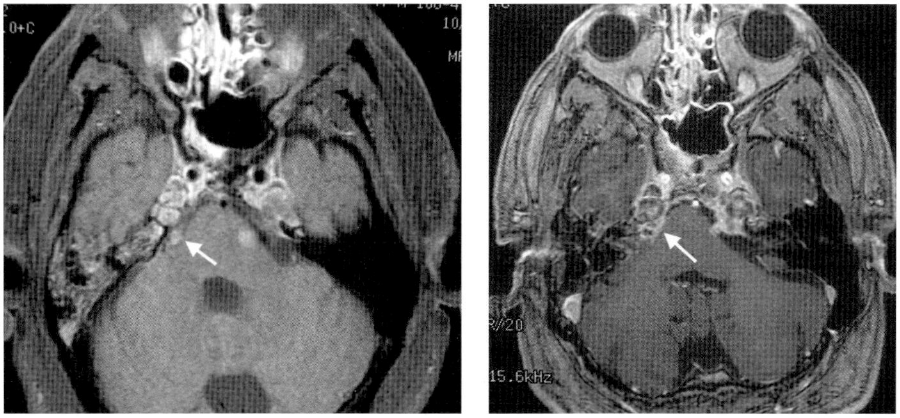

a b

Fig. 4. ***a*** Axial contrast-enhanced MRI showing a clival chordoma (arrow). This patient had undergone two prior skull base resections and one transnasal endoscope tumor resection. ***b*** A 2-year follow-up MRI showing tumor regression.

Table 2. Radiosurgery for benign skull base tumors

References	Technique	Diagnosis	Patients	Mean follow-up months	Tumor control, %	Complications, %
Zabel, et al. [49]	FSRT	glomus tumor	22	67	90	18
Saringer, et al. [50]	GKR	glomus tumor	13	60	100	0
Zhang, et al. [4]	GKR	jugular foramen schwannomas	27	38.7	92.5	0
Mabanta, et al. [6]	LINAC SR	5, 7, 9, 10, 11 schwannomas	18	32	100	22
Nettel, et al. [1]	GKR	trigeminal schwannomas	23	40	91	8
Pollock, et al. [5]	GKR	nonvestibular schwanomas	23	43	96	17
Pan, et al. [2]	GKR	trigeminal schwannomas	46	68	93	8

to microsurgical resection. Eight patients had clinical improvement, 3 remained stable, and 4 died. Two of the 4 patients who died had tumor progression outside of the radiosurgical volumes, but 2 patients died of unrelated disorders. Tumor reduction was noted in 5 of 11 patients. Five patients had defined additional growth and underwent repeat resection [34].

Table 3. Outcomes of radiosurgery for malignant skull base tumors

References	Technique	Diagnosis	Patients	Follow-up months	Tumor control, %	Complications
Debus, et al. [39]	LINAC-SRT	chordomas, chondromas	45	27	82, chondromas 40, chordomas	2
Hug, et al. [40]	Proton beam RT	chordomas, chondromas	58	60	83	6 (12.5%)
Igaki, et al. [41]	Proton beam RT	chordomas	13	69	46 at 5 years	6 (43%)
Muthukumar, et al. [34]	GKR	chordomas, chondromas	15	40	73	0
Kocher, et al. [37]	LINAC-SR	carcinomas, sarcomas	13	NR	61	30%
Cmelak, et al. [48]	LINAC-SR	carcinomas, metastases	47	18	69	8.40%
Miller, et al. [38]	GKR	carcinomas, sarcomas	32	27	91	3%

Invasive Skull Base Cancers

After combined otolaryngological and neurosurgical procedures, we have used adjuvant radiosurgery for invasive skull base cancers (28 patients over the last 17 years). Fourteen patients had adenocarcinomas, 13 squamous cell carcinomas, and 1 patient had a metastatic neuroendocrine tumor. In such cases, radiosurgery has been used as an adjuvant or in combination with external beam fractionated radiation therapy [42, 43]. Many reports have documented the role of radiosurgery as salvage procedure for malignant tumors involving the skull base [38, 44–48] (tables 2, 3).

In chapter 8, the delayed pathological results in a limited number of patients are described. The reason for delayed resection includes persistent neurological symptoms with defined evidence of intracranial growth. Surgeons and referring doctors should be especially cautious about early reoperation for patients with trigeminal nerve sheath tumors which, as noted above, have a much higher tendency to have delayed temporary postradiosurgical swelling and apparent growth, only to show definitive volumetric shrinkage with further observation.

References

1 Nettel B, Niranjan A, Martin JJ, Koebbe CJ, Kondziolka D, Flickinger JC, Lunsford LD: Gamma knife radiosurgery for trigeminal schwannomas. Surg Neurol 2004;62:435–444; discussion 444–446.
2 Pan L, Wang EM, Zhang N, Zhou LF, Wang BJ, Dong YF, Dai JZ, Cai PW: Long-term results of Leksell gamma knife surgery for trigeminal schwannomas. J Neurosurg 2005;102(suppl):220–224.
3 Muthukumar N, Kondziolka D, Lunsford LD, Flickinger JC: Stereotactic radiosurgery for jugular foramen schwannomas. Surg Neurol 1999;52:172–179.
4 Zhang N, Pan L, Dai JZ, Wang BJ, Wang EM, Cai PW: Gamma knife radiosurgery for jugular foramen schwannomas. J Neurosurg 2002;97(suppl 5):456–458.
5 Pollock BE, Foote RL, Stafford SL: Stereotactic radiosurgery: the preferred management for patients with nonvestibular schwannomas? Int J Radiat Oncol Biol Phys 2002;52:1002–1007.
6 Mabanta SR, Buatti JM, Friedman WA, Meeks SL, Mendenhall WM, Bova FJ: Linear accelerator radiosurgery for nonacoustic schwannomas. Int J Radiat Oncol Biol Physics 1999;43: 545–548.
7 Chiou SM, Lunsford LD, Niranjan A, Kondziolka D, Flickinger JC: Stereotactic radiosurgery of residual or recurrent craniopharyngioma, after surgery, with or without radiation therapy. Neuro-Oncol 2001;3:159–166.
8 Hasegawa T, Kondziolka D, Hadjipanayis CG, Lunsford LD: Management of cystic craniopharyngiomas with phosphorus-32 intracavitary irradiation. Neurosurgery 2004;54:813–820; discussion 820–822.
9 Amendola BE, Wolf A, Coy SR, Amendola MA: Role of radiosurgery in craniopharyngiomas: a preliminary report. Med Pediatr Oncol 2003;41:123–127.
10 Ulfarsson E, Lindquist C, Roberts M, Rahn T, Lindquist M, Thoren M, Lippitz B: Gamma knife radiosurgery for craniopharyngiomas: long-term results in the first Swedish patients. J Neurosurg 2002;97(suppl 5):613–622.
11 Chung WY, Pan DH, Shiau CY, Guo WY, Wang LW: Gamma knife radiosurgery for craniopharyngiomas. J Neurosurg 2000;93(suppl 3):47–56.
12 Mokry M: Craniopharyngiomas: a six year experience with Gamma Knife radiosurgery. Stereotact Funct Neurosurg 1999;72(suppl 1):140–149.
13 Pollock BE: Stereotactic radiosurgery in patients with glomus jugulare tumors. Neurosurg Focus 2004;17:E10.
14 Sheehan J, Kondziolka D, Flickinger JC, Lunsford LD: Gamma knife surgery for Glomus Jugulare Tumors: an intermediate report on efficacy and safety. J Neurosurg 2005;102:241–246.
15 Eustacchio S, Leber K, Trummer M, Unger F, Pendl G: Gamma knife radiosurgery for glomus jugulare tumours. Acta Neurochir 1999;141:811–818.
16 Foote RL, Pollock BE, Gorman DA, Schomberg PJ, Stafford SL, Link MJ, Kline RW, Strome SE, Kasperbauer JL, Olsen KD: Glomus jugulare tumor: tumor control and complications after stereotactic radiosurgery. Head Neck 2002;24:332–338; discussion 338–339.
17 Jordan JA, Roland PS, McManus C, Weiner RL, Giller CA: Stereotastic radiosurgery for glomus jugulare tumors. Laryngoscope 2000;110:35–38.
18 Liscak R, Vladyka V, Wowra B, Kemeny A, Forster D, Burzaco JA, Martinez R, Eustacchio S, Pendl G, Regis J, Pellet W: Gamma Knife radiosurgery of the glomus jugulare tumour – early multicentre experience. Acta Neurochir 1999;141:1141–1146.
19 Pollock BE, Foote RL: The evolving role of stereotactic radiosurgery for patients with skull base tumors. J Neuro-Oncol 2004;69:199–207.
20 Lim M, Gibbs IC, Adler JR Jr, Martin DP, Chang SD: The efficacy of linear accelerator stereotactic radiosurgery in treating glomus jugulare tumors. Technol Cancer Res Treat 2003;2: 261–265.
21 Maarouf M, Voges J, Landwehr P, Bramer R, Treuer H, Kocher M, Muller RP, Sturm V: Stereotactic linear accelerater-based radiosurgery for the treatment of patients with glomus jugulare tumors. Cancer 2003;97:1093–1098.
22 Thompson TP, Lunsford LD, Flickinger JC: Radiosurgery for hemangiomas of the cavernous sinus and orbit: technical case report. Neurosurgery 2000;47:778–783.

23 Peker S, Kilic T, Sengoz M, Pamir MN: Radiosurgical treatment of cavernous sinus cavernous haemangiomas. Acta Neurochir 2004;146:337–341; discussion 340.
24 Kida Y, Kobayashi T, Mori Y: Radiosurgery of cavernous hemangiomas in the cavernous sinus. Surg Neurol 2001;56:117–122; discussion 122–123.
25 Nakamura N, Shin M, Tago M, Terahara A, Kurita H, Nakagawa K, Ohtomo K: Gamma knife radiosurgery for cavernous hemangiomas in the cavernous sinus. Report of three cases. J Neurosurg 2002;97(suppl 5):477–480.
26 Chang SD, Meisel JA, Hancock SL, Martin DP, McManus M, Adler JR Jr: Treatment of hemangioblastomas in von Hippel-Lindau disease with linear accelerator-based radiosurgery. Neurosurgery 1998;43:28–34; discussion 34–35.
27 Pan L, Wang EM, Wang BJ, Zhou LF, Zhang N, Cai PW, Da JZ: Gamma knife radiosurgery for hemangioblastomas. Stereotact Funct Neurosurg 1998;70(suppl 1):179–186.
28 Georg AE, Lunsford LD, Kondziolka D, Flickinger JC, Maitz A: Hemangioblastoma of the posterior fossa. The role of multimodality treatment. Arq NeuroPsiquiatr 1997;55:278–286.
29 Niemela M, Lim YJ, Soderman M, Jaaskelainen J, Lindquist C: Gamma knife radiosurgery in 11 hemangioblastomas. J Neurosurg 1996;85:591–596.
30 Patrice SJ, Sneed PK, Flickinger JC, Shrieve DC, Pollock BE, Alexander E 3rd, Larson DA, Kondziolka DS, Gutin PH, Wara WM, McDermott MW, Lunsford LD, Loeffler JS: Radiosurgery for hemangioblastoma: results of a multiinstitutional experience. Int J Radiat Oncol Biol Phys 1996;35:493–499.
31 Chandler HC Jr, Friedman WA: Radiosurgical treatment of a hemangioblastoma: case report. Neurosurgery 1994;34:353–355; discussion 355.
32 Page KA, Wayson K, Steinberg GK, Adler JR Jr: Stereotaxic radiosurgical ablation: an alternative treatment for recurrent and multifocal hemangioblastomas. A report of four cases. Surg Neurol 1993;40:424–428.
33 Jawahar A, Kondziolka D, Garces YI, Flickinger JC, Pollock BE, Lunsford LD: Stereotactic radiosurgery for hemangioblastomas of the brain. Acta Neurochir 2000;142:641–644; discussion 644–645.
34 Muthukumar N, Kondziolka D, Lunsford LD, Flickinger JC: Stereotactic radiosurgery for chordoma and chondrosarcoma: further experiences. Int J Radiat Oncol Biol Phys 1998;41:387–392.
35 Kondziolka D, Lunsford LD, Flickinger JC: The role of radiosurgery in the management of chordoma and chondrosarcoma of the cranial base. Neurosurgery 1991;29:38–45; discussion 45–46.
36 Pamir MN, Kilic T, Ture U, Ozek MM: Multimodality management of 26 skull-base chordomas with 4-year mean follow-up: experience at a single institution. Acta Neurochir 2004;146:343–354; discussion 354.
37 Kocher M, Voges J, Staar S, Treuer H, Sturm V, Mueller RP: Linear accelerator radiosurgery for recurrent malignant tumors of the skull base. Am J Clin Oncol 1998;21:18–22.
38 Miller RC, Foote RL, Coffey RJ, Gorman DA, Earle JD, Schomberg PJ, Kline RW: The role of stereotactic radiosurgery in the treatment of malignant skull base tumors. Int J Radiat Oncol Biol Phys 1997;39:977–981.
39 Debus J, Schulz-Ertner D, Schad L, Essig M, Rhein B, Thillmann CO, Wannenmacher M: Stereotactic fractionated radiotherapy for chordomas and chondrosarcomas of the skull base. Int J Radiat Oncol Biol Phys 2000;47:591–596.
40 Hug EB, Loredo LN, Slater JD, DeVries A, Grove RI, Schaefer RA, Rosenberg AE, Slater JM: Proton radiation therapy for chordomas and chondrosarcomas of the skull base [see comment]. J Neurosurg 1999;91:432–439.
41 Igaki H, Tokuuye K, Okumura T, Sugahara S, Kagei K, Hata M, Ohara K, Hashimoto T, Tsuboi K, Takano S, Matsumura A, Akine Y: Clinical results of proton beam therapy for skull base chordoma. Int J Radiat Oncol Biol Phys 2004;60:1120–1126.
42 Kondziolka D, Lunsford LD: Stereotactic radiosurgery for squamous cell carcinoma of the nasopharynx. Laryngoscope 1991;101:519–522.
43 Firlik KS, Kondziolka D, Lunsford LD, Janecka IP, Flickinger JC: Radiosurgery for recurrent cranial base cancer arising from the head and neck. Head Neck 1996;18:160–165; discussion 166.

44 Chua DT, Sham JS, Kwong PW, Hung KN, Leung LH: Linear accelerator-based stereotactic radiosurgery for limited, locally persistent, and recurrent nasopharyngeal carcinoma: efficacy and complications. Int J Radiat Oncol Biol Phys 2003;56:177–183.
45 Chen HJ, Leung SW, Su CY: Linear accelerator based radiosurgery as a salvage treatment for skull base and intracranial invasion of recurrent nasopharyngeal carcinomas. Am J Clin Oncol 2001;24:255–258.
46 Habermann W, Zanarotti U, Groell R, Wolf G, Stammberger H, Sutter B, Pendl G: Combination of surgery and gamma knife radiosurgery – a therapeutic option for patients with tumors of nasal cavity or paranasal sinuses infiltrating the skull base. Acta Otorhinolaryngol Ital 2002;22:74–79.
47 Lee N, Millender LE, Larson DA, Wara WM, McDermott MW, Kaplan MJ, Sneed PK: Gamma knife radiosurgery for recurrent salivary gland malignancies involving the base of skull. Head Neck 2003;25:210–216.
48 Cmelak AJ, Cox RS, Adler JR, Fee WE Jr, Goffinet DR: Radiosurgery for skull base malignancies and nasopharyngeal carcinoma [see comment]. Int J Radiat Oncol Biol Phys 1997;37:997–1003.
49 Zabel A, Debus J, Thilmann C, Schlegel W, Wannenmacher M: Management of benign cranial nonacoustic schwannomas by fractionated stereotactic radiotherapy. Int J Cancer 2001;96:356–362.
50 Saringer W, Khayal H, Ertl A, Schoeggl A, Kitz K: Efficiency of gamma knife radiosurgery in the treatment of glomus jugulare tumors. Minim Invasive Neurosurg 2001;44:141–146.

L. Dade Lunsford
Department of Neurological Surgery
Suite B-400, University of Pittsburgh Medical Center
200 Lothrop Street
Pittsburgh, PA 15213 (USA)
Tel. +1 412 647 6781, Fax +1 412 647 6483, E-Mail lunsfordld@upmc.edu

Szeifert GT, Kondziolka D, Levivier M, Lunsford LD (eds): Radiosurgery and Pathological Fundamentals. Prog Neurol Surg. Basel, Karger, 2007, vol 20, pp 206–211

10.1.1. Gamma Knife Treatment for Cerebral Arteriovenous Malformations

Andras A. Kemeny, Matthias W.R. Radatz, Jeremy G. Rowe, Lee Walton, Paul Vaughan

National Centre for Stereotactic Radiosurgery, Sheffield, UK

Abstract

One of the earliest indications for Gamma Knife treatment, radiosurgery for cerebral arteriovenous malformations, has stood the test of time. While initially only the ideal cases (small, compact nidus in a non-eloquent site) were chosen, increasingly larger, more complex AVMs were treated. Combination treatment with embolisation and surgery enables most lesions to be treated with success and remarkably low complication rate. This paper is a brief overview of the experience gained in Sheffield.

The first cerebral arteriovenous malformations (AVMs) were treated by Steiner and Backlund in 1970 [1, 2]. In those early presentations and publications the authors established that, when the whole nidus of the malformation received sufficiently high single radiation dose, a thrombo-obliterative process started, leading to an eventual occlusion of the pathological vessels. The histological changes leading to the occlusion are discussed elsewhere in this volume.

The gamma unit in Sheffield was built in 1985 and by the end of 2003 more than 5,000 patients have been treated here [3]. In the first few years the overwhelming majority were treated for vascular indications, and due to this historical practice even in 2003 44% of our annual treatments were for an AVM. This paper is a brief overview of the technique utilised, the results and some of the issues that have arisen over the years using the method.

Material and Methods

Patients

Between September 1985 and December 2003 5,473 patients were treated with the Gamma Knife in Sheffield. Three thousand and ninety-six treatments were for AVM, of which 365 were repeat treatments. The mean age was 36 years (range 1–75). The presentation was haemorrhage (1,918 patients) seizures (370, though another 662 had fits which developed after their bleed), headaches (139) and others including progressive neurological deficits or unrelated symptoms (473). At presentation to us 558 had motor, 277 sensory, 185 cerebellar and 196 visual deficit as a result of their previous haemorrhages and/or surgery. Previous treatments included microsurgery in 21%, endovascular treatment in 13% and both in 5%.

There was a predilection of high-risk territory lesions in our material (14% were in the thalamus or basal ganglia, 3% in the brain stem). The mean nidus size was 4.9 cm^3 (SD 6.9, median 2.3, range 0.1–76 cm^3) but 460 were larger than 10 cm^3. About 64% were Spetzler-Martin (S-M) grade 3 or above.

Radiation Technique

The original RBS Gamma Unit (Nucletec, Switzerland) was replaced with a Gamma Knife Model C (Elekta, Sweden) in 2001. The complexity of planning and thus the conformity to the lesion has increased over the years with the introduction of image corrected digital subtraction angiography, added MRI and the use of GammaPlan (Elekta, Sweden) software.

Median radiation dose to the periphery of the lesion was 25 Gy (range 10–35 Gy). A progressively smaller dose was chosen for larger malformations, in children and after previous radiation treatment to reduce the perceived risk of complications.

The current follow-up protocol is 6-monthly clinical visits supported by MRI/MRA and MRDSA [4] at 2 years, and if no nidus is demonstrated an arterial angiogram. If a residual nidus persists, a second treatment is scheduled at 4 years.

Results

For the purpose of this paper the interim analysis of a smaller subset from 1994 is presented. Of 163 consecutive AVM patients several were abroad and thus not contactable or refused follow-up investigations. We had full data on 122 patients.

Safe obliteration was achieved in 83 of 122 cases (68%), rising to 81% if a later second Gamma Knife treatment was taken into consideration. Substantial reduction but with residual shunt was the result in 25 cases (these were, on the whole, large lesions); 16 were re-treated with the Gamma Knife at a later stage, 13 successfully. Previous embolisation worsened the outcome ($p = 0.017$). The main factor in outcome prediction was size and thus S-M grade. In S-M grade 1 85% of lesions were obliterated by 1 year.

Nine of the 122 (7.4%) had neurological complications (visual field deficit or hemiparesis), but only 5 (4.1%) permanent. In addition, there were 3 non-fatal

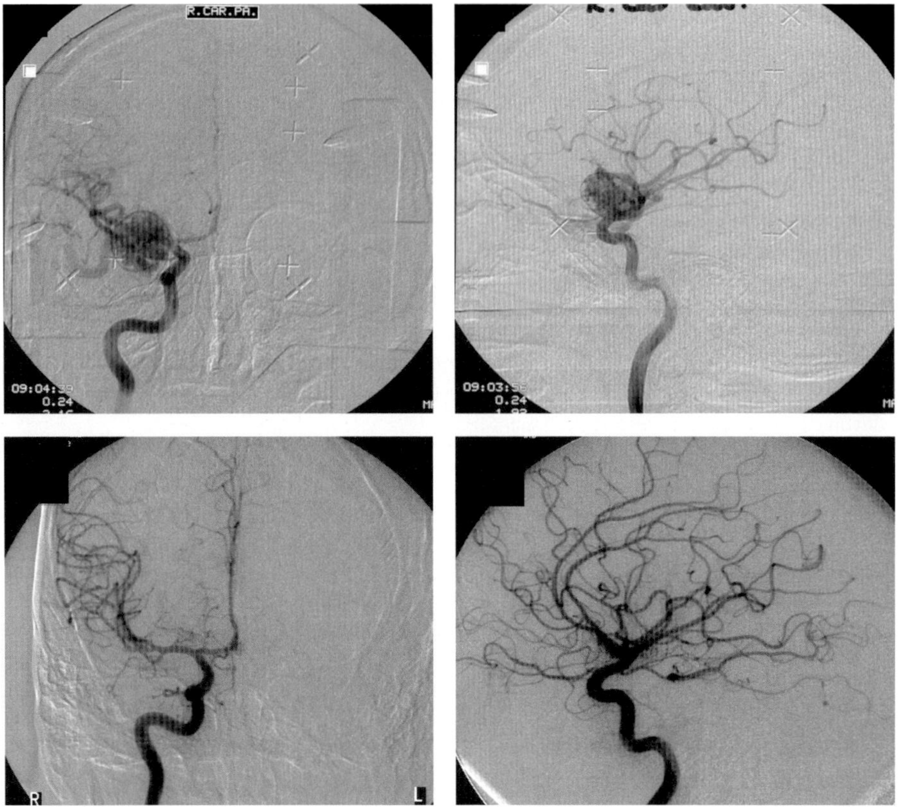

Fig. 1. A typical cerebral AVM with a small and compact nidus. ***a***, ***b*** Appearance on angiography at the time of treatment. ***c***, ***d*** Two-year follow-up result: complete occlusion.

bleeds. There was a 10-year mortality of 2/163 (1.2%), though only one death (0.6%) was due to an AVM bleed and none due to the treatment.

Discussion

The ideal AVM case for radiosurgical treatment is a patient with a small compact and noneloquently placed nidus, particularly if deep seated to make it surgically less attractive (fig. 1).

Since the start of the radiosurgical program increasingly larger and larger malformations were accepted for treatment. Pushing the boundaries upwards, beyond the usually accepted 3-cm diameter, meant a reduction of the dose that could be safely delivered.

The shape of the lesion is an important criterion in patient selection. A craggy irregular lesion is more difficult to plan than a smooth regular one, even though GammaPlan allows intricate plans. The other shape-related factor is the proportion of different diameters. A thin flat nidus does not lend itself to planning when the plan means overlapping several near-spherical treatment fields to match the shape.

It is also important that the margins of the nidus should be readily identifiable. Diffuse malformations are not only difficult to delineate but, because within the outlined target volume some normal parenchyma may be included, the risk of treatment may be higher. The same effect hinders treatment of post-embolisation cases and the outcome seems to be worse. Axial imaging may help to some extent and this effect is under study. We feel that high-quality digital subtraction angiography is necessary even for assessment of suitability for most cases. This allows for the assessment of the nidus and the speed of flow, excluding direct fistulae that would not be expected to respond. For treatment planning we use the combination of angiography and MRI though others reported good experience with axial imaging alone.

The management of small non-eloquent AVMs is controversial. A comparison between an excellent surgical series and a meta-analysis of published radiosurgery results for low surgical risk AVMs [5] found that, if the analysis of the latter included the statistical risk of haemorrhage during the latent period, mortality of surgery appeared better. However, the rate of new or worsened deficits after surgery was 27.4% – a figure many times that of Gamma Knife-treated patients.

Management of large and eloquent AVMs is less controversial: no treatment modality claims high rate of success in isolation. Lesions with high S-M grade have a high neurosurgical risk [6], leading to not infrequent post-surgical remnants particularly with AVMs located in the thalamus, basal ganglia and brainstem [7]. The supportive role of endovascular treatment has been identified over the past decade, aiming at durable and sequential reduction of the nidus. Whereas a few decades ago this was invariably followed by excision of the remnant, increasingly a radiosurgical treatment follows embolisation. At all stages of sequential treatment of these difficult malformations, all three active interventions should be considered [8]. Sequential treatments may require several endovascular interventions followed by one or more radiosurgical treatments and in some the last remnant, particularly if superficial, may be removed surgically.

The outcome of radiosurgery after previous embolisation was significantly worse than without previous treatment, even stratified for size. Surgery has no such negative effect. Similar observation was made by others [9]. The reasons for this include a possible selection bias, a poorer definition of the nidus margin resulting in suboptimal planning and recanalisation of the embolised part, not seen on angiography at the time of treatment. Whether the use of new materials, e.g. Onyx, will prevent these effects, remains to be seen.

The other option for these large lesions is to use sequential radiosurgery without other modalities. First, one can repeat treatment for the remnant after 2–4 years. Second, one could treat the whole lesion with a small number of fractions, though fully fractionated treatment has been largely unsuccessful in the past. Hypofractionation, a small number of fractions, may allow safe delivery of a therapeutic dose without compromising efficacy. A third alternative is to treat different parts of the large nidus each time, leaving a few months between treatments. Good results have been reported with such segmental radiosurgery [10]. Finally, selective radiosensitization of the pathological vessels is being explored.

About 30% of AVM patients have MRI changes adjacent to or within the irradiated volume at a median of 8 months after radiosurgery due to a combination of altered peri-lesional blood flow, the rising of transluminal pressure as the nidus gradually obliterates and the blood brain barrier disruption with transudation of plasma proteins. Clinical side effects are less frequent. About 8% of patients develop neurological sequelae [11], such as focal neurological deficit, cranial nerve abnormalities, seizures. More than half resolve completely although this may take up to 3 years. Delayed malignancy in the treated volume is extremely rare. Formation of a pseudocyst several years after treatment may occur, in our experience approximately in 0.1%, and with careful imaging, planning and targeting it may well be avoidable. Complication rates increase with larger radiation doses and treated volumes. Clinical symptoms depend even more upon the site of the nidus. They are treated with marsupialisation.

The difficulties finding the necessary data for retrospective analysis include lost follow-up as a result of overseas residence, lack of interest by the patients and their physicians to adhere to protocols and patients moving away without forwarding address. However, the most common obstacle is the refusal for patients to undergo the gold standard angiography once they finished a treatment which, at least in their mind and based on axial imaging, has been successful.

Conclusions

Gamma Knife radiosurgery for cerebral AVMs is an important tool in our armamentarium and should be available either locally or by a referral to a specialist centre. It is mandatory that before any treatment (other than emergency surgery for a haematoma) is undertaken, all modalities should be considered by a multidisciplinary team.

Acknowledgements

Gamma Knife radiosurgery in general and the National Centre for Stereotactic Radiosurgery in Sheffield in particular benefited greatly from the pioneering work of David M.C. Forster who was the director of this facility until his retirement in 2001. His vision of the future role of this technique, his enthusiasm, and his dedication to the thoughtful and honest ongoing appraisal of the method are acknowledged by this note.

References

1 Steiner L, Leksell L, Greitz T, Forster DM, Backlund EO: Stereotaxic radiosurgery for cerebral arteriovenous malformations. Report of a case. Acta Chir Scand 1972;138:459–464.
2 Steiner L, Leksell L, Forster DM, Greitz T, Backlund EO: Stereotactic radiosurgery in intracranial arterio-venous malformations. Acta Neurochir 1974;(suppl 21):195–209.
3 Kemeny AA, Radatz MWR, Rowe JG, Walton L, Hampshire A: Gamma knife radiosurgery for cerebral arteriovenous malformations. Acta Neurochir 2004;(suppl)91:55–63.
4 Coley SC, Wild JM, Wilkinson ID, Griffiths PD: Neurovascular MRI with dynamic contrast-enhanced subtraction angiography. Neuroradiology 2003;45:843–850.
5 Schaller C, Schramm J: Microsurgical results for small arteriovenous malformations accessible for radiosurgical or embolisation treatment. Neurosurgery 1997;40:664–672.
6 Morgan MK, Drummond KJ, Grinnel IV, Sorby W: Surgery for cerebral arteriovenous malformation: risks related to lenticulostriate arterial supply. J Neurosurg 1997;86:801–805.
7 Lawton MT, Hamilton MG, Spetzler RE: Multimodality treatment of deep arteriovenous malformations: thalamus, basal ganglia, and brain stem. Neurosurgery 1995;37:29–36.
8 Smith KA, Shetter A, Speiser B, Spetzler RF: Angiographic follow-up in 37 patients after radiosurgery for cerebral arteriovenous malformations as part of a multimodality treatment approach. Stereotact Funct Neurosurg 1997;69:136–142.
9 Pollock BE, Flickinger JC, Lunsford LD, Maitz A, Kondziolka D: Factors associated with successful arteriovenous malformation radiosurgery. Neurosurgery 1998;42:1239–1244.
10 Pollock BE, Kline RW, Stafford SL, Foote RL, Schomberg PJ: The rationale and technique of staged-volume arteriovenous malformation radiosurgery. Int J Radiat Oncol Biol Phys 2000;48: 817–824.
11 Flickinger JC, Kondziolka D, Lunsford LD, et al: A multi-institutional analysis of complication outcomes after arterio-venous malformation radiosurgery. Int J Radiat Oncol Biol Phys 1999;44: 67–74.

Andras A. Kemeny, FRCS, MD
National Centre for Stereotactic Radiosurgery
Royal Hallamshire Hospital, Glossop Road
Sheffield S10 2JF (UK)
Tel. +44 114 271 3572, Fax +44 114 275 4930, E-Mail a.kemeny@shef.ac.uk

Szeifert GT, Kondziolka D, Levivier M, Lunsford LD (eds): Radiosurgery and Pathological Fundamentals. Prog Neurol Surg. Basel, Karger, 2007, vol 20, pp 212–219

10.1.2. Histopathological Changes in Cerebral Arteriovenous Malformations following Gamma Knife Radiosurgery

György T. Szeifert[a], *Walter R. Timperley*[b], *David M.C. Forster*[b], *Andras A. Kemeny*[b]

[a]National Institute of Neurosurgery, and Department of Neurological Surgery, Semmelweis University, Budapest, Hungary; [b]National Centre for Stereotactic Radiosurgery, Department of Neurological Surgery, Royal Hallamshire Hospital, Sheffield, UK

Abstract

Histological, immunohistochemical and electron microscopic investigations were carried out in a series of surgical pathology material that was removed from 7 patients. They were harboring cerebral arteriovenous malformations (AVMs) that had been previously treated with Leksell Gamma Knife radiosurgery, and presented subsequent bleeding 10–52 months after treatment. Light microscopic studies revealed a spindle cell proliferation in the connective tissue stroma and in the subendothelial region of the irradiated AVM vessels. The histological, immunohistochemical and ultrastructural characteristics of the spindle cell population in the Leksell Gamma Knife-treated AVMs are similar to those designated as myofibroblasts in wound healing processes and pathological fibromatoses. Considering that similar cell modifications have not been demonstrated in control, nonirradiated AVM specimens, these myofibroblasts might contribute to the shrinking process and final occlusion of AVMs after radiosurgery.

Arteriovenous malformations (AVMs) of the brain have been regarded as hamartomatous lesions originating from embryonic maldevelopment [1, 2].

Histologically, they are characterized by clusters of abnormal arteries and arterialized veins with irregular vessel wall structure, and without intervening capillary bed. Morphological characteristics of pathological vessels in cerebral AVMs have been studied extensively by previous investigators [1–5], but there is much to learn about the obliteration mechanism in AVMs after radiosurgery. Sophisticated investigational techniques are required. Details of the fine morphological alterations at subcellular level evoked by the ionizing radiation of radiosurgery in AVMs have never been demonstrated. Therefore, the purpose of this study was to present the findings of histological, immunohistochemical and transmission electron microscopic investigations on tissue and ultrastructural architecture of subtotally obliterated AVMs after Gamma Knife surgery (GKS).

Material and Methods

Pathological material was obtained in 7 patients who had undergone GKS for AVMs but who suffered rebleeding 10–52 months after treatment. The resected specimens were fixed in 10% neutral buffered formaldehyde, processed routinely, and embedded in paraffin. Besides the routine HE, elastic van Gieson and Masson trichrome staining, immunohistochemical reactions were performed on 5-μm sections to study desmin (D), vimentin (V), α-smooth muscle actin (A), S100 protein, glial fibrillary acidic protein, and factor VIII-related antigens in the cell populations of malformations after irradiation. Double immunoenzymatic labeling with peroxidase and alkaline phosphatase for A/V, A/D and V/D was also performed to demonstrate the presence of both antigens in the same cell. Tissue samples from five resected AVMs which were not treated with GKS served as nonirradiated controls. For transmission electron microscopic investigations the specimens were reembedded in araldite from the original paraffin-embedded material, cut, and stained with uranyl acetate and lead citrate.

Results

Light microscopy revealed different stages of tissue reactions apparently starting with granulation tissue formation, followed by a spindle cell infiltration, and ending with scar tissue replacement and hyaline degeneration. Both proliferative and degenerative changes were observed in the abnormal vessels' walls and in the connective tissue stroma, which were not seen in the nonirradiated control specimens. The most prominent proliferative change was granulation tissue accumulation infiltrated by inflammatory cells as well as a spindle cell proliferation in the connective tissue stroma and in the subendothelial region of the irradiated AVM vessels (fig. 1a). Vascular channels that had undergone total obliteration were completely replaced by degenerated hyaline scar tissue, and only the vessels' contour was recognizable without any identifiable lumina (fig. 1b).

Immunohistochemical reactions demonstrated marked A positivity in the spindle stromal cells. The V and D reactions were also positive but with less intensity compared to the A activity. Using double labeling V/D positivity was revealed on the same spindle cells (fig. 1c). With the A/V and A/D double reactions, only the A positivity was detected, probably because of the vigorous intensity of this antigen masking the fainter D and V antigen expression. The stromal spindle cell proliferation was closely related to the adventitial layer of the vessels. V positivity was more pronounced in the scar tissue areas. The antigen profile of the subendothelial proliferating spindle cells showed strong A positivity, whereas activity of V and D was less marked. Factor VIII-related antigen was expressed by the lining endothelial cells in a considerably reduced proportion of the vessels. Higher percentage of the vessels did not reveal any endothelial activity at all. Glial fibrillary acidic protein and S100 protein were demonstrated in the glial cells of the surrounding brain parenchyma but not in the stromal cells or vessels of the AVMS. In the early stages after irradiation, granulation tissue formation and spindle cell proliferation were more prominent, whereas in the later stages, collagen production and hyalinization were more pronounced.

Electron microscopy demonstrated different ultrastructural characteristics in the spindle cell population. There were cells demonstrating features of typical conventional resting fibroblasts with oval nuclei and a smooth contour as well as cisterns of endoplasmic reticulum. These cell types were usually surrounded by massive bundles of collagen fibers in the extracellular matrix (fig. 2a). Other cells with similar nuclear morphology contained abundant intracytoplasmic filaments (fig. 2b), and sometimes prominent nucleoli (fig. 2c). Nuclear deformations were connected with abundant cytoplasmic organelles – well-developed rough endoplasmic reticulum (fig 2d). In modified fibroblasts with folds and indentations on the nuclear contour, a striking fibrillary system developed within the cytoplasm, and its peripheral attachment sites were related to an extracellular layer of basement membrane-like material arranged parallel to the cellular border (fig. 2e). These bundles of packed intracytoplasmic fibrils were very similar to those generally expressed by smooth-muscle cells. Also present were unusual fibroblastic cells containing well-developed cisterns of rough endoplasmic reticulum and dense bodies at the periphery of the cytoplasm with wrinkled, irregular nuclei. These ultrastructural characteristics with the abundant intracytoplasmic filamentary system and nuclear deformities reflect morphological consequences of a contractile activity.

Fig. 2. Transmission electron microscopic findings. ***a*** Thick bundles of collagen in the extracellular matrix (×8,000). ***b*** Conventional fibroblast with smooth oval nucleus (×10,000). ***c*** Abundant cytoplasmic filaments and prominent nucleolus (×10,000). ***d*** Modified fibroblast, that is myofibroblast expressing large amounts of intracytoplasmic filaments and irregular folded nucleus (×10,000). ***e*** Modified fibroblast demonstrating well-developed rough endoplasmic reticulum and nuclear deformation (×12,000).

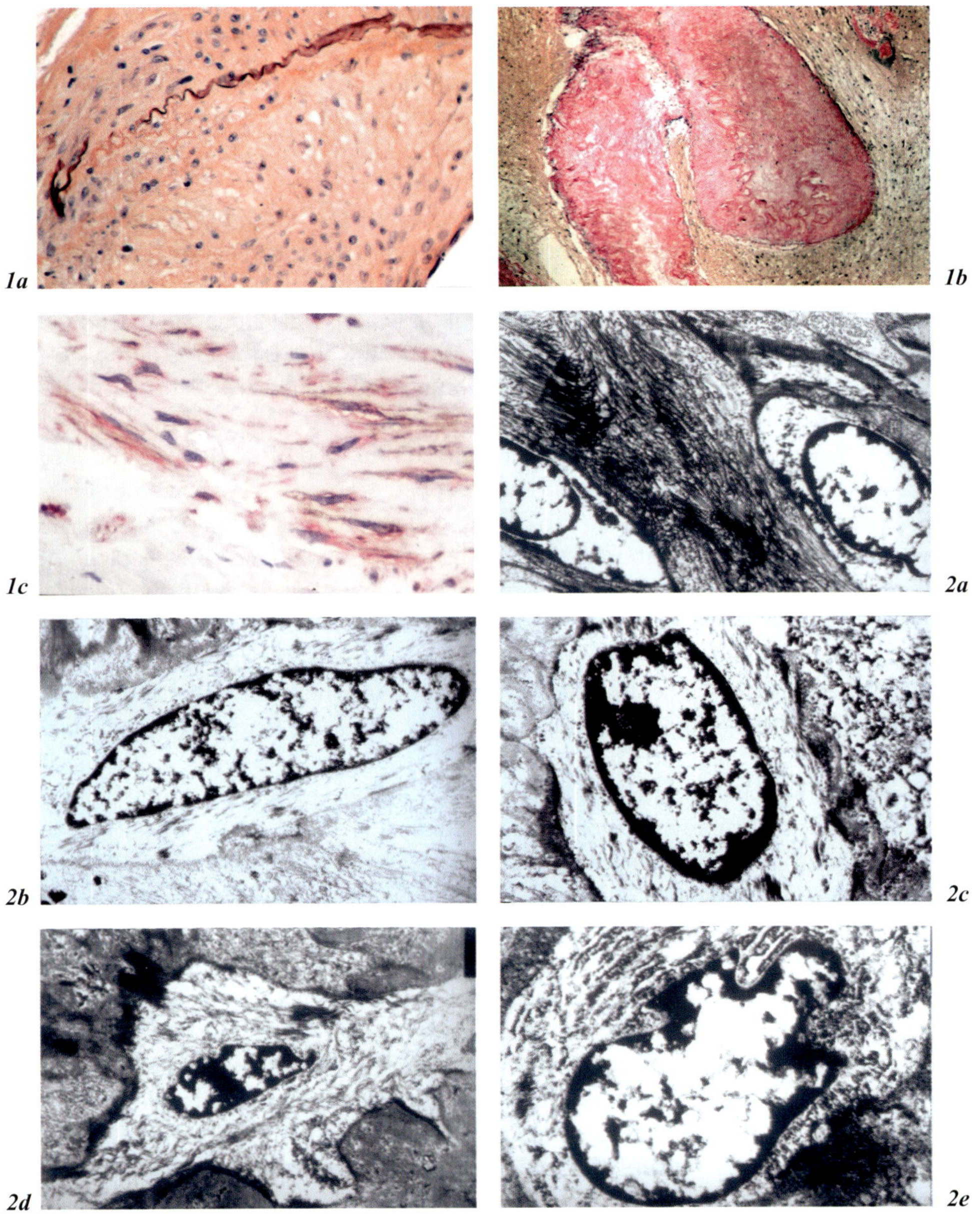

Fig. 1. Light microscopic observations. ***a*** Prominent spindle cell proliferation in the subendothelial region of an AVM vessel's wall (elastic van Gieson, ×200). ***b*** Completely obliterated AVM vessels replaced by hyaline degenerated scar tissue, none with lumen discernible (elastic van Gieson, ×100). ***c*** D/V double immunohistochemical expression on the same spindle cells (brown: D; red: V; blue: nuclear staining); ×400.

Discussion

Since the first report by Steiner et al., in 1972 [6], stereotactic radiosurgery has become an effective and widely accepted method for the treatment of selected cerebral AVMs when using either the Leksell Gamma Knife [7], or a linear accelerator [8]. The goal of stereotactic radiosurgery in the management of cerebral AVMs is to obliterate the nidus completely to eliminate the risk of hemorrhage. Radiosurgery was originally invented to treat functional disorders [9]. Soon after its development AVMs became one of the major indications, providing a new tool for the treatment of brain lesions in regions where surgical access was unacceptably risky [10, 11]. MRI and angiographic studies have documented that 65–87% of AVMs are obliterated, and that 75% shrink in volume 2–5 years after radiosurgery [12].

Following Virchow's fundamental work on the pathological description of vascular brain lesions [13], the current histopathological classification of cerebral vascular malformations into AVMs, cavernomas, teleangiectasias and venous anomalies was elaborated by McCormick [14]. Although the histology of abnormal vessels in AVMs has been demonstrated previously, relatively little has been known about the pathological response of AVMs to a single high-dose ionizing radiation treatment. Recently a few authors have described histopathological changes in the vessels of cerebral AVMs following radiosurgery [15–19]. According to these light microscopic studies, there are various parenchymal stages of vessel occlusion and connective tissue stroma changes in AVMs. It seems that both proliferative and degenerative changes contribute to the obliteration process. The early reaction from the connective tissue stroma of an AVM is formation of granulation tissue infiltrated by chronic inflammatory cells. Later, a spindle cell population follows the granulation tissue and, in turn, is replaced by a hypocellular, hyaline degenerated scar tissue, which is the stable end result of the obliteration process. The parenchymal vessel occlusion starts with endothelial destruction followed by subendothelial and perivascular spindle cell proliferation. These spindle cells express immunohistochemical characteristics resembling those of myofibroblasts, and they have a contractile capacity through smooth-muscle actin production. In later stages conventional resting fibroblasts and fibrocytes produce collagen bundles to replace the myofibroblasts. The collagen fibers undergo hyaline degeneration and form scar tissue, which supplements and stabilizes the AVM vessels, thus obliterating the lumen 'safely'. The hyalinized scar tissue does not have a propensity for neovascularization.

The findings of the present electron microscopic study underscore and extend previous light microscopic observations regarding the origin and nature of the spindle cell population in AVM parenchymal vessels and connective tissue stroma, which contribute to the obliteration process following radiosurgery.

The ultrastructural characteristics of these spindle cells are similar to those of modified fibroblasts or myofibroblasts. They have a dual capacity to produce collagen fibers and contractile elements such as smooth-muscle actin as well. The nuclear morphology and fine architecture of these cells also suggest contractile activity. They could be transformed from conventional resting fibroblasts triggered by the ionizing energy of high-dose irradiation. The contractile capacity can promote vessel occlusion and final volume reduction. The collagen production undergoing hyaline degeneration might complete and stabilize AVM obliteration after radiosurgery.

As stated previously, there is a latent interval of some years between treatment and occlusion of an AVM. It is still not clear from the different series whether there is a significant change in the risk of hemorrhage during the latency period. The risk is higher for larger AVMs and for older patients, and is lower when higher-dose radiation is used [20, 21]. Another issue is that the total obliteration of the nidus verified on negative angiography has been until recently considered definitive evidence of cure after radiosurgical treatment of an AVM [22, 23]. In newer studies, a few cases have been reported with recurrent hemorrhage after angiographic confirmation of AVM occlusion [24–26].

Indirectly, the results of the current study might suggest how this could happen. During the obliteration process there might be thrombus evolution, which plugs the lumen and precludes the filling of the vessel at the time of angiography. This occlusion could be responsible for the normal angiogram, and the patient might be thought to be 'cured'; however, thrombi may undergo recanalization. The newly formed vessels usually possess an abnormal, disorganized, thin, fragile wall structure which might serve as a pathological basis for potential rupture and rebleeding contrary to the normal-appearing angiograms. Therefore, these vessels might be regarded as 'nonsafely' obliterated channels as long as the organization of thrombi has not been completed by granulation tissue followed by scar tissue replacement. It is emphasized that it is hyalinization of the scar tissue that finally stabilizes the thrombo-obliteration process.

Regular neurological and radiological follow-up examination (contrast-enhanced MRI and MR angiography at 6-month intervals until the disappearance of contrast enhancement) is recommended for radiosurgery-treated patients with AVMs. The abundant capillary content of the granulation tissue probably supplies background for the arterial blush on control angiograms and for the contrast enhancement on the CT and MR images as well. The proliferation of granulation tissue might also explain the increased metabolic activity of the AVM region after radiosurgery because an increase in activity has been detected by PET [25]. Its disappearance indicates the maturation of the scar-forming process. The role of combined MRI and PET follow-up examinations should be considered in the future. This sensitive imaging technique provides independent metabolic data that are complementary to the anatomical information of angiography, CT, or MRI [27, 28]. With these sophisticated methods, we might be able to detect metabolic activity of angiographically occult, invisible, but as yet unsafe and only seemingly obliterated AVMs.

Conclusions

Histopathological, immunohistochemical and electron microscopic studies suggest that after GKS a proliferation of myofibroblastic-like cells develops with contractile properties. The cytoskeletal and ultrastuctural characteristics of these cells closely resemble the appearance of conventional myofibroblasts [29], and their contractility may contribute to AVM occlusion and final volume reduction.

References

1 Dandy W: Arteriovenous aneurysm of the brain. Arch Surg 1928;17:190–243.

2 Olivecrona H, Landenheim J: Congenital Arteriovenous Aneurysms of the Carotid and Vertebral Arterial Systems. Berlin, Springer, 1957.

3 Isoda K, Fukuda H, Takamura N, et al: Arteriovenous malformation of the brain: histological study and micrometric measurement of abnormal vessels. Acta Pathol Jpn 1981;31:883–893.

4 Mandybur TI, Nazek M: Cerebral arteriovenous malformations: a detailed morphological and immunohistochemical study using actin. Arch Pathol Lab Med 1990;114:970–973.

5 Wong JH, Awad IA, Kim JH: Ultrastructural pathological features of cerebrovascular malformations: a preliminary report. Neurosurgery 2000;46:1454–1459.

6 Steiner L, Leksell L, Greitz T, et al: Stereotaxic radiosurgery for cerebral arteriovenous malformations. Report of a case. Acta Chir Scand 1972;138:459–464.

7 Lunsford LD, Kondziolka D, Flickinger JC, et al: Stereotactic radiosurgery for arteriovenous malformations of the brain. J Neurosurg 1991;75:512–524.

8 Friedman WA, Bova FJ: Linear accelerator radiosurgery for arteriovenous malformations. J Neurosurg 1992;77:832–841.

9 Leksell L: Cerebral radiosurgery. I. Gamma thalamotomy in two cases of intractable pain. Acta Chir Scand 1968;134:585–595.

10 Marujama K, Kondziolka D, Niranjan A, et al: Stereotactic radiosurgery for brainstem arteriovenous malformations: factors affecting outcome. J Neurosurg 2004;100:407–413.

11 Massager N, Regis J, Kondziolka D, et al: Gamma knife radiosurgery for brainstem arteriovenous malformations: preliminary results. J Neurosurg 2000;93(suppl 3):102–103.

12 Szeifert GT, Major O, Fazekas I, et al: Effects of radiation on cerebral vasculature: a review. Neurosurgery 2001;48:452–453.

13 Virchow R: Die krankhaften Geschwülste: Dreissig Vorlesungen, gehalten während des Wintersemesters 1862–1863 an der Universität zu Berlin. Berlin, Hirschwald, 1863.

14 McCormick WF: The pathology of vascular ('arteriovenous') malformations. J Neurosurg 1966;24: 807–816.

15 Schneider BF, Eberhard DA, Steiner LE: Histopathology of arteriovenous malformations after gamma knife radiosurgery. J Neurosurg 1997;87:352–357.

16 Szeifert GT: Radiosurgery and AVM histopathology. J Neurosurg 1998;88:356–357.
17 Szeifert GT, Kemeny AA, Timperley WR, et al: The potential role of myofibroblasts in the obliteration of arteriovenous malformations after radiosurgery. Neurosurgery 1997;40:61–65; discussion 65–66.
18 Yamamoto M, Jimbo M, Ide M, et al: Gamma knife radiosurgery for cerebral arteriovenous malformations: an autopsy report focusing on irradiation-induced changes observed in nidus-unrelated arteries. Surg Neurol 1995;44:421–427.
19 Yamamoto M, Jimbo M, Kobayashi M, et al: Long-term results of radiosurgery for arteriovenous malformation: neurodiagnostic imaging and histological studies of angiographically confirmed nidus obliteration. Surg Neurol 1992;37:219–230.
20 Friedman WA, Blatt DL, Bova FJ, et al: The risk of hemorrhage after radiosurgery for arteriovenous malformations. J Neurosurg 1996;84:912–919.
21 Karlsson B, Lax I, Soderman M: Risk for hemorrhage during the 2-year latency period following gamma knife radiosurgery for arteriovenous malformations. Int J Radiat Oncol Biol Phys 2001;49: 1045–1051.
22 Levrier O, Manera L, Regis J, et al: Advances in the contributions of imaging to stereotaxic localization of cerebral arteriovenous malformations for radiosurgery. Neurochirurgie 2001;47:201–211.
23 Lindquist C, Steiner L: Stereotactic radiosurgical treatment of arteriovenous malformations; in Lunsford LD (ed): Modern Stereotactic Neurosurgery. Boston, Nijhoff, 1988, pp 491–505.
24 Lindqvist M, Karlsson B, Guo WY, et al: Angiographic long-term follow-up data for arteriovenous malformations previously proven to be obliterated after gamma knife radiosurgery. Neurosurgery 2000;46:803–808; discussion 809–810.
25 Szeifert GT, Salmon I, Baleriaux D, et al: Immunohistochemical analysis of a cerebral arteriovenous malformation obliterated by radiosurgery and presenting with re-bleeding. Case report. Neurol Res 2003;25:718–721.
26 Yamamoto M, Jimbo M, Hara M, et al: Gamma knife radiosurgery for arteriovenous malformations: long-term follow-up results focusing on complications occurring more than 5 years after irradiation. Neurosurgery 1996;38:906–914.
27 Levivier M, Wikier D, Goldman S, et al: Integration of the metabolic data of positron emission tomography in the dosimetry planning of radiosurgery with the gamma knife: early experience with brain tumors. Technical note. J Neurosurg 2000;93(suppl 3):233–238.
28 Levivier M, Wikler D Jr, Massager N, et al: The integration of metabolic imaging in stereotactic procedures including radiosurgery: a review. J Neurosurg 2002;97:542–550.
29 Gabbiani G, Ryan GB, Majno G: Presence of modified fibroblasts in granulation tissue and their possible role in wound contraction. Experientia 1971;27:549–550.

György T. Szeifert, MD, PhD
Centre Gamma Knife, Hôpital Académique Erasme, Université Libre de Bruxelles
Route de Lennik 808
BE–1070 Brussels (Belgium)
Tel. +32 2 555 3174, Fax +32 2 555 3176, E-Mail gyorgyszeifert@yahoo.com

Szeifert GT, Kondziolka D, Levivier M, Lunsford LD (eds): Radiosurgery and Pathological Fundamentals. Prog Neurol Surg. Basel, Karger, 2007, vol 20, pp 220–230

10.2.1. Radiosurgery for Cavernous Malformations

Douglas Kondziolka[a,b,d], *John C. Flickinger*[a,b,d], *L. Dade Lunsford*[a–d]

Departments of [a]Neurological Surgery, [b]Radiation Oncology and [c]Radiology and [d]The Center for Image-Guided Neurosurgery, University of Pittsburgh, Pittsburgh, Pa., USA

Abstract

The role of radiosurgery for cavernous malformations of the brain remains to be fully defined. We have used Gamma Knife radiosurgery for selected patients with symptomatic, hemorrhagic malformations in high-risk brain locations. Indications, techniques, and results are presented.

The management of patients with brain cavernous malformations (angiographically occult vascular malformations, cavernous angiomas, cavernomas) remains controversial. Since the mid 1980s there has been an improved understanding of their natural history [1, 9, 15, 18, 24, 30, 33, 36], as well as documented experience with surgical resection [3, 5, 10, 31, 35, 37]. In the case of an arteriovenous malformation (AVM), the elimination of the angiographically identifiable anatomic shunt can be demonstrated on imaging and correlates highly with cure. However, since a cavernous malformation cannot be defined by angiography, complete obliteration of the malformation vessels cannot be confirmed with imaging. Because some patients have cavernous malformations that are not amenable to surgical resection with acceptable risk, alternative strategies are sought. When such malformations repeatedly bleed they warrant management. Radiosurgery is the only potential alternative to resection.

Stereotactic radiosurgery can provide a reduction in hemorrhage risk after an initial latency interval [2, 6, 8, 12–14, 17, 19, 22, 23, 29] for patients with high-risk cavernous malformations. Our observations confirm the hypothesis that

Table 1. Locations of 112 cavernous malformations selected for radiosurgery

Location	Malformations
Pons/midbrain	62
Thalamus	12
Medulla	10
Temporal lobe	6
Parietal lobe	5
Basal ganglia	8
Frontal lobe	4
Cerebellum	4
Occipital lobe	1

radiosurgical intervention reduces subsequent bleeding rates. The microvasculature of a cavernous malformation ultimately responds to radiosurgery in the same way AVMs respond [20]. However, unlike with AVMs, there is little pathological material that has been studied. Without an imaging correlate of risk elimination, clinical follow-up remains the standard by which radiosurgery must be judged.

University of Pittsburgh Experience

High-risk cavernous malformations were managed with stereotactic radiosurgery at the University of Pittsburgh between 1987 and 2004 in a total of 112 patients. The mean age was 39 years (range 4–81 years). Almost all patients had multiple hemorrhages (range 2–9, mean = 2.6), while some suffered a single imaging-confirmed hemorrhage but had a subsequent stepwise decline in neurological function. A hemorrhage was defined as a symptomatic, ictal event that consisted of new neurological symptoms or deficits and imaging confirmation of new blood on MRI or CT. Patients were selected for radiosurgery when the malformation caused functional deterioration due to hemorrhage. Four patients had seizures. In general, the lesions tended to be located in critical brain regions as demonstrated in table 1. Prior to radiosurgery, 30% of patients had surgical interventions that included attempted malformation resection, clot evacuation, biopsy, or shunt placement. One patient had proton beam irradiation and Gamma Knife radiosurgery prior to care at our Center.

Radiosurgical Technique

Prior to radiosurgery, all patients underwent MRI to ensure that the lesion was a typical cavernous malformation. Typically, MRI showed mixed signal change within an outer hemosiderin ring of low signal intensity [25, 32] (fig. 1).

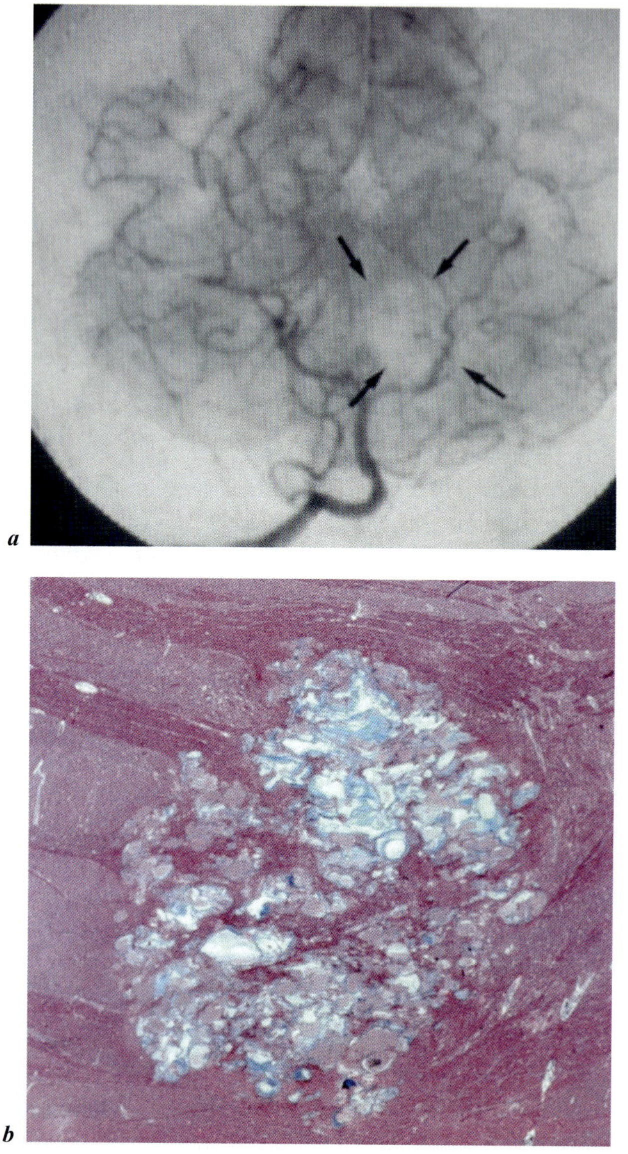

Fig. 1. ***a*** Vertebral artery angiogram showing a region of absent perfusion (arrows) indicating the presence of a cavernous malformation. ***b*** Histological preparation showing a cavernous malformation within the pons.

If there was any question about the diagnosis, angiography was performed to exclude an AVM or associated venous malformation.

Radiosurgery was performed with the use of the Leksell Model G stereotactic frame (Elekta Instruments, Atlanta, Ga., USA). The frame was applied after mild sedation and local anesthesia was administered. General anesthesia was reserved for patients under 12 years of age. After frame application, all patients had stereotactic imaging. CT was used for planning in all patients prior to 1990. Patients treated from 1988 through 1992 had both CT and MRI. Since 1992, stereotactic MRI alone has been utilized, because MRI was superior to CT in defining cavernous malformations and equally accurate. A sagittal short-repetition time (TR) scout image acquisition was obtained, followed by axial short- and long-TR images obtained at 3-mm image intervals. Finally, repeat axial and coronal short-TR images with volume acquisitions (1- to 1.5-mm slices) and contrast enhancement were obtained.

Images were transferred to the dose planning workstation of the Gamma Knife (GammaPlan®, Elekta Instruments, Atlanta, Ga., USA). Single or multiple isocenter (range 1–9) plans were constructed to give a conformal and selective irradiation volume for the cavernous malformation margin (fig. 2). The mean number of isocenters was 3.3. The target nidus was defined as the region characterized by mixed signal change within the outer hemosiderin ring, typically of low signal intensity. Hematoma eccentric from the malformation was excluded from dose planning. In all patients in this series, the 50% isodose or greater was used for the target margin. The average radiosurgery dose was lower than that used for AVMs, but dependent on the location and volume of the cavernous malformation [12, 17]. The mean volume was 2.37 ml (range 0.12–9.5 ml), while the mean maximum and marginal doses were 30 Gy (maximum = 40 Gy) and 16 Gy (maximum = 20 Gy), respectively. Radiosurgery was performed with a 201-source cobalt-60 Leksell Gamma Knife, Models U, B, or C (Elekta Instruments, Atlanta, Ga., USA). After radiosurgery, all patients received 40 mg methylprednisolone and were discharged from the hospital within 24 h.

Follow-up

Clinical follow-up data were obtained from either the patients or their referring physicians if they lived at a distance from Pittsburgh. Where necessary, patients were contacted by telephone to update their outcome for the purposes of this study. Imaging follow-up was requested at 6-month intervals for the first 2 years after radiosurgery, and then annually. The following equation was used to determine hemorrhage rates: rate = total hemorrhages observed/total patient-years observed.

Hemorrhage rates were compared before and after radiosurgical intervention using a paired t test. A hemorrhage was defined as a new neurological symptom or sign associated with new blood detected on MRI.

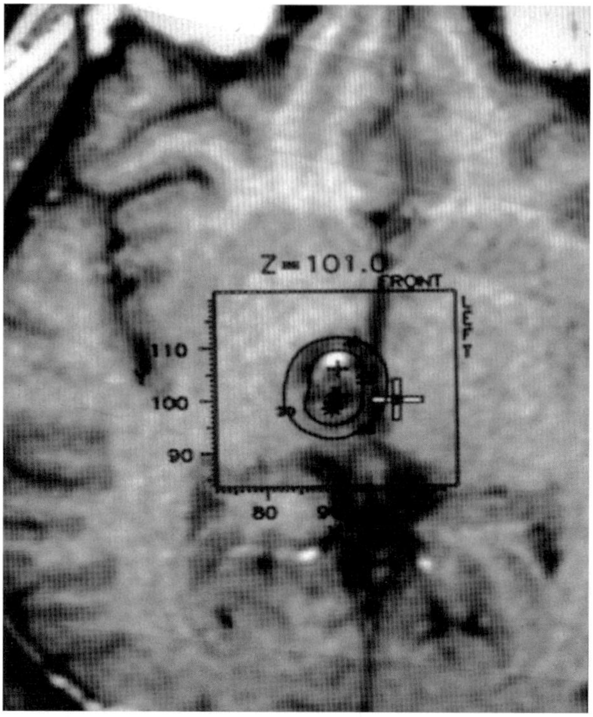

Fig. 2. Axial MRI at radiosurgery in a young man who had two prior thalamic hemorrhages from a cavernous malformation. Gamma Knife radiosurgery was performed with three 8-mm isocenters. Ten years after radiosurgery, he has had no further hemorrhages or additional neurologic symptoms.

Preradiosurgery Hemorrhage Rates

Preradiosurgical patient observation began with the first symptomatic, image-documented hemorrhage and ended with radiosurgery. At our last comprehensive review, a total of 446 patient-years were observed by this definition, giving a mean observation time of 3.98 years per patient (range 0.17–20 years). During this period, 290 hemorrhages (2.58 per patient) were observed. We excluded the first hemorrhage in our analysis. This gave an annual hemorrhage rate of 39.9%, a rate that remained fairly stable over five separate annual observations. Previously, we studied the annual rehemorrhage rate after the first bleed, and found in years 1 through 5 that the incidence was 52, 35, 39, 24, and 32%.

Postradiosurgery Hemorrhage Rates

The mean postradiosurgical follow-up was 4.92 years per patient (range 0.42–16 years), with a total of 552 patient-years of follow-up. During this period,

21 hemorrhages were identified, for an overall hemorrhage rate of 3.8%. Of these hemorrhages, 19 occurred during the first 2 years after radiosurgery, representing 195 patient-years of observation, for an annual hemorrhage rate of 9.7% per year. After the expected latency period, two hemorrhages were identified during 357 patient-years of observation, giving a 0.56% per year hemorrhage rate from years 2–16. One patient had neurological deterioration accompanied by increased edema on T_2-weighted MRI and increased high signal on T_1-weighted MRI, suggestive of new blood, at 5 years. The other patient's bleed was asymptomatic, but follow-up imaging at 10 years showed an increase in size and high signal intensity in T_1-weighted imaging. There was no significant difference between the maximum dose received, the margin dose received, the number of isocenters, or the number of hemorrhages prior to treatment between the group who rehemorrhaged after radiosurgery and those who remained hemorrhage free.

The mean number of hemorrhages per patient was significantly reduced after radiosurgery (2.43 vs. 0.22, $p < 0.0001$) as well as after the 2-year latent interval (0.19 vs. 0.02, $p < 0.01$). We compared a group of 52 patients who had their first hemorrhage more than 2 years before radiosurgery (group 1) to 30 patients who had their first symptomatic bleed within 2 years of radiosurgery (group 2). During years 0–2 after radiosurgery, the annual bleeding rates were 16.6 and 4.2% for groups one and two, respectively. After 2 years following radiosurgery, the rates were 1.1 and 0%. These data indicated that the hemorrhage rate after radiosurgery was independent of the time from the first hemorrhage [12].

Morbidity of Radiosurgery

Eighteen patients (18.8%) had new neurological symptoms without hemorrhage after radiosurgery (12.4%). Such new symptoms are suspected to be adverse radiation effects (AREs). AREs have been uncommon since 1992, when we instituted lower margin doses and switched exclusively to MR-based targeting. Eight of the new deficits were minor and seven of these were temporary. All suspected AREs were seen within a year of radiosurgery. Patients with AREs received a small, but significantly higher marginal dose (17.45 vs. 16.05, $p < 0.03$) delivered by a lower number of isocenters (1.64 vs. 3.06, $p < 0.01$), and tended to have more previous hemorrhages (3.18 vs. 2.32, $p < 0.001$). There were more complications observed with malformations in the brainstem or diencephalon compared to other sites.

Morbidity after radiosurgery is higher when the malformation is located in an area of critical brain function, and this series includes mainly deep brain locations. Patients were chosen for radiosurgery because they had progressively symptomatic cavernous malformations, located in areas that are associated with unacceptable surgical risk of morbidity. In general, they did not present at a pial or ependymal surface. We suspect that AREs are related to the hemosiderin ring surrounding the malformation, corresponding to a region of normal brain stained with iron pigment which is a potential radiation sensitizer. The use of MRI (in comparison to CT) facilitates recognition of the hemosiderin rim. The target lies within this volume. Small isocenters and high conformality of dose delivery also make higher selectivity (i.e. dose reduction to the surrounding brain).

The Goal of Radiosurgery: Reduction in Hemorrhage Risk

We believe that radiosurgery on such high-risk, cavernous malformations must improve outcomes compared to the natural history of these vascular malformations. Any therapeutic modality must rely on clinical follow-up to demonstrate its effectiveness and justify its use. Studies of the natural history of asymptomatic cavernous malformations have suggested that they have a relatively low yearly risk of hemorrhage [1, 9, 15, 18, 24, 30, 33, 36]. A study at the University of Pittsburgh [18] concluded that the overall annual risk of hemorrhage was 2.6%. However, when these patients were stratified into those who had previously suffered a hemorrhage and those who had not, the former group appeared to be at higher risk. Patients with one previous hemorrhage had a yearly 4.5% risk of hemorrhage, while those without had a 0.6% yearly risk. Patients with two or more hemorrhages had a bleeding rate of approximately 30% per year [19]. It was for this reason that the patients with prior hemorrhage were chosen for radiosurgery. It follows, then, that their results may differ from the former groups at lower risk. Barker et al. [4] hypothesized that symptomatic cavernous malformation hemorrhage may occur in a pattern of temporal clustering. They noted a 2.4-fold decline in the hemorrhage rate after 2.5 years, and suggested that this alone may be responsible for the reduced bleeding rate seen after radiosurgery. These data were derived from a series of 141 patients who had resection or proton beam irradiation of their malformation over an 18-year period. However, only 63 patients even had a second hemorrhage. This series is different from ours in that most patients were not observed to see if they would rebleed without treatment.

We believe that the observed 39.9% yearly risk of hemorrhage prior to radiosurgery in our series defined a high risk subpopulation who warranted intervention. Within 2 years of radiosurgery, this risk of hemorrhage was reduced to 9.7% per year. After the anticipated 2-year latency interval, the yearly risk of hemorrhage was further reduced to 0.56%. This risk approximated the 0.6% yearly rate [18] of hemorrhage seen in patients who harbored asymptomatic cavernous malformations. Radiosurgery was associated with a greater than 30-fold reduction in the baseline risk of symptomatic bleeding.

The Radiobiological Effect of Radiosurgery

It is not clear why the risk for hemorrhage is reduced after radiosurgery. Our hypothesis is that the endothelial-lined channels undergo progressive hyalinization leading to thickening and eventual luminal closure, perhaps via the chronic inflammatory response typical of radiation-induced vasculopathy [15, 19, 34]. Unfortunately, there are few reports about the histology of cavernous malformations after radiation. Gewirtz et al. [11] reported pathological changes in 11 patients who underwent surgical resection after irradiation. Of these lesions, 8 were identified as cavernous malformations, while one was identified as a true AVM and two were not identified adequately. No malformation was completely thrombosed, a not surprising finding since most had rebled necessitating surgical resection. Six lesions showed a combination of marked vessel fibrosis, fibrinoid necrosis, and ferrugination. In addition, Karlsson et al. [13] noted a patient whose cavernous malformation was resected after Gamma Knife radiosurgery; more than 70% of the lesion had been obliterated.

Chang et al. [6] reported 57 patients with surgically inaccessible cavernous malformations treated by helium ion or linear accelerator radiation techniques. They found an annual hemorrhage rate of 9.4% that was reduced to 1.6% after 36 months after radiosurgery. Complications included symptomatic radiation changes (7%), necrosis (2%), and increased seizures (2%). Amin-Hanjani et al. [3] reported 95 patients with 98 cavernous malformations who were managed with stereotactic Bragg-peak proton beam therapy. They found that the annual hemorrhage rate was reduced from 17.3% before irradiation to 4.5% after a latency period of 2 years with a 16% incidence of permanent neurological deficit and a 3% mortality rate. Karlsson et al. [13] reported a postradiosurgery hemorrhage rate of 8%, but cautioned on the use of this technique because of side effects (27%). Some of their patients had radiosurgery without MR guidance, and at doses that presently would be considered excessive. Some may have had associated venous anomalies.

Kida and Hasegawa [14] reported their experience in 152 patients, the majority having malformations in critical brain locations. They delivered a mean margin dose of 14.9 Gy. The hemorrhage rate in the 5 years before radiosurgery was 31.8%. This rate decreased 3.2%/year/patient, to approximately one tenth the bleeding rate at 5 years after radiosurgery. The hemorrhage rate was 8% in the 1st year, 5% in the 2nd, and 0 at year 7. Rebleeding after radiosurgery occurred in 13% of patients, and symptomatic perimalformation imaging changes were observed in 11%. Twenty-three patients had radiosurgery rather than resection for an intractable seizure disorder. Results were not consistent, with significant improvement in seizures noted in 12 patients.

Compared with surgical resection, the obvious disadvantage of radiosurgery is the latency interval necessary to achieve a reduction in the bleeding rate. This disadvantage is outweighed by the lower risk of radiosurgery for hemorrhagic malformations completely located within critical brain parenchyma. Although Pollock et al. [29] reported a reduction in the bleeding rate after radiosurgery in their series of 17 patients (reduced from 40% before radiosurgery to 2.9% 2 years later), they found a radiation-related morbidity rate of 41%. This may have been due to the high median margin dose of 18 Gy, leading to higher doses in the adjacent hemosiderin-stained brain.

It is still unclear whether radiosurgery should be offered to a patient after one symptomatic hemorrhage. Good clinical decision-making is difficult in this group since their overall yearly hemorrhage rate is approximately 4–5% per year [18]. Any intervention for this group must have a lower overall morbidity associated with it and offer a clear benefit. Perhaps the best patient for radiosurgery after a single bleed is a younger patient whose first hemorrhage caused disabling symptoms. Since the morbidity of radiosurgery for cavernous malformations may be much lower than previously thought, and the rate of hemorrhagic risk reduction dramatic, we think that radiosurgery after a single bleed is reasonable for selected patients. A decision analysis model should help to elucidate the crossover points of morbidity and hemorrhage rate that would make radiosurgery an appropriate treatment strategy for patients with a first hemorrhage from a cavernous malformation.

References

1 Aiba T, Tanaka R, Koike T, Kameyama S, Takeda N, Komata T: Natural history of intracranial cavernous malformations. J Neurosurg 1995;83:56–59.

2 Amin-Hanjani S, Ogilvy CS, Canadia G, Lyons S, Chapman PH: Stereotactic radiosurgery for cavernous malformations: Kjellberg's experience with proton beam therapy in 98 cases at the Harvard cyclotron. Neurosurgery 1998;42:1229–1237.

3 Amin-Hanjani S, Ogilvy CS, Ojemann RG, Crowell RM: Risks of surgical management for cavernous malformations of the nervous system. Neurosurgery 1998;42:1220–1228.

4 Barker FG II, Amin-Hanjani S, Butler WE, Lyons S, Ojemann RG, Chapman PH, Ogilvy CS: Temporal clustering of hemorrhages from untreated cavernous malformations of the central nervous system. Neurosurgery 2001;49:15–25.

5 Bertalanffy H, Gilsbach JM, Eggert HR, Seeger W: Microsurgery of deep-seated cavernous angiomas: report of 26 cases. Acta Neurochir (Wien) 1991;108:91–99.

6 Chang SD, Levy RP, Adler JR, Martin DP, Krakovitz PR, Sternberg GK: Stereotactic radiosurgery of angiographically occult vascular malformations: fourteen years experience. Neurosurgery 1998;43:213–221.

7 Clatterbuck RE, Moriarity JL, Elmaci I, Lee R, Breiter SN, Rigamonti D: Dynamic nature of cavernous malformations: a prospective magnetic resonance imaging study with volumetric analysis. J Neurosurg 2000;93:981–986.

8 Coffey RJ, Lunsford LD: Radiosurgery of cavernous malformations and other angiographically occult vascular malformations; in Awad AI, Barrow DL (eds): Cavernous Malformations. Park Ridge Ill: American Association of Neurological Surgeons, 1993, pp 187–200.

9 Curling OD, Kelly DL, Elster AD, Craven TE. An analysis of natural history of cavernous angiomas. J Neurosurg 1991;75:702–708.
10 Davis DH, Kelly PJ. Stereotactic resection of occult vascular malformatons. J Neurosurg 1990;72: 698–702.
11 Gewirtz RJ, Steinberg GK, Crowly R, Levy RP: Pathological changes in surgically resected angiographically occult vascular malformations after radiation. Neurosurgery 1998;42:738–743.
12 Hasegawa T, McInerney J, Kondziolka D, Lee JYK, Flickinger J, Lunsford LD. Long term results after stereotactic radiosurgery for patients with cavernous malformations. Neurosurgery 2002;50: 1190–1198.
13 Karlsson B, Kihlstrom L, Lindquist C, Ericson K, Steiner L: Radiosurgery for cavernous malformations. J Neurosurg 1998;88:293–297.
14 Kida Y, Hasegawa T: Radiosurgery for cavernous malformations: results of long-term follow-up. Radiosurgery 2004;5:153–160.
15 Kim DS, Park YG, Choi JU, Chung SS, Lee KC: An analysis of the natural history of cavernous malformations. Surg Neurol 1997;48:9–18.
16 Kondziolka D, Lunsford LD, Flickinger JC: The radiobiology of radiosurgery. Neurosurg Clin N Am 1999;10:157–166.
17 Kondziolka D, Lunsford LD, Coffey RJ, Bissonette DJ, Flickinger JC: Stereotactic radiosurgery of angiographically occult vascular malformations: indications and preliminary experience. Neurosurgery 1990;27:892–900.
18 Kondziolka D, Lunsford LD, Flickinger JC: The natural history of cerebral cavernous malformations. J Neurosurg 1995;83:820–824.
19 Kondziolka D, Lunsford LD, Flickinger JC, Kestle JR: Reduction of hemorrhage risk after stereotactic radiosurgery for cavernous malformations. J Neurosurg 1995;83:825–831.
20 Lunsford LD, Kondziolka D, Flickinger JC, Bissonette DJ, Jungreis CA, Maitz AH, Horton JA, Coffey RJ: Stereotactic radiosurgery for arteriovenous malformations of the brain. J Neurosurg 1991;75:512–524.
21 Maesawa S, Flickinger JC, Kondziolka D, Lunsford LD: Repeated radiosurgery for incompletely obliterated arteriovenous malformations. J Neurosurg 2000;92:961–970.
22 Maesawa S, Kondziolka D, Lunsford LD: Stereotactic radiosurgery for management of deep brain cavernous malformations. Neurosurg Clin N Am 1999;10:503–511.
23 Mitchell P, Hodgson TJ, Seaman S, Kemeny AA, Forster DMC: Stereotactic radiosurgery and the risk of haemorrhage from cavernous malformations. Br J Neurosurg 2000;14:96–100.
24 Moriarity JL, Wetzel M, Clatterbuck RE, Javedan S, Sheppard J-M, Hoenig-Rigamonti K, Crone NE, Breiter SN, Lee RR, Rigamonti D: The natural history of cavernous malformations: a prospective study of 68 patients. Neurosurgery 1999;44:1166–1173.
25 Muras I, Confronti R, Scuotto A: Cerebral cavernous angioma: diagnostic considerations. J Neuroradiol 1993;20:34–41.
26 Ondra SL, Troupp H, George ED, Schwab K: The natural history of symptomatic arteriovenous malformations of the brain: a 24-year follow-up assessment. J Neurosurg 1990;73:387–391.
27 Pollock BE, Flickinger JC, Lunsford LD, Bissonette DJ, Kondziolka D: Hemorrhage risk after stereotactic radiosurgery of cerebral arteriovenous malformations. Neurosurgery 1996;38: 652–659.
28 Pollock BE, Flickinger JC, Lunsford LD, Maitz A, Kondziolka D: Factors associated with successful arteriovenous malformation radiosurgery. Neurosurgery 1998;42:1239–1247.
29 Pollock BE, Garces YI, Stafford SL, Foote RL, Schomberg PJ, Link MJ: Stereotactic radiosurgery for cavernous malformations. J Neurosurg 2000;93:987–991.
30 Porter PJ, Willinsky RA, Harper W, Wallace MC: Cerebral cavernous malformations: natural history and prognosis after clinical deterioration with or without hemorrhage. J Neurosurg 1997;87: 190–197.
31 Pozzati E: Thalamic cavernous malformations. Surg Neurol 2000;53:30–40.
32 Rigamonti D, Drayer BP, Johnson PC, Hadley MN, Zabramski J, Spetzler RF: The MRI appearance of cavernous malformations (angiomas). J Neurosurg 1987;67:518–524.
33 Robinson JR, Awad IA, Little JR. Natural history of cavernous angioma. J Neurosurg 1991;75: 709–714.

34 Schneider BF, Eberhard DA, Steiner LE: Histopathology of arteriovenous malformations after gamma knife radiosurgery. J Neurosurg 1997;87:352–357.
35 Steinberg GK, Chang SD, Gewirtz RJ, Lopez JR: Microsurgical resection of brainstem, thalamic, and basal ganglia angiographically occult vascular malformations. Neurosurgery 2000;46: 260–271.
36 Zabramski JM, Wascher TM, Spetzler RF, Johnson B, Gofinos J, Dryer BP, Brown B, Rigamonti D, Brown G: The natural history of familial cavernous malformations: results of an ongoing study. J Neurosurg 1994;80:422–432.
37 Zimmerman RS, Spetzler RF, Lee KS, Zabramski JM, Hargraves RW: Cavernous malformations of the brain stem. J Neurosurg 1991;75:32–39.

Douglas Kondziolka, MD
Professor of Neurological Surgery
Suite B-400, UPMC, 200 Lothrop St.
Pittsburgh, PA 15213 (USA)
Tel. +1 412 647 6782, Fax +1 412 647 0989, E-Mail kondziolkads@upmc.edu

Szeifert GT, Kondziolka D, Levivier M, Lunsford LD (eds): Radiosurgery and Pathological Fundamentals. Prog Neurol Surg. Basel, Karger, 2007, vol 20, pp 231–234

10.2.2. Pathological Considerations to Irradiation of Cavernous Malformations

István Nyáry, Ottó Major, Zoltán Hanzély, György T. Szeifert

National Institute of Neurosurgery and Department of Neurological Surgery, Semmelweis University, Budapest, Hungary

Abstract

Stereotactic radiosurgery is a controversial treatment modality in the management of cerebral cavernous malformations (CVMs). Systematic pathological studies of irradiated specimens probably could help to resolve the controversy. Light microscopic investigation of a surgically resected thalamic CVM 1 year after 40-Gy irradiation revealed endothelial cell destruction in the cavernous channels, and marked fibrosis with scar tissue formation in the connective stroma of the lesion. These histopathological findings were similar to those described in arteriovenous malformations after Gamma Knife surgery, and suggest that the ionizing effect of radiation energy evokes vascular and connective tissue stroma changes in CVMs as well.

The role of irradiation in the management of cerebral cavernous malformations (CVMs) is controversial [1, 2]. The problem of management arises in part because of the scarcity of available microscopic morphological investigation data on CVMs after radiation therapies [3, 4]. It has been suggested that systematic pathological investigations could help resolve this controversy. The purpose of this study was to present the histopathological findings 1 year after 40-Gy irradiation.

Case History

This 26-year-old man was admitted to another hospital with sudden headaches, vomiting, and deterioration of consciousness. A CT scan revealed a hemorrhagic lesion in the posterior part of the diencephalon (fig. 1a). The lesion was diagnosed as a thalamic tumor, and the patient was treated with 40-Gy of fractionated external-beam radiotherapy. Following the

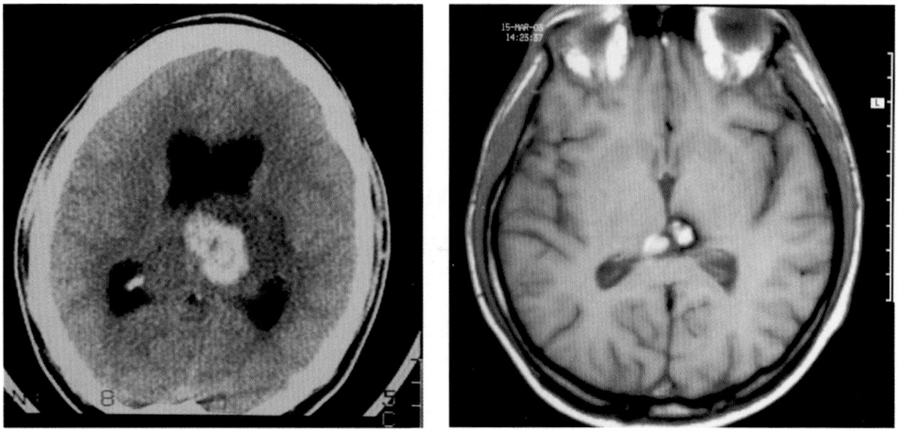

a b

Fig. 1. ***a*** Cranial CT demonstrating the original lesion diagnosed as a thalamic tumor. ***b*** One year after 40-Gy fractionated radiotherapy the left thalamic lesion was reconsidered to be a CVM based on MRI.

radiotherapy, ventricular enlargement developed and a ventriculoperitoneal shunt was inserted. One year after radiotherapy, the patient was admitted to our Department. A new MR image was obtained, and the diagnosis was revised to a CVM in the light of our findings (fig. 1b). The CVM was removed via an open transcallosal approach.

Pathological Findings

Histological examination of the surgical specimen revealed a typical CVM with postirradiation changes. In addition to HE staining, elastic van Gieson, Prussian blue and Masson trichrome staining were performed. Immunohistochemical reactions for Factor VIII and CD34 antigens, as vascular endothelial cell markers, were also carried out on 5-μm paraffin-embedded sections.

The specimens were compared with CVM tissue obtained from nonirradiated control CVM samples (fig. 2). This comparison indicated that there was endothelial cell destruction in the caverns, accompanied by marked fibrosis with hyaline degeneration and scar tissue formation in the connective tissue stroma of the 40-Gy-treated CVM (fig. 3a, b). Most of the vessels were obliterated in the irradiated tissue samples; however, granulation tissue with a large number of newly formed thin-walled channels, that is precapillary arterioles, capillaries, and postcapillary venules were observed. Hemosiderin pigmentation intermingled with recent foci of hemorrhage was also demonstrated (fig. 3c, d).

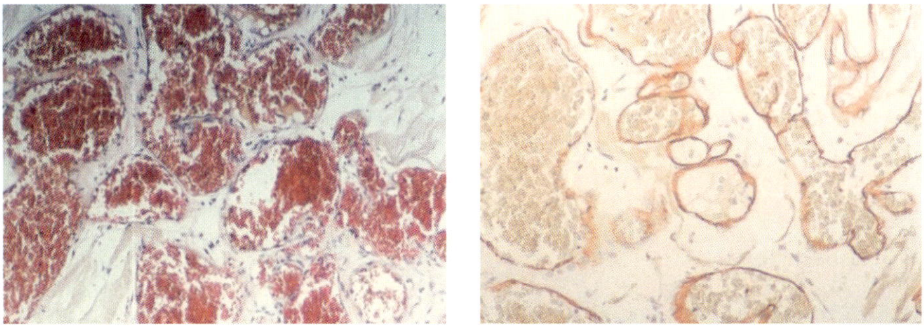

a *b*

Fig. 2. ***a*** Photomicrograph of a control nonirradiated CVM specimen with dilated, blood-filled vessels (caverns). HE, ×200. ***b*** Photomicrograph showing vigorous CD34 positivity in the lining endothelial cells. CD34, ×200.

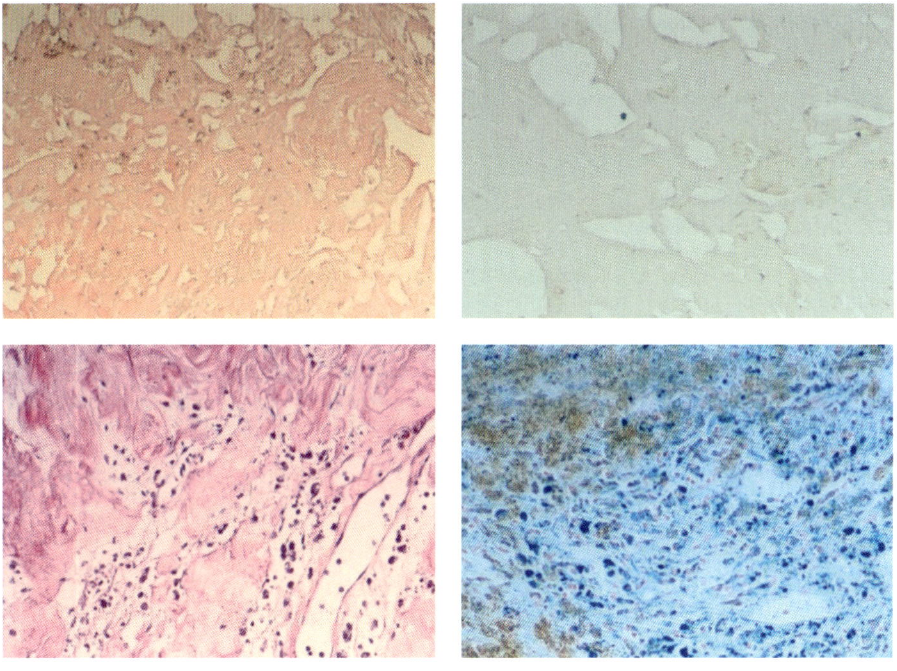

a *b* *c* *d*

Fig. 3. ***a*** Marked scar tissue formation in the stroma after 40-Gy irradiation. HE, ×200. ***b*** Total destruction of endothelial cell layer after irradiation. CD34, ×200. ***c*** Most of the vessels are obliterated by connective tissue in the irradiated CVM, but some open lumina containing blood cells in thin-walled channels are still present. Elastic van Gieson, ×200. ***d*** Prominent hemosiderin pigmentation is seen, which suggests microhemorrhages from the newly formed capillaries of granulation tissue following irradiation. Prussian blue, ×200.

These pathological findings are similar to those described in subtotally obliterated arteriovenous malformations after Gamma Knife surgery [5, 6]. Results of the present study suggest that the radiation treatment evokes similar morphological changes in CVMs, which would enable the same therapeutic effect that is seen in AVMs [7].

Conclusions

This case study suggests that cavernous malformations undergo occlusive changes similar to those seen in AVMs. More histopathological studies are necessary to determine the consistency of the findings in this report.

References

1 Karlsson B, Kihlstrom L, Lindquist C, Ericson K, Steiner L: Radiosurgery for cavernous malformations. J Neurosurg 1998;88:293–297.

2 Maesawa S, Kondziolka D, Lunsford LD: Stereotactic radiosurgery for management of deep brain cavernous malformations. Neurosurg Clin N Am 1999;10:503–511.

3 Gewirtz RJ, Steinberg GK, Crowley R, Levy RP: Pathological changes in surgically resected angiographically occult vascular malformations after radiation. Neurosurgery 1998;42:738–742; discussion 42–43.

4 Hasegawa T, McInerney J, Kondziolka D, Lee JY, Flickinger JC, Lunsford LD: Long-term results after stereotactic radiosurgery for patients with cavernous malformations. Neurosurgery 2002;50: 1190–1197; discussion 97–98.

5 Szeifert GT, Kemeny AA, Timperley WR, Forster DM: The potential role of myofibroblasts in the obliteration of arteriovenous malformations after radiosurgery. Neurosurgery 1997;40:61–65; discussion 65–66.

6 Schneider BF, Eberhard DA, Steiner L: Histopathology of arteriovenous malformations after gamma knife radiosurgery. J Neurosurg 1997;87:352–357.

7 Nyary I, Major O, Hanzely Z, Szeifert GT: Histopathological findings in a surgically resected thalamic cavernous hemangioma 1 year after 40-Gy irradiation. J Neurosurg 2005;102(suppl): 56–58.

Prof. István Nyáry, MD, PhD
National Institute of Neurosurgery
Amerikai út 57
HU–1145 Budapest (Hungary)
E-Mail nyary@oiti.hu

Szeifert GT, Kondziolka D, Levivier M, Lunsford LD (eds): Radiosurgery and Pathological Fundamentals. Prog Neurol Surg. Basel, Karger, 2007, vol 20, pp 235–243

11.1.1. Radiosurgery for Trigeminal Neuralgia

Nicolas Massager, José Lorenzoni, Daniel Devriendt, Marc Levivier

Gamma Knife Center, Erasme Hospital and Jules Bordet Institute, Brussels, Belgium

Abstract

Radiosurgery has recently emerged as a suitable treatment of pharmacologically resistant idiopathic trigeminal neuralgia. Results and complications of this treatment are related to parameters of the dosimetry, i.e. the dose and the target. We found that the irradiation dose delivered to the brainstem, the distance between the target and the brainstem, and the occurrence of facial numbness after radiosurgery are related to a better pain outcome.

Trigeminal neuralgia (TN) is defined as brief paroxysms of pain that are limited to the facial distribution of the trigeminal nerve and precipitated by stimuli to sensory endings in the trigeminal receptive area [1]. The diagnosis depends strictly on clinical criteria, such as those established by the International Headache Society in 1988 [1]. The overall incidence rate is estimated to be approximately 3–5 cases per year per 100,000 persons, and this number increases with the age of the patients [2]. The median age at diagnosis is 67 years [2]. Clinical experience with the natural history of TN suggests that the paroxysmal pain worsens over time [2]. TN may develop in patients with multiple sclerosis, after a herpes zoster infection, after a surgical or dental procedure, or secondary to an intracranial tumor; however, the majority of cases of TN are idiopathic [1]. The pathophysiological mechanism of TN remains uncertain, but the role of a vascular compression of the trigeminal nerve is currently well established. The most accepted pathophysiological theory is that vascular compression induces focal demyelination of the damaged trigeminal root, leading to the hyperexcitability of nerve fibers; as a result, normal sensory impulses stimulate adjacent pain fibers to discharge, resulting in paroxysms of facial pain [1, 2].

Drug therapy is considered to be the first line of treatment of TN [1]. Unfortunately, medical treatment does not initially provide satisfactory pain relief for 25% of patients; moreover, the relief provided by drug therapy generally decreases over time and the increased dosage of these medications is limited because of side effects [1, 2]. Several surgical options are available for patients with medically intractable TN, including microvascular decompression (the Jannetta procedure), radiofrequency-induced rhizotomy, glycerol-induced rhizotomy, balloon compression, and, more recently, radiosurgery [1].

Historical Background of Radiosurgery for TN

Lars Leksell performed the first radiosurgical treatment of TN in 1953 [3, 4]. The narrow beam of ionizing radiation was generated from a modified orthovoltage X-ray tube that was mounted on a conventional stereotactic frame system. Because the aim of this procedure was the selective blocking of pain conduction in the trigeminal ganglion, the radiation beam was targeted at the gasserian ganglion, which was located using plain skull radiographs. For the procedure of 'radioganglionectomy' developed by Leksell, an X-ray tube was used with approximately 20 portals of entry on the convexity of the head, in order to deliver a total dose of radiation that was estimated to range between 16.5 and 22 Gy to the gasserian ganglion. The excellent clinical results obtained by Leksell in the first 2 patients treated with this method have encouraged others to irradiate the trigeminal ganglion by using the Gamma Knife (GK) [3]. A later report by Lindquist et al. [5] on the use of stereotaxic radiogangliotomy, as performed by Leksell on 46 patients with TN, showed that approximately 50% of the patients initially become pain free, but that most of these patients noticed a recurrence of their neuralgia several years after the radiosurgical procedure. The unpredictable and relatively short-term pain control obtained with the use of this target motivated some teams to find another target of irradiation. Rand et al. [6] and Lindquist et al. [5] first tried to target the nerve more proximally, at the trigeminal root near its entry into the pons. The initial results attained using this target were reported in the beginning of the 1990s. At the same period, Régis et al. [7] started to irradiate the distal portion of the trigeminal root, which is immediately posterior to the gasserian ganglion. Using this modified target, that group reported a high rate of effective pain control and very low morbidity. A multicenter study involving 5 GK centers was conducted to evaluate the clinical outcome and morbidity related to the use of this treatment with various radiation doses [8]. The publication of the results of this study in 1996 has been the cause of the worldwide increasing use of this treatment for medically intractable TN. More recently, linear accelerators have started to be used for the radiosurgical treatment of TN [9, 10].

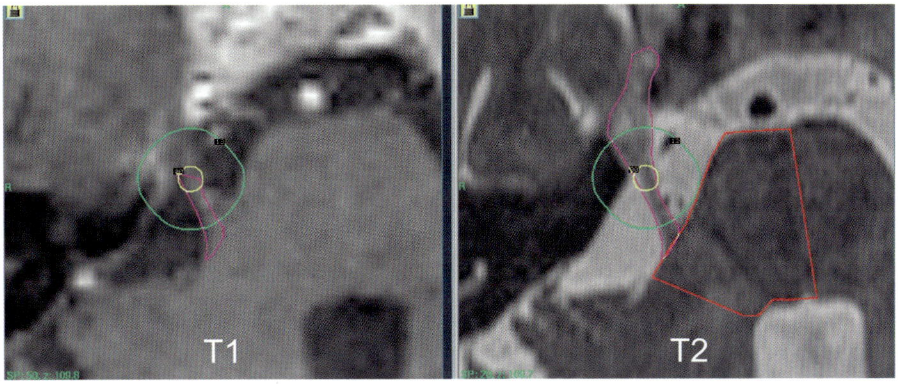

Fig. 1. Radiosurgical planning for GK treatment of a right-sided TN using an anterior target. The cisternal part of the trigeminal nerve is contoured (pink line) on axial MR sequences. The 90% isodose (yellow line) is positioned on the cisternal part of the nerve. The right side of the brainstem, previously contoured (red line) to provide a dose-volume histogram, comes into contact with the 12 Gy isodose (green line).

Material and Methods

Between January 2000 and January 2004, 93 GK procedures were performed in patients with pharmacologically resistant TN at the Gamma Knife Center of Brussels, Belgium. Eighty patients suffered from idiopathic TN and 13 patients had secondary TN, 5 patients with TN associated with multiple sclerosis, 2 patients with tumor-related TN, 4 patients with TN that had been induced by surgical or dental procedures, and 2 patients with postherpetic TN. The median age of the patients was 68 years (range 35–87 years). There were 39 women and 54 men. The TN was on the right side in 55 patients and on the left side in 38 patients. For 63 patients, GK radiosurgery was the first surgical option undertaken to treat their TN.

Radiosurgical Procedure

The Leksell G stereotactic frame (Elekta Instruments AB) was attached to the patient's head after a local infiltration anesthetic agent with a mild intravenous sedative had been administered in a standard manner. The frame was applied as close as possible to the plane of the intracisternal trigeminal nerve root. We obtained stereotactic axial T_1-weighted MR slices without and with gadolinium-contrast enhancement, and three-dimensional T_2-weighted volume acquisitions divided into 1-mm slices, followed by stereotactic CT densitometric imaging acquisition. Treatment planning was performed using Leksell GammaPlan (version 5.31; Elekta Instruments, AB). The cisternal portion of the trigeminal nerve was contoured. A single 4 mm isocenter was positioned on the cisternal portion of the nerve (fig. 1); some centers used a proximal target located 2–4 mm from the REZ and others used a more anterior target located immediately posterior to the gasserian ganglion [7]. A maximum dose of 70–90 Gy is currently used. In our center, for the patients described here, we used a very anterior target, located immediately posterior to the gasserian ganglion as originally described by Régis et al. [7], and a maximum dose of 90 Gy. The brainstem was contoured and a dose-volume histogram was generated to verify that 1 mm^3 or less of the brainstem received a dose of less than 15 Gy, and that 10 mm^3 or less received a dose of less than 12 Gy. When the dose delivered to the brainstem exceeded those values, beam channel blocking is used. The treatment can be performed using LGK Model U, B or C.

Results

Pain Control

The results of GK in terms of pain control are usually evaluated after a period of 6–12 months following the irradiation. Pain outcome can be classified into 4 categories: excellent (100% pain relief and no medication), good (90–99% pain reduction and medication stopped or reduced), fair (50–89% pain reduction) and poor (<50% pain reduction). For data analysis, patients with excellent or good outcomes were sometimes gathered into one group described as 'satisfactory pain reduction', and patients with fair or poor pain control were put together in one group described as 'unsatisfactory pain reduction'.

From a series of 80 patients treated for idiopathic TN, 62 patients had a clinical and radiological follow-up of minimum 6 months. The initial pain relief was excellent in 45 patients (73%), good in 8 patients (13%), fair in 3 patients (5%) and poor in 6 patients (9%); thus, satisfactory pain control (excellent + good pain relief) was achieved in 53 patients (86%). The follow-up period of those 62 patients ranged from 6 to 42 months (mean 19 months); the Kaplan-Meier actuarial curve of pain relief demonstrated that 74% of patients had satisfactory pain reduction, including 63% of patients with excellent pain relief, 42 months after the radiosurgical procedure (fig. 2).

Morbidity

No acute complication occurred after the radiosurgical procedure. During the clinical follow up, 4 patients (6%) complained of bothersome facial numbness, which appeared between 2 and 6 months after radiosurgery. When specifically asked about the occurrence of a facial sensory disturbance following the radiosurgical procedure, 21 patients (34%) reported experiencing mild, trouble-free facial numbness. We found no other complication related to the GK treatment; particularly, no patient experienced significant facial paresthesia, jaw weakness, decreased corneal sensation (dry eye syndrome [11]), deafferentation pain, or any other neurological dysfunction.

Prognostic Factors of Pain Control

We have conducted a prospective study to evaluate the influence of some data on pain outcome after GK radiosurgery. Fifteen potential prognostic factors of

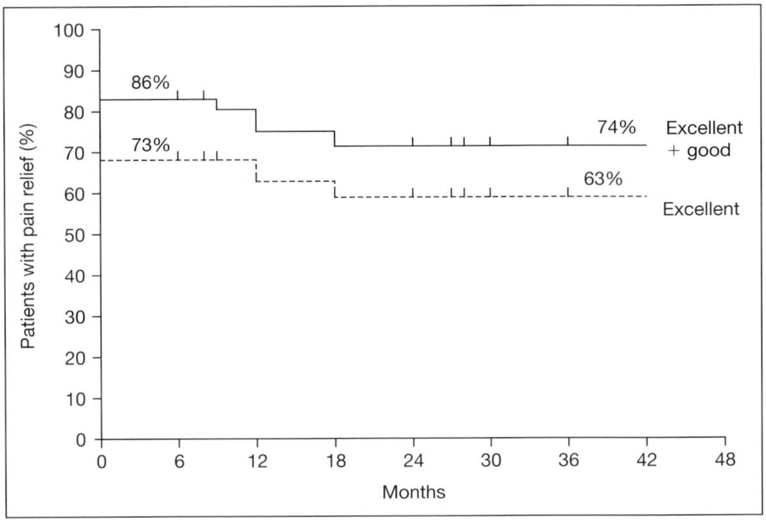

Fig. 2. Kaplan-Meier actuarial curves showing the pain relief rate in our population.

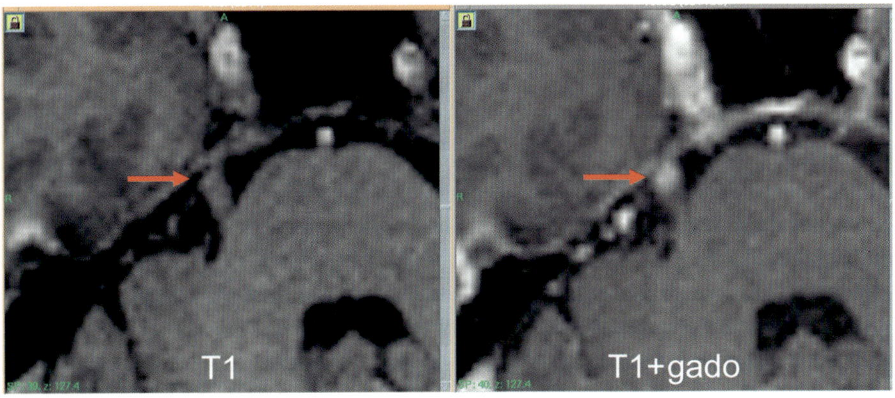

Fig. 3. Enhancement on the trigeminal nerve at the radiosurgical target on MRI T_1 sequences with gadolinium performed 6 months after the radiosurgical procedure.

effective pain control after radiosurgery have been analyzed: patient's age, sex, size and location of trigeminal pain, number of roots reached, previous surgical procedure for TN, neurovascular conflict on MRI, distance between the target and brainstem, use of plugs, dose rate, dose received by 1 and 10 mm^3 of the brainstem, contrast enhancement on MRI 6 months after radiosurgery (fig. 3), and postoperative development of mild or bothersome facial sensory disturbance.

Four prognostic factors were found to be significantly associated with pain outcome: the distance between the target and the brainstem, the dose received by the first 1 and 10 mm^3 of the brainstem, and the occurrence of mild facial sensory disturbance. In other words, a shorter distance between the target and brainstem, a higher irradiation dose delivered to the brainstem, and the development of mild facial numbness are statistically significant factors of effective pain control.

Discussion

Results of Radiosurgery for TN

Pain outcome is related to the irradiation dose used; a dose of more than 65 Gy is mandatory to obtain a significant pain reduction [8]. Depending on the target and some other dosimetric parameters, a dose of 70–90 Gy at the 100% isodose is currently used for GK radiosurgery. The pain control rates in the series published recently show that 35–74% of patients have excellent pain outcome, and 54–87% of patients have satisfactory pain outcome. Analysis of the actuarial pain outcome after the radiosurgical procedure has been performed in some series. A pain relapse rate of 5–20% is noticed in the first 3 years following the radiosurgical procedure.

Complications related to the radiosurgical treatment of TN depend on the radiosurgical tool [12] and dosimetric parameters used [13]. Morbidity after radiosurgery includes mainly facial numbness; corneal weakness, dysgeusia, anesthesia dolorosa and motor weakness of the 5th nerve root have also been reported. As others [14], we have found that GK radiosurgery performed with a distal intracisternal target seems to have a lower rate of complications compared with the use of a proximal target with the same irradiation dose [13]. Pollock et al. [15] has shown that the use of a maximal dose of 90 Gy and a proximal target is associated with a significantly higher rate of complications and should be avoided.

Following the results of a prospective study performed in our Center and recently published [13], we currently use a maximum dose of 90 Gy for all patients and the shot is located on the intracisternal part of the nerve root, at a distance between 5 and 8 mm from the brainstem. Actually, patients treated with those dosimetric parameters obtained the highest pain control rate and the lowest morbidity rate.

Prognostic Factors of Pain Relief

We have analyzed 15 demographic or dosimetric factors that may influence pain outcome. We have found that the position of the target along the intracisternal part of the nerve root is significantly associated with the results of radiosurgery. Our results also stated that the occurrence of facial numbness after the radiosurgical procedure seems to be associated with pain control, as found by others [16]. Interestingly, enhancement on the trigeminal nerve at the radiosurgical target on MRI T_1 sequences with gadolinium performed 6 months after the radiosurgical procedure (fig. 3) are associated neither with pain outcome nor facial numbness.

Second Radiosurgical Procedure for TN

Some radiosurgical centers have started to retreat patients with TN relapse [17, 18]. In our Center, we have performed a second GK treatment in 9 patients; all had had an excellent pain control in the following months after the radiosurgical procedure before the trigeminal pain relapsed. We have used a maximal dose of 70 Gy for all patients and a target more proximal than the first one along the intracisternal portion of the nerve root. Preliminary results of this procedure show a pain control rate of >70%; induced facial numbness has occurred in 80% of our patients. Our results are in accordance with those published in the literature [17, 18].

Future Improvement in Radiosurgery for TN

The search for the optimal target and dose for the radiosurgical dosimetry is still in progress. Prospective, multicenter studies comparing the different targets and doses used in the radiosurgical centers are needed to better define the optimal dosimetric radiosurgical procedure for TN. Also, the influence of the brainstem irradiation on pain control and morbidity after TN radiosurgery requires further investigation. An analysis of the relationship between the occurrence and side of a neurovascular conflict and the results of radiosurgery is in progress in our Center.

In order to better understand the structural effect of GK radiosurgery on the trigeminal nerve root, experimental models will be of great interest. Until now, only one experimental model has been used to better understand the effect of TN radiosurgery, using baboons [19]. Further experimental studies are highly warranted.

Recently, TN radiosurgery has been performed with the new generation of linear accelerator, such as the Novalis Micro-Multileaf [9] and the CyberKnife [10]. Results are promising, but a longer follow-up and a larger population are required to compare pain outcome and morbidity with those obtained with the GK [12].

Conclusions

GK radiosurgery is currently the least invasive surgical technique for the treatment of pharmacoresistant TN. This procedure is safe and efficient, and must be part of the therapeutic armamentarium for the physician as well as the therapeutic choice for the patient. A better knowledge of the pathophysiology of TN and the therapeutic effect of the radiosurgical procedure are warranted to optimize the results of this therapy.

References

1 Joffroy A, Levivier M, Massager N: Trigeminal neuralgia. Pathophysiology and treatment. Acta Neurol Belg 2001;101:20–25.
2 Kitt CA, Gruber K, Davis M, Woolf CJ, Levine JD: Trigeminal neuralgia: opportunities for research and treatment. Pain 2000;85:3–7.
3 Leksell L: Stereotaxic radiosurgery in trigeminal neuralgia. Acta Chir Scand 1971;137:311–314.
4 Leksell L: The stereotaxic method and radiosurgery of the brain. Acta Chir Scand 1951;102: 316–319.
5 Lindquist C, Kihlstrom L, Hellstrand E: Functional neurosurgery: a future for Gamma Knife? Stereotact Funct Neurosurg 1991;57:72–81.
6 Rand RW, Jacques DB, Melbye RW: Leksell Gamma Knife treatment of tic douloureux. Stereotact Funct Neurosurg 1993;61(suppl 1):93–102.
7 Régis J, Bartolomei F, Metellus P, Rey M, Genton P, Dravet C, Bureau M, Semah F, Gastaut JL, Peragut JC, Chauvel P: Radiosurgery for trigeminal neuralgia and epilepsy. Neurosurg Clin N Am 1999;10:359–377.
8 Kondziolka D, Lunsford LD, Flickinger JC, Young RF, Vermeulen S, Duma CM, Jacques DB, Rand RW, Régis J, Péragut JC, Manera L, Epstein MH, Lindquist C: Stereotactic radiosurgery for trigeminal neuralgia: a multi-institutional study using the gamma unit. J Neurosurg 1996;84: 940–945.
9 Goss BW, Frighetto L, DeSalles AA, Smith Z, Solberg T, Selch M: Linear accelerator radiosurgery using 90 Gy for essential trigeminal neuralgia: results and dose volume histogram analysis. Neurosurgery 2003;53:823–828.
10 Romanelli P, Heit G, Chang SD, Martin D, Pham C, Adler J: Cyberknife radiosurgery for trigeminal neuralgia. Stereotact Funct Neurosurg 2003;81:105–109.
11 Matsuda S, Serizawa T, Sato M, Ono J: Gamma Knife radiosurgery for trigeminal neuralgia: the dry-eye complication. J Neurosurg 2002;97(suppl 5):525–528.
12 Massager N, Levivier M: Linear accelerator radiosurgery using 90 Gray for essential trigeminal neuralgia: results and dose volume histogram analysis. Neurosurgery 2003;53:829–830.
13 Massager N, Lorenzoni J, Devriendt D, Desmedt F, Brotchi J, Levivier M: Gamma Knife radiosurgery for idiopathic trigeminal neuralgia performed using a far-anterior cisternal target and a high dose of radiation. J Neurosurg 2004;100:597–605.
14 Régis J: High-dose trigeminal neuralgia radiosurgery associated with increased risk of trigeminal nerve dysfunction. Neurosurgery 2002;50:1401–1402.
15 Pollock BE, Phuong LK, Foote RL, Stafford SL, Gorman DA: High-dose trigeminal neuralgia radiosurgery associated with increased risk of trigeminal nerve dysfunction. Neurosurgery 2001;49: 58–62.
16 Pollock BE, Phuong LK, Gorman DA, Foote RL, Stafford SL: Stereotactic radiosurgery for idiopathic trigeminal neuralgia. J Neurosurg 2002;97:347–353.
17 Brisman R: Repeat Gamma Knife radiosurgery for trigeminal neuralgia. Stereotact Funct Neurosurg 2003;81:43–49.

18 Herman JM, Petit JH, Amin P, Kwok Y, Dutta PR, Chin LS: Repeat gamma knife radiosurgery for refractory or recurrent trigeminal neuralgia: treatment outcomes and quality-of-live assessment. Int J Radiot Oncol Biol Phys 2004;59:112–116.
19 Kondziolka D, Lacomis D, Niranjan A, Mori Y, Maesawa S, Fellows W, Lunsford LD: Histological effects of trigeminal nerve radiosurgery in a primate model: implications for trigeminal neuralgia radiosurgery. Neurosurgery 2000;46:971–976.

Nicolas Massager, MD
Gamma Knife Center, University Hospital Erasme
Route de Lennik 808
BE–1070 Brussels (Belgium)
Tel. +32 2 555 31 74, Fax +32 2 555 31 76, E-Mail nmassage@ulb.ac.be

Szeifert GT, Kondziolka D, Levivier M, Lunsford LD (eds): Radiosurgery and Pathological Fundamentals. Prog Neurol Surg. Basel, Karger, 2007, vol 20, pp 244–248

11.1.2. Pathological Findings following Trigeminal Neuralgia Radiosurgery

György T. Szeifert[b], Isabelle Salmon[a], José Lorenzoni[a], Nicolas Massager[a], Marc Levivier[a]

[a]Centre Gamma Knife, Hôpital Académique Erasme, Université Libre de Bruxelles, Brussels, Belgium; [b]National Institute of Neurosurgery and Department of Neurological Surgery, Semmelweis University, Budapest, Hungary

Abstract

Autopsy, 3D MRI and histopathological findings are presented in a patient who had suffered from trigeminal neuralgia and was treated two times by radiosurgery. The first treatment was performed with 90 Gy at the distal part of the nerve. Because of recurrent pain, a second irradiation was carried out delivering 70 Gy at a more proximal segment of the nerve 10 months later. The patient died from a hemorrhagic stroke 26 days following the second intervention. Autopsy revealed a neurovascular conflict close to the second radiosurgery shot. Histopathology demonstrated acute and chronic stage radiation-induced lesions in the trigeminal nerve.

Trigeminal neuralgia (TN) is characterized by paroxysms of shooting pain into the face, affects about 5 per 100,000 persons per year, and this number increases with the age of patients [1]. Usually, drug therapy is the first choice of treatment; however, it has an initial failure of pain control in 25% of the cases. This ratio has been growing according to addiction to increasing doses of medication. Treatment protocols in drug-resistant TN include thermocoagulation or balloon compression of the gasserian ganglion, glycerol-induced rhizotomy, microvascular decompression of the nerve root and more recently radiosurgery. The first patient suffering from TN was treated with radiosurgery by Lars Leksell in 1953 [2]. Since then, it has become a successful treatment modality in the management of drug-resistant TN. The intervention is a bloodless 1-day surgery service, and pain relief is achieved 4–6 weeks after irradiation.

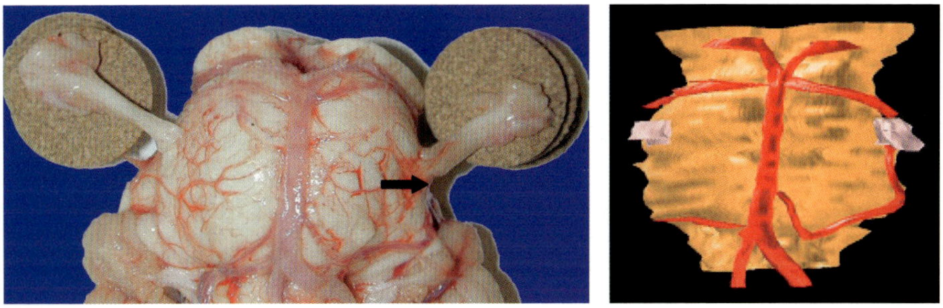

a b

Fig. 1. ***a*** The neurovascular conflict (arrow) at the left trigeminal nerve entry zone in the autopsy specimen. ***b*** 3D reconstruction of high-resolution dynamic MRI demonstrates the same pathology.

The number of cases treated with radiosurgery has been increasing rapidly, but a longstanding debate exists about the optimal placement of the irradiation shot. Some radiosurgery centers prefer targeting the proximal region of the nerve near the entry zone [3], while others aim at the distal part of the nerve, close to the plexus triangularis [4]. We have found that targeting the cisternal portion of the nerve root at a fixed distance of 5–8 mm from the brainstem, and a high radiation dose offers satisfactory pain relief with a low risk of morbidity [1].

Animal experiments have suggested that an irradiation dose less than 100 Gy should be used to avoid permanent trigeminal dysfunction [5]. There is no human pathological study exploring basic histological changes and pathophysiological mechanism of radiosurgery-treated TN. Dosimetric data have been extrapolated to human radiosurgery practice from animal experiments and from clinical experience. A better understanding of the biological and morphological effects of high-dose irradiation may help decide where to place the treatment shot to improve pain control, and maintain low morbidity rates after radiosurgery.

Case Report and Pathological Findings

We have investigated the autopsy material of a case that had been treated two times with Gamma Knife radiosurgery because of drug-resistant left-sided idiopathic TN. The first treatment was performed with a dose of 90 Gy at the distal part of the nerve near the plexus triangularis. A second irradiation was carried out delivering 70 Gy for the proximal segment of the nerve closer to the root entry zone because of recurrent pain 10 months later. The patient died from a hemorrhagic stroke not related to radiosurgery 26 days following the second intervention.

Postmortem examination supported the neurovascular conflict by a loop of the left anterior inferior cerebellar artery at the nerve entry zone (fig. 1a); it was compared with the

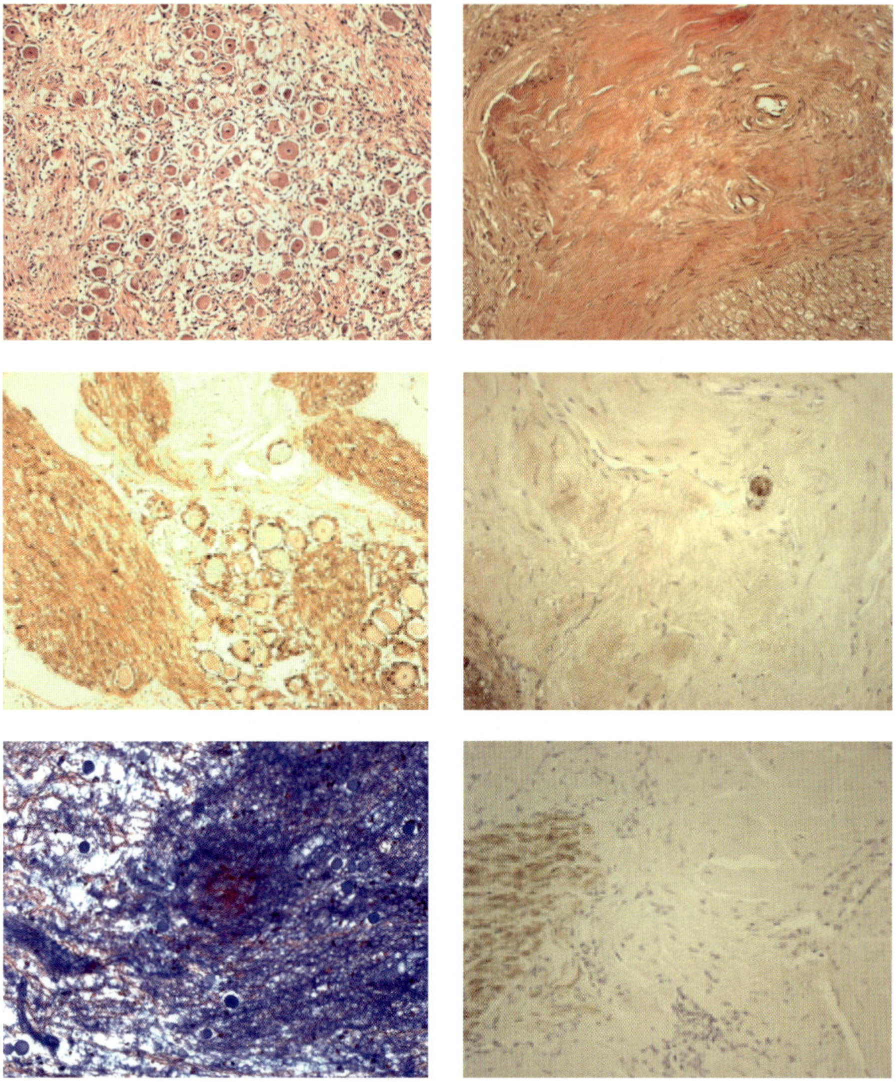

Fig. 2. ***a*** Distal part of the nonirradiated control trigeminal nerve at the gasserian ganglion (HE, ×100). ***b*** Marked fibrotic lesion in the same region of the radiosurgery-treated nerve 11 months following a 90 Gy shot (van Gieson, ×100). ***c*** S100 positivity in the distal part of the control nonirradiated nerve (×100). ***d*** Some S100 positivity at the edge of the gamma radiolesion, but not inside 11 months after the 90 Gy shot (×100). ***e*** Well-circumscribed fibrinoid necrotic lesion at the proximal part of the nerve 26 days following a 70 Gy shot (Masson trichrome, ×100). ***f*** S100 reaction revealed no surviving nerve fibers inside the lesion (×100).

3D reconstruction of dynamic serial high-resolution MRI studies as well (fig. 1b). Histological study revealed acute and chronic-stage, sharply demarcated lesions towards the surrounding trigeminal nerve fibers according to the steep radiation fall-off at the edge of shots that characterizes radiosurgery [6]. A well-circumscribed, hypocellular, fibrotic lesion with hyaline degenerated collagen bundles and scattered fibrocytes were demonstrated at the place of the first (distal) treatment with 90 Gy, 11 months after radiosurgery (fig. 2a, b). These findings are consistent with chronic-stage, radiation-induced pathological changes, and could be regarded as late consequences of radiosurgery. Immunohistochemistry for S100 protein did not reveal any surviving nerve fibers inside the fibrotic area, but around it residual positivity demonstrated that radiosurgery effect was localized according to the position of the shot (fig. 2c, d). There was a sharply demarcated necrotic center, containing fibrinoid material and tissue debris, encircled by surviving nerve bundles at the region of the second (proximal) treatment with 70 Gy, 26 days following irradiation (fig. 2e, f). S100 positivity was intense in the surrounding trigeminal fibers, but stopped at the periphery of the lesion markedly. These alterations correspond to acute-stage radiation-induced changes, and belong to the early consequences of radiosurgery. The nontreated, right-sided trigeminal nerve served as nonirradiated control. Radiation-induced changes could not be explored, and S100 reaction was vigorous in this nerve.

Conclusions

It has been generally accepted that in most of the cases with idiopathic TN a neurovascular conflict between the nerve and an arterial loop is the underlying pathological condition for the disorder. This anatomical conflict constitutes the indication for microvascular decompression surgery in drug-resistant cases [7]. Radiosurgery has become an effective and successful alternative treatment modality in the management of TN through the intact skull, without damaging the surrounding normal tissues. High-resolution, powerful, dynamic MRI studies elucidate and localize the pathological neurovascular conflict, and may help decide where to place the shot. Histological and immunohistochemical investigations supported that 90 Gy irradiation produced an effective pathological lesion, free from fibers, in the trigeminal nerve.

References

1 Massager N, Lorenzoni J, Devriendt D, De Smedt F, Brotchi J, Levivier M: Gamma knife surgery for idiopathic trigeminal neuralgia performed using a far-anterior cisternal target and a high dose of radiation. J Neurosurg 2004;100:597–605.

2 Leksell L: Sterotaxic radiosurgery in trigeminal neuralgia. Acta Chir Scand 1971;137:311–314.

3 Kondziolka D, Lunsford LD, Flickinger JC, et al: Stereotactic radiosurgery for trigeminal neuralgia: a multiinstitutional study using the gamma unit. J Neurosurg 1996;84:940–945.

4 Régis J, Bartolomei F, Metellus P, et al: Radiosurgery for trigeminal neuralgia and epilepsy. Neurosurg Clin N Am 1999;10:359–377.

5 Kondziolka D, Lacomis D, Niranjan A, et al: Histological effects of trigeminal nerve radiosurgery in a primate model: implications for trigeminal neuralgia radiosurgery. Neurosurgery 2000;46: 971–976; discussion 976–977.

6 Larsson B, Leksell L, Rexed B, Sourander P, Mair W, Andersson B: The high-energy proton beam as a neurosurgical tool. Nature 1958;182:1222–1223.

7 Jannetta PJ: Outcome after microvascular decompression for typical trigeminal neuralgia, hemifacial spasm, tinnitus, disabling positional vertigo, and glossopharyngeal neuralgia. Review. Clin Neurosurg 1997;44:331–383.

György T. Szeifert, MD, PhD
National Institute of Neurosurgery and Department of Neurological Surgery
Semmelweis University
Amerikai út 57
HU–1145 Budapest (Hungary)
Tel. +36 1 2512 999, Fax +36 1 2515 678, E-Mail gyorgyszeifert@yahoo.com

Szeifert GT, Kondziolka D, Levivier M, Lunsford LD (eds): Radiosurgery and Pathological Fundamentals. Prog Neurol Surg. Basel, Karger, 2007, vol 20, pp 249–266

11.2. Movement Disorder Radiosurgery – Planning, Physics and Complication Avoidance

Christopher M. Duma

Department of Neurosurgery, Hoag Memorial Hospital Presbyterian, Newport Beach, Calif., USA

Abstract

Gamma Knife radiosurgical thalamotomy is an effective and useful alternative to invasive radiofrequency techniques for patients at high surgical risk. The mechanical accuracy of the gamma unit combined with the anatomical accuracy of high-resolution MRI make radiosurgical lesioning safe and precise. Higher radiosurgical doses are more effective than lower ones at eliminating or reducing tremor, and are generally without complications. The results from radiosurgical pallidotomy, as opposed to those of gamma thalamotomy, have been disappointing. A 50% complication rate in the former (homonymous field cuts, hemipareses and dysphagias) combined with a poor success rate has led us to reevaluate the indications for this procedure in the face of the excellent results from radiofrequency pallidotomy with physiological monitoring and deep brain stimulation. Perhaps experience with lowered radiosurgical prescription doses will improve the complication rate. There appears to be a differential sensitivity of the pallidum to radiation, anatomically, than the thalamus. Age-related or anatomy-related susceptible blood supply to the area may lead to hypoxia after single-fraction radiosurgery, in a nuclear complex known to be especially susceptible to hypoxia. In addition, varying levels of iron deposition within the pallidum may catalyze free radical formation in the elderly only to be further exacerbated by tissue hypoxia. Although reported, the success of radiosurgical caudatotomy, subthalamotomy and lesioning of the VL nucleus remains to be further elucidated.

With the advent of deep brain stimulation (DBS) technology, movement disorder stereotactic neurosurgery has taken on a life of its own. There is no question that implantation of an electrode with subsequent control via an implanted generator has many advantages over historical lesioning techniques. These techniques include radiofrequency ablation, cryoablation and radiosurgical lesioning. The advantage of the latter, however is that it is a 'closed-skull' technique and may be preferable for patients who are infirm, on blood-thinners, etc. Thus, stereotactic radiosurgery is being used to create functional lesions in patients with movement disorders that were once only created with 'open' stereotactic neurosurgical techniques. Patients with Parkinson's disease (PD), essential tremor (ET), dystonias, and tremors of other origins have been and are being treated worldwide using such technology [1–7].

Recent history has shown, however, that our attempt to make this type of brain surgery less and less invasive has its risks. Without intraoperative physiologic feedback the radiosurgical lesion is targeted based on anatomy alone, which is obviously variable between patients. Furthermore, unlike the latitude that DBS affords through programming and reversibility, the radiosurgical lesion, like radiofrequency ablation, is finite and irreversible [8–16]. Finally, as will be discussed, the radiosurgical lesion can vary from patient to patient in its size and edemagenic potential, sometimes leading to severe complications depending on target location.

Various conditions may predispose patients to having radiosurgery versus other invasive techniques. Such conditions are chronic use of anticoagulants and severe cardiac or respiratory disease, very elderly and noncompliant patients, and simply those who may voluntarily choose a less invasive alternative to open stereotactic technique at the expense of a lower success rate. These patients are often left with no other option but to tolerate markedly disabling symptoms of the disease. The advantages of radiosurgery are obvious. Radiosurgery involves no opening of the cranium and no incisions. The risk of hemorrhage from passing an electrode to the depths of the thalamus is eliminated and so is the potential risk of meningitis.

The Gamma Knife and Dose Selection

To date there is no reported experience using LINAC technique for the treatment of movement disorders; however, accurate lesions to 3 mm in the vervet monkey subthalamic nucleus and substantia nigra using a dedicated Novalis® (BrainLAB Inc.) system has been reported [1]. The preferred radiosurgical tool for treatment of movement disorders, as supported in the literature, is the Gamma Knife (GK). The gamma unit's supreme mechanical accuracy made its adaptation to the field of 'functional stereotactic radiosurgery' an easy one. The unit is capable of focusing cobalt-derived photon energy through 201 separate 4 mm collimator openings. At their target, these beams usually create a well-circumscribed lesion measuring 5–6 mm at the

50% isodose line lending themselves perfectly to the goal of noninvasive destruction of aberrant neural pathways, either by direct cell kill, or protein and DNA destruction [2–5].

Based on pathological and radiographic analysis, Leksell and Lindquist described necrotic lesions from their early experience with functional radiosurgery [2–6]. Doses of 160–200 Gy maximum were felt to be effective at creating a permanent necrotic lesion; however, large collimators were to be avoided based on complications experienced in their early work. More modern reports describe single-fraction doses varying between 110 and 200 Gy, which means treatment times would vary from about 45 min to up to 2 h depending upon the age of the cobalt. The selection of dose has been guided by a dose-volume analysis of prior experience with parenchymal tolerance to GK radiosurgery. Of those with the largest experience, a final target dose of 130 Gy has become the norm [11–14]. Immediately after radiosurgery, all patients are given a single intravenous dose of 10 mg of dexamethasone. The treatment is usually performed as an outpatient procedure.

MRI and Target Planning

Concerns about spatial inaccuracies of MRI, particularly for functional cases, have all but vanished. Prior concerns were based on perturbations of the MR field due variations in the metals used in a certain stereotactic frame. Bednarz et al. [7] studied the impact of geometric distortions on the spatial accuracy of MRI-guided localization for GK functional radiosurgery. Accuracy was evaluated by comparing stereotactic coordinates of intracranial targets, fiducials and anatomic structures defined by MRI and CT using a skull phantom. The average difference between the two modalities was only one pixel (or approximately 1 mm^3) along the x, y and z axes. They concluded that the spatial accuracy of an MRI-based localization system can be comparable to that of CT with the added benefit of MRI resolution.

At our institution, regardless of target, we use a whole brain RAGE algorithm with 1 mm slice thickness and T_1-weighted sequences (TR 11, TE 4.4) to define the AC-PC line. We use a different series (in coronal and axial planes) to define our targets: T_2-weighted STIR sequences, 6,000 TR, 30 TE, TI 300, flip angle 180, 24 FOV, 256 – squared matrix, and 2-mm-thick slices.

Others have used axial images with 2 mm slices obtained from the top to the bottom of the head by the FASE method with similar axial and coronal slices taken using proton density MR sequences [8].

Target Planning

Targeting the VIM Nucleus of the Thalamus

Radiofrequency thermocoagulation of the VIM nucleus of the thalamus has been the mainstay of the treatment of the tremor of PD and ET [9–31]. More recently, DBS has been used as well, and may become the standard of care for this pathology.

Our intraoperative experience with radiofrequency thalamotomies has shown that rarely do our planned targets and actual lesion targets differ [22]. If they do differ, it is only by a few millimeters, clearly within the margin of error of a single 4 mm collimated shot. It is this fact that justified our using anatomical landmarks only for the treatment of this select population of patients.

Target localization of the VIM nucleus of the thalamus is determined by coordinates based on the position of the nucleus relative to the AC/PC line, anatomical information gathered from very high resolution MRI and subjective surgeon correlation with the Schaltenbrand atlas [32]. Computer atlases referenced to the size of the patient's brain, the AC-PC line and floor of the 3rd ventricle can also be helpful [33, 34]. The x, y, and z coordinates are determined for the target using SurgiPlan® (Elekta Inc., Atlanta, Ga., USA). These coordinates are then transcribed to GammaPlan® (Elekta). Using this software, we place the 50% isodose line of the 4 mm collimator at the edge of the contralateral internal capsule (IC) medially. At a level 4 mm above the AC-PC line, the 50% isodose line of the 4 mm collimator lies in the angle of a line drawn parallel to the medial aspect of the posterior limb of the IC and a line drawn between the posterior limits of the globus pallidi (fig. 1a, 'Duma's lines'). The target is at a point midway along the length of the posterior limb of the IC and just above the line joining the tips of the most posterior aspects of both globus pallidi (fig. 1b). The average target coordinates for all thalamotomies in this series was x = 15 mm lateral to the AC/PC line, y = 6 mm posterior to the midpoint of the AC/PC line, and z = 4 mm superior to the AC/PC line. The same target is used for patients with ET.

Ohye et al. [35] used the lateral part of VIM as their ideal target. According to these authors, the VIM nucleus lies 7–8 mm anterior to the PC, 3–4 mm superior to the level of the PC and 2 mm medial to the lateral border of the thalamus. They then describe placing the shot using GammaPlan, so that the IC and the VC nucleus lay outside the 30% isodose line of a single 4 mm collimator. This usually brings the target approximately 1–2 mm more medial and anterior than a similar target point for radiofrequency thermocoagulation. Of note, the treatment strategy was the same for patients with ET. In a more recent report, the same authors changed their targeting strategy calculating the lateral VIM nucleus at a point 45% of the distance posteriorly from the anterior tip of the

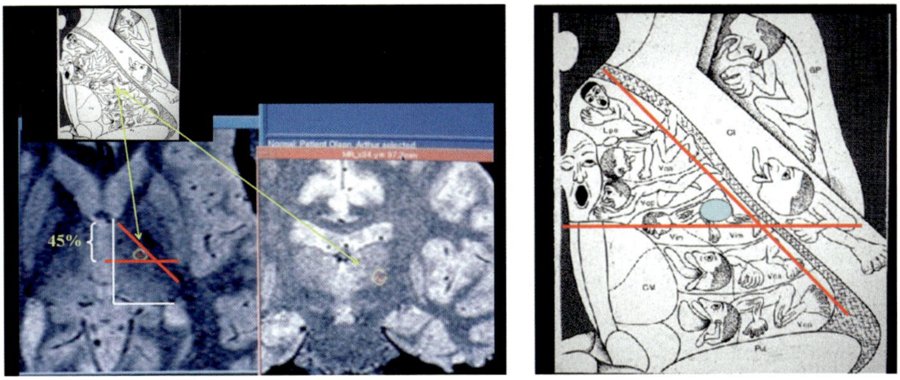

a *b*

Fig. 1. ***a*** Radiosurgical target localization of the VIM nucleus. Average coordinates in the series of successfully treated patients: x = 15 mm lateral to the AC/PC line; y = 6 mm posterior to mid-AC/PC line; z = 4 mm superior to AC/PC line. 'Duma's lines': 50% isodose line of the 4 mm collimator lies at the medial aspect of the posterior limb of IC – target is at the angle formed by a line parallel to the posterior limb of the IC and a line joining the tips of the most rostral aspects of the globus pallidi. ***b*** Coronal MRI targeting of the VIM nucleus.

thalamus along the AC-PC line. If the primary disturbance was rigidity, then they targeted 2–3 mm more anteriorly to cover the VO nucleus. If the target appeared too close to the IC laterally or VC posteriorly, it was modified or corrected. They also described using plugging patterns to avoid the IC, but we have not found this to be clinically important. Finally, from their experience with microelectrode recording in failed GK patients, they found that normal neuronal activity was seen in the high signal zone of the radiosurgical lesion. Thus, they no longer moved their target to avoid the VC and IC. The 50% isodose line was kept at the edge of VC and IC as in our series [8].

Targeting the Globus Pallidus, Subthalamic, Caudate and VL Nuclei

Target localization of globus pallidus interna (GPi) was determined by coordinates based on anatomical information gathered from very high resolution MRI and subjective surgeon correlation with the Schaltenbrand atlas [32]. The 50% isodose line of a single or double isocenter 4 mm collimator plan was placed at the center of GPi. In our series of 19 patient treated with radiosurgical pallidotomy, all targets were to the center of GPi using similar target planning strategies to that of thalamotomy.

In the first-ever reported case of radiosurgical subthalamotomy, Keep et al. [36] used a primary target of 13 mm lateral to, 2 mm posterior to the midpoint of, and 5 mm inferior to the AC-PC line. This was altered using atlas reference and experience.

Friehs et al. [37, 38] reported targeting the center of the heads of the caudate nuclei bilaterally to treat the bradykinesia and rigidity of parkinsonism, and Pan et al. [37] targeted the anterior portion of the VL nucleus for dystonia.

VIM Radiosurgical Thalamotomy

We have previously reported our experience with the treatment of ET and PD tremor using GK radiosurgery [38]. Between March 1991 and September 2002, 42 patients (25 males and 17 females) with disabling tremor from PD or ET recalcitrant to medical therapy underwent radiosurgical VIM thalamotomy using the 201-source cobalt-60 GK. Four patients had bilateral procedures separated by 6 months for a total of 46 lesions. Thirty lesions were left sided for right-sided tremor. No patients had prior surgery for their Parkinson's symptoms. Patient's ages ranged from 60 to 84 years old (median 72).

Patients were accepted for radiosurgery if they did not satisfy the criteria for invasive radiofrequency pallidotomy or thalamotomy: poor surgical or anesthetic risk, advanced age, use of anticoagulants, or personal choice. The United Parkinson's Disease Rating Scale (UPDRS) [39] was used to assess the patients pre- and postoperatively. Only patients with UPDRS grade 3 or 4 tremor, bradykinesia and/or rigidity were chosen for treatment.

Independent neurologist evaluations and UPDRS scoring of patient response to treatment were obtained at regular clinical follow-up intervals particular to the referring neurologists. Patients underwent 1-, 3-, and 6-month and semi-annual follow-up examinations by the treating neurosurgeons, but these evaluations were not used in the outcome data. Patients were also asked to subjectively rate the percentage improvement of their symptoms on a 'UPDRS-correlated' improvement scale. Statistical correlation between patient and independent neurologist assessment of outcome was made using the Pearson correlation analysis. Patient clinical outcome per low dose versus high dose groups was statistically analyzed using the Wilcoxon nonparametric test.

'Mild' improvement was categorized as a change of one UPDRS grade per independent neurologist evaluation and a subjective patient response of 1–33% improved. 'Good' improvement was categorized as a change of two UPDRS grades and 34–66% subjective patient response improvement, and 'excellent' improvement was categorized as a change of three UPDRS grades and a subjective patient response score of 67–99% improvement (table 1).

Follow-up MRI was performed at 3-month intervals for the first 6 months and at 6-month intervals thereafter. MRI protocols included 2 mm high-resolution axial and coronal T_2-, and T_1-weighted images with and without gadolinium (fig. 2).

Table 1. Correlation of independent neurologist evaluations and patient self-assessment scores

Δ UPDRS score as reported by independent neurologists	Subjective improvement as reported by the patients
0	none
1	mild (1–33% relief)
2	good (34–66%)
3	excellent (67–99%)
3 or 4	absent tremor

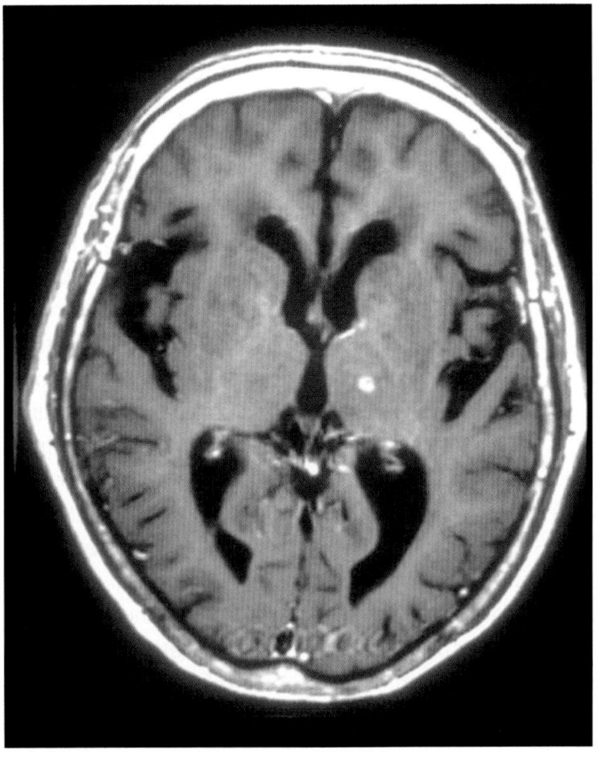

Fig. 2. T_1 gadolinium-enhanced MRI: 6-month follow-up radiosurgical lesion (4 mm collimator, maximum dose 160 Gy).

Clinical and radiological follow-up ranged from 6 to 90 months (median 30 months) Changes in clinical tremor as determined by the delta UPDRS scoring by the neurologists, and by the objective scoring by the patients were highly correlative: 0.89 (Pearson correlation coefficient, $p < 0.001$).

No change in tremor occurred in 4 GK thalamotomies (8.6%), 'mild' improvement was seen in 4 (8.6%), 'good' improvement was seen in 13 (28%), and 'excellent' improvement in 13 (28%). In 12 thalamotomies (26%), the tremor was eliminated completely. The high-dose (160 Gy mean maximum dose) thalamotomy lesion was more effective at reducing tremor (78% mean improvement) than the low-dose (120 Gy mean maximum dose) lesion (56% mean improvement, $p < 0.04$, Wilcoxon nonparametric test).

Median time of onset of improvement was 2 months (range 1 week to 8 months). Three patients who underwent unilateral thalamotomy had bilateral improvement of their tremors. Two patients who had initial improvement in their tremors but who eventually returned to baseline in their follow-up were included in the treatment failure group. All other patients maintained their level of improvement throughout the course of the follow-up. The 4 patients who received bilateral thalamotomies separated by a 6-month interval had no subjective cognitive or performance changes other than improvement in their tremors.

Seven patients underwent formal testing of general tests of overall function. The 'observed activity' scores after GK thalamotomy were improved ($p < 0.02$), as were the 'activity by history' scores ($p < 0.05$). The 'time to walk 20 feet' scores and the '20-second timed test' scores did not statistically differ between the patients.

One patient, after bilateral treatment, suffered a mild acute dysarthria 1 week after GK thalamotomy, which has persisted at follow-up. There were no other objective or subjective adverse changes in motor or cognitive functions as a result of treatment. MRI showed a well-circumscribed spherical lesion which enhanced with gadolinium on T_1-weighted images at a median of 3 months after radiosurgical lesioning, and a mildly diffuse T_2 signal change which usually followed white matter tracts, at a median of 4.5 months following treatment, representing what is felt to be edema or 'radiation change'.

The average T_1-weighted, gadolinium enhancing lesion size was no different for the low and high dose groups and ranged from 3 to 6 mm (mean 5.0) at a median follow-up of 6 months. This lesion was present on follow-up scans as far out as 72 months.

The average T_2-weighted lesion size was no different for the low and high dose groups and ranged from 6 to 22 mm (mean 9.2) at a median of 6 months follow-up. This lesion also persisted on future MRIs. Although there was a trend toward more edema in the 160 Gy treatment group, the differences in the T_1- and T_2-weighted images of the thalamic lesions between the two groups did not differ significantly.

Ohye et al. [35] reported 36 gamma thalamotomies in 31 patients. Twenty-two patients had parkinsonian tremor (2 of these had repeat procedures),

5 patients had ET (1 had repeat procedure, another had a contralateral procedure), 2 had intention tremor (1 had a repeat procedure); 1 had posttraumatic tremor, and 1 had dystonia. Maximum dose was 150 Gy in the first 6 cases, which was subsequently reduced to 130 Gy. In 2 patients undergoing repeat procedures, the dose was decreased to 120 Gy. In all cases except one, a single 4 mm isocenter was used. Repeat lesions were made in 3 of 4 patients to enlarge previous radiofrequency lesions. Their longest follow-up period was 6 years. Reduction of tremor usually occurred by 1 year and rapidly progressed after that. Their earliest response was 3 months. In only 1 patient did the tremor worsen prior to improving.

In their 15 cases with more than 2 years of follow-up, a clinically good result was seen in 87%, with no noticeable side effects. Good results have lasted 3–5 years with no sign of recidivism. In a more recent paper, these same authors have followed a total of 53 patients for nearly 8 years. Thirty-five of them were followed for more than 2 years. A satisfactory outcome was described as tremor reduction to <25% of the preoperative state and was achieved in 80% of cases [8].

They too found a clinically insignificant variance in lesion size over the course of their experience. On follow-up imaging, the authors noted two different patterns of postradiosurgical lesions. One was a simple round punched out lesion with enhancing borders with good symmetry, 7–8 mm in diameter to the enhancing edges, which maintained the same shape and size over up to 5 years of follow-up. The second type of lesion seen extended to the surrounding areas including the capsule with 'rail-like' high signal along the border of the thalamus and GP. The smaller lesion measured an average of 200 mm^3 and the larger lesion measuring 400–500 mm^3. Of note, there was no correlation between the two types of lesion and the clinical effect on tremor. Those with the larger, 'extended' lesion had no ill effects. In 2 patients the tremor remained after the follow-up period, and these underwent radiofrequency thalamotomy with microelectrode recording. Normal neuronal activity was found 2–3 mm outside the necrotic zone [8].

Young et al. [40] in a large series of patients reviewed their use of GK thalamotomy for the treatment of tremor; a series which includes some of our previously reported results [38]. Hundred and two patients with parkinsonian tremor, 52 patients with ET, and 4 patients with tremor of other etiology were treated with a single 4 mm collimator with doses varying from 110–160 Gy. Median follow-up was 52.5 (range 11–93) months for patients with parkinsonian tremor and 74 patients have been followed for more than 4 years. At the time of reporting, 76.5% were tremor free, and 11.8% were 'nearly free of tremor' and these results were consistently maintained in patients followed for 4 years or longer. Thus there was failure in 11.8%. In 52 patients with disabling ET, median follow-up was 26 months. Seventeen patients were followed for more than 48 months. At 1 year, 92.1% were completely or nearly tremor free, after 4 years of follow-up this percentage decreased to 88.2%. No patients required medication for tremor after GK.

One patient experienced a transient complication of contralateral balance disturbance, 1 patient had mild contralateral paresthesias in the face and upper extremity without detectable sensory deficit and no impairment of function. A third patient had a mild weakness and dysphasia. All complications were felt to be due to lesions which became larger than expected as described in this text. The overall complication rate was 1.3%. Lesion sizes ranged from 0 to 2,030 mm^3 as far out as 3 years.

In the above reports, complications were few (<2%) and minimal in clinical significance. Siderowf et al. [41] reported a case of a 59-year-old patient with ET who developed a complex, disabling movement disorder following GK thalamotomy. Their conclusion was that there was a need for long-term follow-up to fully evaluate the potential for complications following radiosurgery.

Radiosurgical GPi Pallidotomy

Between March 1991 and August 1995, 18 patients with medically recalcitrant and disabling symptoms of PD underwent stereotactic radiosurgical pallidotomy using the 201-source cobalt-60 GK at our institution [38]. Patient ages ranged from 59 to 85 years at time of treatment, median 73 years old. No patients had had prior surgery for their Parkinson's symptoms.

Patients were accepted for radiosurgery if they did not satisfy the criteria for invasive radiofrequency pallidotomy: poor surgical or anesthetic risk, advanced age, use of anticoagulants, or personal choice. The UPDRS [39] was used to assess the patients pre- and postoperatively. All were tested both off and on levodopa (challenge test), and were accepted for treatment only if responsive to levodopa.

Fifteen patients were treated using a single 4 mm collimator with a median maximum prescription dose of 160 (range 90–165) Gy. Three patients were treated using a combination of two 4 mm shots with a dose of 160 Gy.

Independent neurologist evaluations and UPDRS scoring of patient response to treatment were obtained at regular clinical follow-up intervals particular to the referring neurologists. Patients underwent 1-, 3-, and 6-month and semi-annual follow-up examinations by the treating neurosurgeons, but these evaluations were not used in the outcome data. Patients were also asked to subjectively rate the percentage improvement of their tremor on a 'UPDRS-correlated' improvement scale.

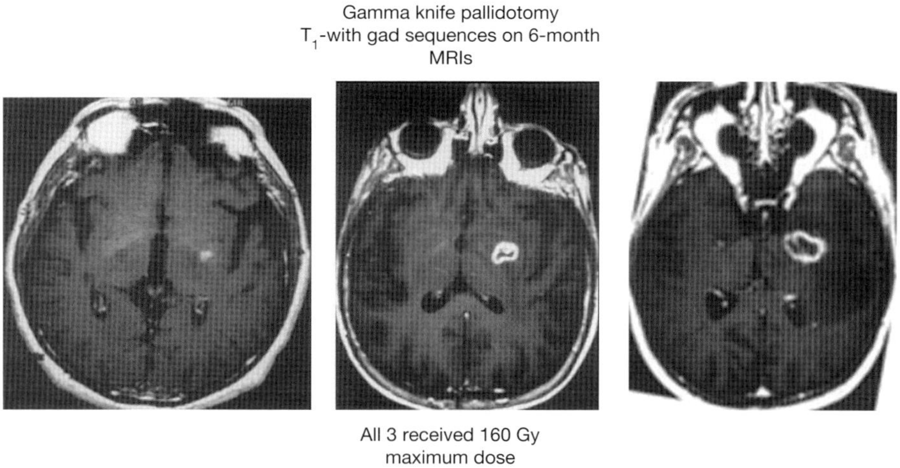

Fig. 3. Variability in gadolinium-enhanced T_1-weighted 8-month follow-up MRIs between 3 different patients who received the same 160 Gy maximum prescription dose with a single 4 mm collimator.

The results were not good. Only 6 patients (33%) showed improvement in rigidity and dyskinesia. Three patients (17%) were unchanged, and 9 patients (50%) were worsened by the treatment. Of the 6 patients with improvement, 2 exhibited visual field deficits. Overall, 4 (22%) patients had a visual field deficit, 3 patients had speech and/or swallowing difficulties, 3 had worsening of their gait, and 1 had numbness in the contralateral hemibody. Nine patients (50%) had one or more complications related to treatment.

The explanation for the complication rate of 50% in our series is no doubt due to the variability and unpredictability of the lesion size when the globus pallidus serves as the target. This unpredictability and variability was not seen in the VIM thalamotomy series and probably represents anatomical susceptibility to very small venous or arterial infarction in the area of GPi. For the same dose at similar follow-up intervals (160 Gy maximum dose at 8 month follow-up) lesion sizes varied from 6 to 30 mm on T_1-weighted MR sequences with gadolinium enhancement (fig. 3). Immeasurable variability in edema patterns was visible at the same follow-up intervals on T_2-weighted MR sequences (fig. 4). Over time, lesion sizes tended to decrease slightly but in general were consistent throughout the course of follow-up.

Others have reported their experience with GK pallidotomy [42, 43]. Okun et al. [43] echoed our complications of GK pallidotomy in a report describing 8 patients seen in an 8-month period referred for complications of GK

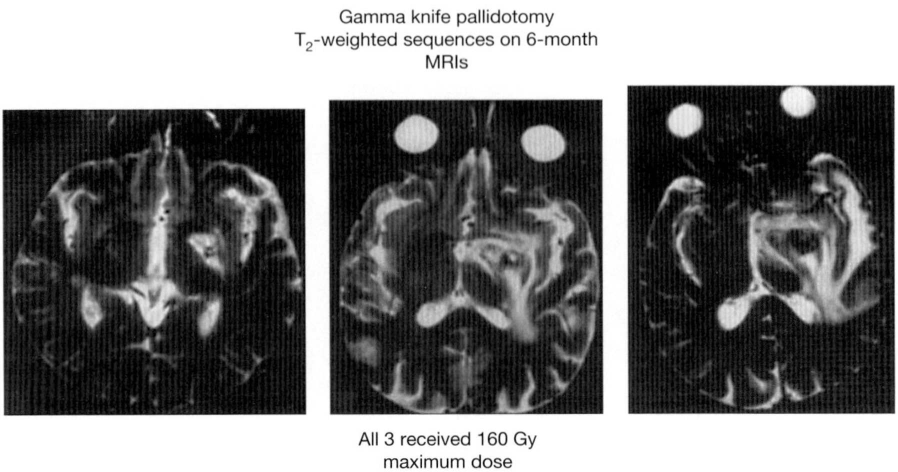

Fig. 4. Extreme edema variability in T_2-weighted 8-month follow-up MRIs between 3 different patients who received the same 160 Gy maximum prescription dose with a single 4 mm collimator.

radiosurgery. Complications included hemiplegia, homonymous field cut, weakness, dysarthria, hypophonia, aphasia, hemihypesthesia and pseudobulbar laughter. They described the lesions as 'off target'. One of these 8 patients subsequently died secondary to dysphagia and aspiration pneumonia.

The experience of Friedman et al. [44] is also similar to ours. They described their results in 4 patients using GK pallidotomy in advanced disease. The selected target was that of GPi as described by Laitinen [45, 46]. All 4 patients exhibited a response to levodopa prior to inclusion in the treatment. A single 4 mm collimator with a maximum dose prescription of 180 Gy was used to make the lesion in all patients. No patient improved in a significant manner within the follow-up interval of 18 months. One patient experienced an improvement in his dyskinesia, but also became transiently psychotic and demented. The other 3 patients suffered no adverse effects. Follow-up MRI scans at 1 year revealed accurately placed lesions, but with variable and unpredicted sizes.

Bonnen et al. [47] in a single case report, described a permanent contralateral homonymous hemianopsia and transient paresis in a patient treated with GK pallidotomy. The resulting lesion size was greater than expected.

One group studied the effects of GK thalamotomy (GKT) on Parkinson disease-related tremor and ET before and after reloading of radioactive cobalt. A maximum dose of 130 Gy was delivered to the target by using a single isocenter with the 4 mm collimator. The course after GKT was compared between the 25 cases with PD treated before reloading and the 35 cases treated after reloading. In the majority (80–85%) treated after reloading, tremor and rigidity were reduced around 6 months after GKT. In the cases treated before reloading, this effect took approximately 1 year. The thalamic reaction on MRI showed the same two lesion types in both series: a restricted and a diffuse. After reloading, the restricted lesion was more frequent and the lesion volume was smaller. They concluded that the shorter delay in clinical improvement and smaller lesion size may have been related to an increased radiation dose [48].

Radiosurgical Caudatotomy

Friehs et al. [49] reported the efficacy of GK radiosurgery caudatotomy for the treatment of the bradykinesia and rigidity of parkinsonism. One month after treatment, 6 of 10 patients showed clear benefit from bilateral 4 mm head of caudate lesions without any treatment-related complications.

Radiosurgical Subthalamotomy

Keep et al. [36] reported the first radiosurgical subthalamotomy using the GK in a single case report. The 73-year-old patient received 120 Gy to the 100% isodose line using the 4 mm collimator helmet. At 2 weeks, she was able to reduce her Sinemet dose. At 5 weeks, she had no tremor, rigidity or dyskinesia and walked easily with improved balance while using only a one-point cane for support. At 3 months, she had partial return of increased motor tone and cogwheel rigidity. At 1 year, after medication adjustments, she was able to move with ease and had no tremor. At 42 months, motor tone was normal as were finger-tapping and rapid alternating movements. No patient exhibited tremor. Imaging at 42 months showed a well-demarcated signal focus corresponding to the subthalamotomy.

Radiosurgery for Torsion Spasm

Pan et al. [37] reported on 2 patients who underwent radiosurgery for torsion spasm to evaluate the efficacy of GKS as an alternative treatment. The first patient was a 33-year-old woman with severe right-sided lower-limb torsion dystonia. The second patient was a 20-year-old man with right-sided upper-limb torsion dystonia. The target was located at the anterior portion of the ventrolateral nucleus. The maximum doses were 150 and 145 Gy, respectively.

Double isocenters with a 4 mm collimator were used. Follow-up lasted for 18 and 8 months, respectively. Both patients had excellent clinical improvement 2–3 months after GKS, respectively. The authors concluded that GKS may be a safe and efficient treatment for torsion spasm.

Discussion

This work represents the largest review of patients treated using stereotactic radiosurgery for the treatment of movement disorders. We have found that GK radiosurgical thalamotomy is a safe and effective alternative to invasive radiofrequency or DBS techniques for patients at high surgical risk. The mechanical accuracy of the gamma unit combined with the anatomical accuracy of high-resolution MRI makes radiosurgical lesioning safe and precise. Higher radiosurgical doses are more effective than lower ones at eliminating or reducing tremor, and are generally without complications.

This is not the case with radiosurgical pallidotomy. The sheer paucity of reports in the literature reflects a deserved lack of faith in the procedure. The posteroventral lesion location has been the target in a large number of radiofrequency-treated PD patients and has consistently demonstrated very good results with rigidity and bradykinesia, as well as control of tremor in many reports [45, 50–57]. Even within the posteroventral pallidum, however, subtle differences in lesion targeting have the potential to affect outcome. Without physiologic feedback, differentiation of internal and external globus pallidus was impossible during gamma pallidotomy, and the advantages gained by electrophysiologic unit-cell recording during radiofrequency lesioning was lost. The lack of clinical improvement may therefore have been attributable to 'sloppy' or inaccurate physiological lesioning within the GP without physiological monitoring.

The explanation for the profoundly high complication rate of 50% in our pallidotomy series is no doubt due to the variability and unpredictability of the lesion size when the globus pallidus serves as the target. This unpredictability and variability was not seen in the VIM thalamotomy series and probably represents anatomical susceptibility to very small vessel venous or arterial infarction in the area of GPi. It is entirely possible that GK pallidal lesioning with a lower prescription dose could reduce or eliminate these complications and at the same time, be clinically effective. Friehs et al. [49] studied the reproducibility and consistency of the GK radiosurgical lesion produced during the treatment of functional disorders. They studied the T_1 gadolinium-enhanced MR images of 140 lesions made with varying doses and numbers of isocenters in different targets at various postradiosurgical intervals. They concluded that as one strayed from a single isocenter treatment with doses greater than 160 Gy, lesion size became unpredictable.

Interestingly, we had minimal to no complications in our large series of GK thalamotomies. This has led us to believe that there is a differential sensitivity to radiation between these two locations. Historically, the pallidum has exhibited a 'supersensitivity' to hypoxia, and this may indeed be the reason for our complications. Bilateral pallidal lesions from carbon monoxide (CO) poisoning are well understood. The affinity of CO for the hemoglobin molecule impairs oxygen transport and release. Oxygen and CO are competitors for the same binding sites on the hemoglobin molecule. Therefore, the pallidum is sensitive to relative hypoxia. Other areas of the brain such as the hippocampus and cerebellum are also sensitive to ischemia and hypoxia, but the pallidum seems particularly so.

This special sensitivity of the pallidum has also been borne out in case reports of hypoxic injury from inhalation pneumopathy, cardiac arrest, and sepsis where patients have exhibited movement disorders upon resuscitation and bilateral pallidal lesions on MRI [58].

'Postcardiac surgery choreic syndrome' occurs usually in children as a complication of cardiac surgery requiring deep hypothermia and bypass. Clinically, the children have choreoathetosis and on MRI and CT scans they exhibit bilateral selective globus pallidus injuries [59].

Hallervorden-Spatz disease, a rare fatal disorder, characterized by choreoathetoid movements and 'tiger's eye' appearance on MRI due to pallidal necrosis, is yet another disorder suggestive of the susceptibility of the pallidum to metabolic disease [60].

Finally, the pallidum is known to contain high levels of iron, and these levels typically rise with age. It has been hypothesized that the presence of iron within this structure may catalyze free radical reactions causing toxicity to the aging brain [61].

The above evidence for special sensitivity of the pallidum to hypoxia and perhaps free radical formation speaks to the possible explanation for the high complication rate of injury to the pallidum with single-fraction radiosurgery. The tapering end-artery distribution of the lenticulostriate supply may be more susceptible to radiation vascular effects, which in turn could cause infarct and edema seen in this series. With a maximum dose of 160 Gy, the 10% isodose line (16 Gy) of a 4 mm collimator may measure 12 mm in diameter. It is entirely possible that radionecrosis or tissue hypoxia or vascular damage may occur within that isodose volume at that dose.

This would also explain why certain patients had no adverse effects related to the dose. Perhaps less iron composition in their pallidum (causing less free radical formation), or better blood supply to the area, counteracted the effects of the single fraction radiosurgery.

References

1 De Salles AA, Melega WP, Lacan G, Steele LJ, Solberg TD: Radiosurgery performed with the aid of a 3-mm collimator in the subthalamic nucleus and substantia nigra of the vervet monkey. J Neurosurg 2001;95:990–997.

2 Leksell L: The stereotaxic method and radiosurgery of the brain. Acta Chir Scand 1951;102: 316–319.

3 Leksell L: Cerebral radiosurgery. I. Gammathalanotomy in two cases of intractable pain. Acta Chir Scand 1968;134:585–595.

4 Leksell L: Modern Concepts in Pshchiatric Surgery. Amsterdam, Elsevier, 1979.

5 Lindquist C, Kihlstrom L, Hellstrand E: Functional neurosurgery – a future for the gamma knife? Stereotact Funct Neurosurg 1991;57:72–81.

6 Lindquist C, Steiner L, Hindmarsh T: Gamma Knife Thalamotomy for Tremor: Report of Two Cases. New York, Raven Press, 1992.

7 Bednarz G, Downes MB, Corn BW, Curran WJ, Goldman HW: Evaluation of the spatial accuracy of magnetic resonance imaging-based stereotactic target localization for gamma knife radiosurgery of functional disorders. Neurosurgery 1999;45:1156–1161; discussion 61–63.

8 Ohye C, Shibazaki T, Zhang J, Andou Y: Thalamic lesions produced by gamma thalamotomy for movement disorders. J Neurosurg 2002;97(suppl):600–606.

9 Boecker H, Wills AJ, Ceballos-Baumann A, et al: Stereotactic thalamotomy in tremor-dominant Parkinson's disease: an H2(15)O PET motor activation study. Ann Neurol 1997;41:108–111.

10 Brophy BP, Kimber TJ, Thompson PD: Thalamotomy for parkinsonian tremor. Stereotact Funct Neurosurg 1997;69(pt 2):1–4.

11 Cooper IS, Bravo G: Chemopallidectomy and chemothalamectomy. J Neurosurg 1958;15: 244–250.

12 Cooper IS, Bravo GJ: Implications of a five-year study of 700 basal ganglia operations. Neurology 1958;8:701–707.

13 Fox MW, Ahlskog JE, Kelly PJ: Stereotactic ventrolateralis thalamotomy for medically refractory tremor in post-levodopa era Parkinson's disease patients. J Neurosurg 1991;75:723–730.

14 Goldman MS, Kelly PJ: Stereotactic thalamotomy for medically intractable essential tremor. Stereotact Funct Neurosurg 1992;58:22–25.

15 Hua SE, Lenz FA, Zirh TA, Reich SG, Dougherty PM: Thalamic neuronal activity correlated with essential tremor. J Neurol Neurosurg Psychiatry 1998;64:273–276.

16 Jankovic J, Cardoso F, Grossman RG, Hamilton WJ: Outcome after stereotactic thalamotomy for parkinsonian, essential, and other types of tremor. Neurosurgery 1995;37:680–686; discussion 6–7.

17 Keller TM, Tcheng TK, Burkhard PR, Richard H, Tamas LB: Stereotactically guided thalamotomy for treatment of parkinsonian tremor isolated to the lower extremity. Case report. J Neurosurg 1998;89:314–316.

18 Kelly PJ, Ahlskog JE, Goerss SJ, Daube JR, Duffy JR, Kall BA: Computer-assisted stereotactic ventralis lateralis thalamotomy with microelectrode recording control in patients with Parkinson's disease. Mayo Clin Proc 1987;62:655–664.

19 Koller W, Pahwa R, Busenbark K, et al: High-frequency unilateral thalamic stimulation in the treatment of essential and parkinsonian tremor. Ann Neurol 1997;42:292–299.

20 Lenz FA, Normand SL, Kwan HC, et al: Statistical prediction of the optimal site for thalamotomy in parkinsonian tremor. Mov Disord 1995;10:318–328.

21 Lenz FA, Tasker RR, Kwan HC, et al: Single unit analysis of the human ventral thalamic nuclear group: correlation of thalamic 'tremor cells' with the 3–6 Hz component of parkinsonian tremor. J Neurosci 1988;8:754–764.

22 Limousin P, Speelman JD, Gielen F, Janssens M: Multicentre European study of thalamic stimulation in parkinsonian and essential tremor. J Neurol Neurosurg Psychiatry 1999;66: 289–296.

23 Linhares MN, Tasker RR: Microelectrode-guided thalamotomy for Parkinson's disease. Neurosurgery 2000;46:390–395; discussion 5–8.

24 Moriyama E, Beck H, Miyamoto T: Long-term results of ventrolateral thalamotomy for patients with Parkinson's disease. Neurol Med Chir (Tokyo) 1999;39:350–356; discussion 6–7.
25 Ohye C: Selective Thalamotomy for Movement Disorders: Microrecording Stimulation Techniques and Results. Boston, Martinus Nijhoff Publishing, 1988.
26 Ohye C, Hirai T, Miyazaki M, Shibazaki T, Nakajima H: Vim thalamotomy for the treatment of various kinds of tremor. Appl Neurophysiol 1982;45:275–280.
27 Pahwa R, Lyons KL, Wilkinson SB, et al: Bilateral thalamic stimulation for the treatment of essential tremor. Neurology 1999;53:1447–1450.
28 Schuurman PR, Bosch DA, Bossuyt PM, et al: A comparison of continuous thalamic stimulation and thalamotomy for suppression of severe tremor. N Engl J Med 2000;342:461–468.
29 Shahzadi S, Tasker RR, Lozano A: Thalamotomy for essential and cerebellar tremor. Stereotact Funct Neurosurg 1995;65:11–17.
30 Tasker RR, DeCarvalho GC, Li CS, Kestle JR: Does thalamotomy alter the course of Parkinson's disease? Adv Neurol 1996;69:563–583.
31 Zirh A, Reich SG, Dougherty PM, Lenz FA: Stereotactic thalamotomy in the treatment of essential tremor of the upper extremity: reassessment including a blinded measure of outcome. J Neurol Neurosurg Psychiatry 1999;66:772–775.
32 Schaltenbrand G: Atlas for Stereotaxy of the Human Brain. Chicago, Stuttgart, Year Book Medical Publishers, Inc., Georg Thieme Publishers; 1977.
33 Otsuki T, Jokura H, Takahashi K, et al: Stereotactic gamma-thalamotomy with a computerized brain atlas: technical case report. Neurosurgery 1994;35:764–767; discussion 7–8.
34 Patil AA, Falloon T, Hahn F, Cheng J, Wang S: Direct identification of ventrointermediate nucleus of the thalamus on magnetic resonance and computed tomography images. Surg Neurol 1999;51:674–678.
35 Ohye C, Shibazaki T, Ishihara J, Zhang J: Evaluation of gamma thalamotomy for parkinsonian and other tremors: survival of neurons adjacent to the thalamic lesion after gamma thalamotomy. J Neurosurg 2000;93(suppl 3):120–127.
36 Keep MF, Mastrofrancesco L, Erdman D, Murphy B, Ashby LS: Gamma knife subthalamotomy for Parkinson disease: the subthalamic nucleus as a new radiosurgical target. Case report. J Neurosurg 2002;97(suppl):592–599.
37 Pan L, Zhang N, Dai JZ, Wang EM: Gamma knife radiosurgery for torsion spasm. Report of two cases. J Neurosurg 2000;93(suppl 3):189–190.
38 Duma CM, Jacques DB, Kopyov OV, Mark RJ, Copcutt B, Farokhi HK: Gamma knife radiosurgery for thalamotomy in parkinsonian tremor: a five-year experience. J Neurosurg 1998;88:1044–1049.
39 Fahn S, Elton RL: Members of the UPDRS Development Committee. Recent Developments in Parkinson's Disease. Florham Park, New Jersey, MacMillan Healthcare Information, 1987.
40 Young RF, Jacques S, Mark R, et al: Gamma knife thalamotomy for treatment of tremor: long-term results. J Neurosurg 2000;93(suppl 3):128–135.
41 Siderowf A, Gollump SM, Stern MB, Baltuch GH, Riina HA: Emergence of complex, involuntary movements after gamma knife radiosurgery for essential tremor. Mov Disord 2001;16:965–967.
42 Friedman JH, Epstein M, Sanes JN, et al: Gamma knife pallidotomy in advanced Parkinson's disease. Ann Neurol 1996;39:535–538.
43 Okun MS, Stover NP, Subramanian T, et al: Complications of gamma knife surgery for Parkinson disease. Arch Neurol 2001;58:1995–2002.
44 Friedman DP, Goldman HW, Flanders AE, Gollomp SM, Curran WJ Jr: Stereotactic radiosurgical pallidotomy and thalamotomy with the gamma knife: MR imaging findings with clinical correlation – preliminary experience. Radiology 1999;212:143–150.
45 Laitinen LV, Bergenheim AT, Hariz MI: Leksell's posteroventral pallidotomy in the treatment of Parkinson's disease. J Neurosurg 1992;76:53–61.
46 Laitinen LV: Brain targets in surgery for Parkinson's disease. Results of a survey of neurosurgeons. J Neurosurg 1985;62:349–351.
47 Bonnen JG, Iacono RP, Lulu B, Mohamed AS, Gonzalez A, Schoonenberg T: Gamma knife pallidotomy: case report. Acta Neurochir (Wien) 1997;139:442–445.
48 Ohye C, Shibazaki T, Sato S: Gamma knife thalamotomy for movement disorders: evaluation of the thalamic lesion and clinical results. J Neurosurg 2005;102(suppl):234–240.

49 Friehs GM, Noren G, Ohye C, et al: Lesion size following Gamma Knife treatment for functional disorders. Stereotact Funct Neurosurg 1996;66(suppl 1):320–328.
50 Bakay RA, DeLong MR, Vitek JL: Posteroventral pallidotomy for Parkinson's disease. J Neurosurg 1992;77:487–488.
51 Giller CA, Dewey RB, Ginsburg MI, Mendelsohn DB, Berk AM: Stereotactic pallidotomy and thalamotomy using individual variations of anatomic landmarks for localization. Neurosurgery 1998;42:56–62; discussion 5.
52 Guiot G, Brion S: Treatment of abnormal movement by pallidal coagulation. Rev Neurol (Paris) 1953;89:578–580.
53 Iacono RP, Shima F, Lonser RR, Kuniyoshi S, Maeda G, Yamada S: The results, indications, and physiology of posteroventral pallidotomy for patients with Parkinson's disease. Neurosurgery 1995;36:1118–1125; discussion 25–27.
54 Iacono RP, Lonser RR, Oh A, Yamada S: New pathophysiology of Parkinson's disease revealed by posteroventral pallidotomy. Neurol Res 1995;17:178–180.
55 Lehman RM, Mezrich R, Sage J, Goldbe L: Peri- and postoperative magnetic resonance imaging localization of pallidotomy. Stereotact Funct Neurosurg 1994;62:61–70.
56 Lozano AM, Lang AE, Galvez-Jimenez N, et al: Effect of GPi pallidotomy on motor function in Parkinson's disease. Lancet 1995;346:1383–1387.
57 Lozano A, Hutchison W, Kiss Z, Tasker R, Davis K, Dostrovsky J: Methods for microelectrode-guided posteroventral pallidotomy. J Neurosurg 1996;84:194–202.
58 Feve AP, Fenelon G, Wallays C, Remy P, Guillard A: Axial motor disturbances after hypoxic lesions of the globus pallidus. Mov Disord 1993;8:321–326.
59 Kupsky WJ, Drozd MA, Barlow CF: Selective injury of the globus pallidus in children with post-cardiac surgery choreic syndrome. Dev Med Child Neurol 1995;37:135–144.
60 Malandrini A, Fabrizi GM, Bartalucci P, et al: Clinicopathological study of familial late infantile Hallervorden-Spatz disease: a particular form of neuroacanthocytosis. Childs Nerv Syst 1996;12: 155–160.
61 Bartzokis G, Beckson M, Hance DB, Marx P, Foster JA, Marder SR: MR evaluation of age-related increase of brain iron in young adult and older normal males. Magn Reson Imaging 1997;15:29–35.

Christopher M. Duma, MD
Medical Director, Hoag/UCI Gamma Knife Program
351 Hospital Road, Suite 401
Newport Beach, CA 92663 (USA)
Tel. +1 949 642 6787, Fax +1 949 642 4833, E-Mail cduma@hoaghospital.org

Szeifert GT, Kondziolka D, Levivier M, Lunsford LD (eds): Radiosurgery and Pathological Fundamentals. Prog Neurol Surg. Basel, Karger, 2007, vol 20, pp 267–278

11.3.1. Epilepsy

Jean Régis, Fabrice Bartolomei, Patrick Chauvel

Departments of Functional Neurosurgery and Neurophysiology and Epileptology, Timone University Hospital, Marseille, France

Abstract

The first Gamma Knife radiosurgery for mesial temporal lobe epilepsy was performed in Marseille in March 1993. Since then, around 130 patients have undergone epilepsy surgery using Gamma Knife at Marseille Timone University Hospital. The majority of epilepsy surgeries in our epilepsy surgery program in Marseille are performed conventionally because we still consider epilepsy radiosurgery as underevaluated. All epilepsy patients in Marseille are treated in the context of a successive prospective controlled trial, and we are convinced that few of the radiosurgical indications have been scrutinized and evaluated with more rigorous methodology. Some other centers (Madrid, San Diego, San Francisco) have now treated patients with comparable results.

The Marseille Historical Experience

A strong rationale for radiosurgery in epilepsy already existed in 1993.

Firstly, the effect of radiation on the epileptic cortex had been studied in animal models [51]. These pioneer works led Talairach et al. [50] in the 1950s to propose the 'surgical use of radiation' for the treatment of drug-resistant mesial temporal lobe epilepsy (MTLE). Radiosurgery of tumors [46] or vascular malformations [13, 16, 28, 38] in human have been demonstrated to be efficient for the associated epilepsy. In line with these observations and some complementary animal studies [14, 15, 35], in the 1980s Barcia Salorio et al. [3, 4] and Lindquist et al. [30] attempted to treat various kinds of epilepsies with disappointing results. Several recent animal studies have confirmed the antiepileptic effect of radiosurgery and enhanced our understanding of the role of radiation dose on seizure reduction probability [9, 29, 32, 33, 36, 49].

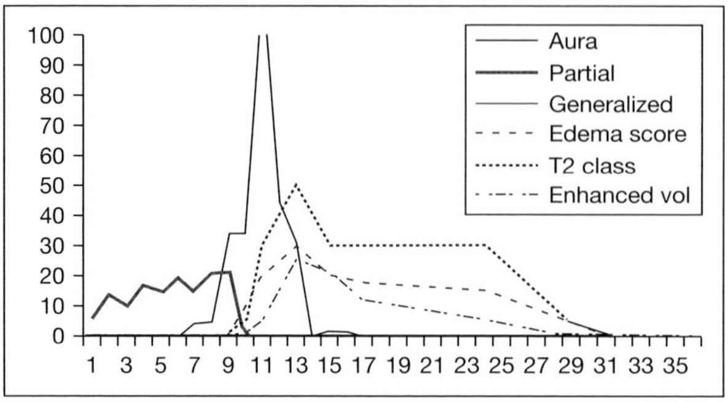

Fig. 1. Timetable of clinical and MR changes in a typical case.

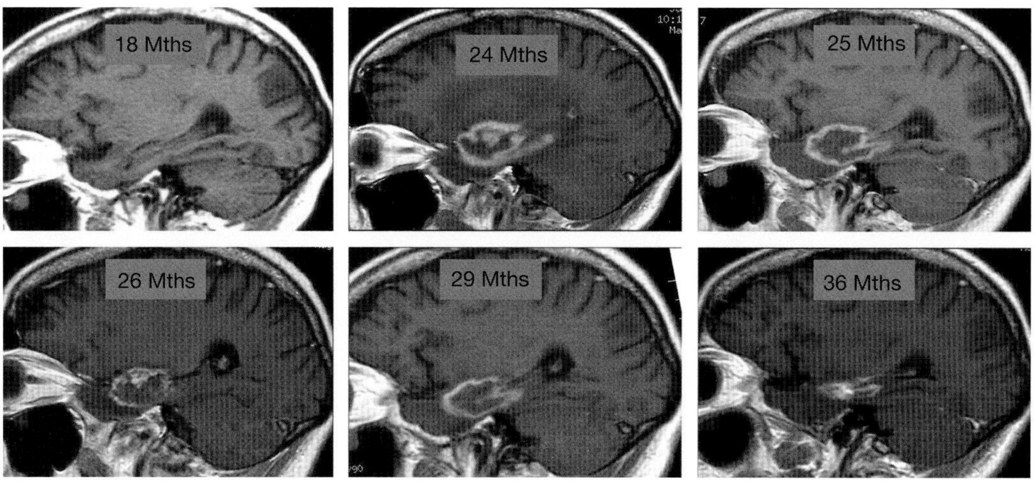

Fig. 2. Typical time course of the radiological events.

As early as 1994, we described a very specific timetable of events [39, 43, 45] several months after epilepsy radiosurgery (fig. 1). This sequence of events includes a trend for shorter seizures, more frequent seizures with no or brief loss of consciousness, delayed peak of seizures followed by a dramatic reduction in frequency and then seizure cessation. Radiologically, some discreet transient high T_2 signals are occasionally observed in the target area during the first weeks after Gamma Knife surgery (GKS) (fig. 2). Delayed (median 10.5 months; range 7–22 months) radiation affects include contrast enhancement in the region of 50% isodose line, high T_2 signal spreading outside the target through the temporal lobe and eventually going beyond its limits and a mass effect locally or even - outside the temporal lobe [39, 40]. These very impressive MR changes appear suddenly and quickly reach their maximum. Over time, these regress partly or totally. The temporal relationship between clinical and radiological changes is not constant. It is not uncommon to notice the peak of aura and or the seizure cessation before the onset of the dramatic MR changes. These changes were further delayed in the subgroup treated with a lower regimen of doses (18–20 Gy) [42].

Later, a dose de-escalation study demonstrated a close relationship between the marginal dose and the probability of seizure cessation [19, 42]. Dose reduction at the margin from 24 to 20 or 18 was associated with a significantly lower probability of seizure cessation at 3 years [19, 42]. Subsequent studies confirmed these results [11, 27, 48].

MTLE radiosurgery is associated with a high short middle term safety and efficacy. Since 1993, we have organized several strictly controlled prospective clinical trials studying the safety and efficacy of radiosurgery in patients harboring MTLE without associated space-occupying lesion [39, 44]. All these studies have established good safety and efficacy of GKS for this new indication. However, these studies have also shown the importance of a cautious patient selection, a very careful selection of the dosimetric parameters, and target delineation. In fact, this is the most detailed and careful surgical strategy ever proposed to this group of patients. Consequently, the precise definition of the real extent of the epileptogenic zone and the selection of patients demonstrating a very circumscribed epileptogenic zone has become mandatory. If the patient selection, dosimetry and clinical management are not strictly controlled, the risk of failure increases dramatically. Microsurgical resection of the epileptogenic zone in hypothalamic hamartomas is associated with very significant risks due to the close relationship with highly critical brain structures (mammillary bodies, hypothalamus, fornix, visual pathways) and vicinity of the important major vessels and perforators in the surrounding cisterns. The delay of the radiosurgery effect on epilepsy is related to an additional risk of sudden unexpected death in epilepsy but perhaps a reduced risk of severe postoperative depression.

More recently, we have observed a very low impact of radiosurgery on neuropsychological outcome and especially on verbal mnesic function when the dominant side was treated [44]. The preliminary results of the multicenter study in the US support our results [2]. An intriguing animal study performed in Pittsburgh provided additional evidence that radiosurgery could not spare the mnesic function when directed toward the mesial temporal lobe structures [32].

Acute MR changes do not correspond to a necrotic phenomenon! The arguments that initially led to hypothesize the absence of tissue necrosis in the majority of patients and the existence of a neuromodulation effect accounting

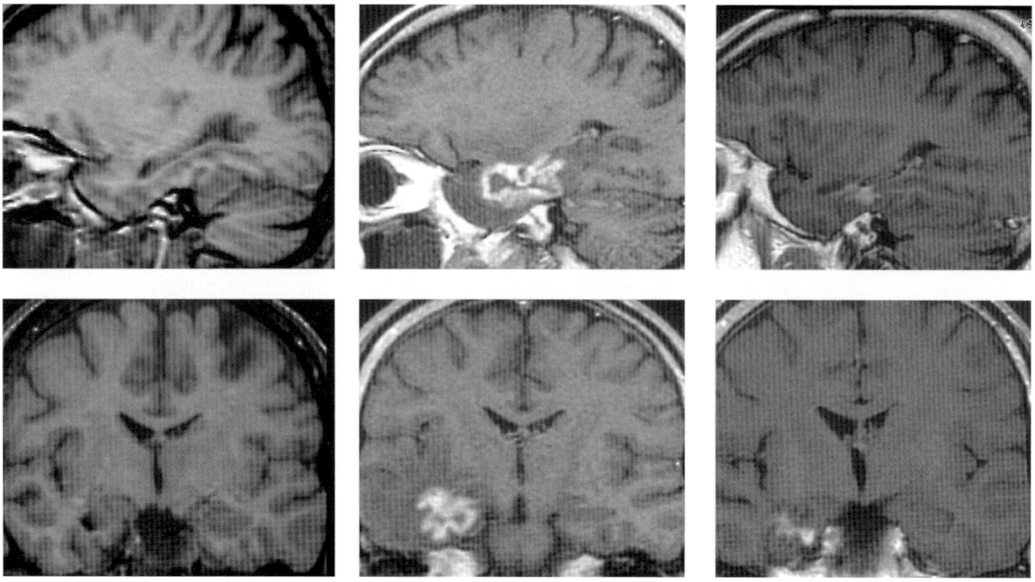

Fig. 3. Late MR aspect compared with preradiosurgical changes. The late aspect is very close to the preradiosurgical aspect, especially when the extent of the MR changes is taken into account.

for the antiepileptic efficacy have been summarized in 2002 [37]. A longer follow-up has confirmed these observations (fig. 3). The latter certainly account for the better mnesic function sparing after radiosurgery as compared to microsurgical removal. Additionally, a recent PET study comparing the long-term outcome in patients operated microsurgically and radiosurgically has demonstrated that the worsening of the hypometabolism (18FDG) was more severe and widespread after selective amygdalohippocampectomy (SAH) than after GKS [31].

Eighteen adult patients with drug-resistant MTLE associated with unilateral hippocampal sclerosis were included. Ten patients were treated by SAH (group 1) and 8 by GK radiosurgery (group 2). PET using ^{18}F-fluorodeoxyglucose (FDG) and MRI were performed before surgery and at least 1 year later. Group analysis of PET imaging was performed using statistical parametric mapping software (SPM99). The comparison between preoperative and postoperative FDG-PET scans demonstrated a statistically significant worsening of the hypometabolism after both surgical procedures. In group 1, we found a significant decrease in the metabolism after SAH in the ipsilateral temporal pole, in the caudate nucleus and in the thalamus and a worsening of the hypometabolism in the medial temporal lobe. In group 2, we found a worsening of the hypometabolism in the ipsilateral temporal pole and in the medial temporal lobe. The comparison of metabolic data after both surgical procedures showed a similar worsening of the hypometabolism in the ipsilateral temporal pole. The worsening of the hypometabolism was less severe after GK than after SAH in the medial temporal lobe and similar in the ipsilateral temporal pole.

The reversal of the epileptic encephalopathy associated with hypothalamic hamartomas has been demonstrated to be achievable [41] if radiosurgery is performed early enough. Cognitive decline can be halted and even reversed as sometimes some children are able to go back to a normal rhythm of acquisition. Frequently, psychiatric assessment shows diverse levels of heteroaggressivity, clear attention deficit and hyperactivity disorder, marked oppositional defiant disorder. Selective sustained attention and control of impulsivity are frequently poor. These symptoms are frequently improved or even normalized especially in children treated at a very young age. Our first results indicate that GKS is as effective as microsurgical resection and much safer. GKS avoids the vascular risk related to radiofrequency lesioning or stimulation. The disadvantage of radiosurgery is its delayed action. Longer follow-up is mandatory for a serious evaluation of the role of GKS. Results are faster and more complete in patients with smaller lesions inside the 3rd ventricle (type 2). The early effect on subclinical discharges plays a major role in the dramatic improvement of sleep quality, behavior, and developmental acceleration at school.

The mechanism of the antiepileptic effect is not clearly understood. Seizure cessation some months after the radiosurgical treatment of arteriovenous malformations in highly functional areas (i.e. primary motor area) with no functional deficit is a common observation. This demonstrates the capability of low-dose (usually 24-Gy) radiosurgery to render the cortex of the epileptogenic area no longer epileptic while sparing its function. This kind of clinical observations have led us to speculate that radiosurgery, under certain conditions, can act as a neuromodulatory therapy [37]. This 'nonlesional' antiepileptic effect of radiosurgery is especially interesting for future indications in functional brain surgery. In MTLE patients, we have until now observed no objective neuropsychological worsening. After microsurgical cortectomy, especially when the dominant side is operated, verbal mnesic deficits have been reported [10, 17, 18, 20]. This fact has even led us to accept to treat some patients with MTLE contraindicated for a cortectomy due to Wada test failure (prediction of a verbal mnesic deficit). Until now, none of these patients have experienced verbal memory decline. Of course, Wada test prediction has imperfect reliability. In MTLE, radiosurgery is systematically associated with important MR changes some (8–26) months after GKS. These MR changes are very suggestive of a radioinduced necrosis and have been considered so for a long time [10, 17, 18, 20, 45]. However, systematic radiological follow-up of these patients demonstrated a progressive disappearance of these aspects.

Several years after mesial temporal radiosurgery, the images are either comparable to the preoperative ones or demonstrate slight retractive change confined to the location corresponding to the center of the dosimetry. Finally, in the large majority of patients presenting with hypothalamic hamartomas radiosurgical treatment of epilepsy does not induce any kind of, even transient, MR change. This is, in our opinion, a specially convincing demonstration that radiosurgery can make the epileptogenicity of the cortex disappear with no major histological changes.

Dosimetry strategy in epilepsy radiosurgery is very difficult. The goal is to obtain a high probability of seizure cessation without inducing any necrotic effect and especially functional worsening. The precise definition of the target, and the selection of the appropriate reference dose for the selected target volume still requires more experimental data and clinical evaluation.

What Is the Target ? The Key Role of the Entorhinal Cortex

The dose issue is especially difficult to address in absence of a clear definition of the target boundary. Thus, comparison of patient groups treated with different regimens of marginal dose is not achievable. Even more, the best suited target is probably not the same for all the patients presenting features of the so-called 'MTLE syndrome' [7, 34]. Thus, it is classically thought that the hippocampus is the most important structure generating MTLE seizures. However, there is increasing evidence that mesial temporal structures other than the hippocampus participate in seizure generation; in particular, the entorhinal cortex (EC) [6, 47]. Recently, several neuroradiological studies demonstrated diminution in the volume of EC ipsilateral to the epileptic side in patients with TLE. The rate of patients exhibiting a significant reduction in EC volumes ranges from 52 to 96% [8, 26]. A recent study shows a correlation between the degree of EC atrophy and the epileptogenicity of this structure [5].

In patients with MTLE, the EC may be early involved by a tonic epileptic discharge, and the role of the EC could be different depending on the type of the interictal to ictal transition. Two classical patterns of seizure onset have been described [52].

In the first one (type 1), the seizure onset is characterized by the emergence of a low-frequency (<2 Hz); high-amplitude rhythmic spiking followed by a tonic discharge in one or several mesial structures. In the second one (type 2), the seizure onset is characterized by the emergence of a tonic discharge in one or several mesial structures without prior spiking activity. We have recently studied the involvement of three major mesial structures (amygdala, hippocampal head and EC) in these types of seizure onset. The role of each structure was evaluated by quantifying the degree of synchrony and the direction of couplings between the signals recorded from these three structures. We found that the EC was never the leader in the two other structures in type 1, but was the leader in more than 50% of the patients displaying a type 2 pattern of ictal discharge [7]. In a second study, we measured the volume of the EC in these patients and in a control group of same age. The volume of the EC on the side of the epilepsy was significantly reduced. We also found a correlation between the atrophy of the EC and its involvement in seizures, particularly in type 2 seizures [5]. This data reinforce the idea that the so-called MTLE syndrome is a heterogeneous condition and includes different subtypes specially distinguished by a different role of the EC. Perhaps this kind of tiny distinction has few practical consequences when all MTLE patients operated receive a quite large cortectomy including the pole, the mesial structures including the parahippocampal cortex, and the anterior aspect of the basal and the lateral temporal lobe cortex. From an anatomical point of view, the EC corresponds to the ambiens gyrus situated just anteriorly to the intralimbicus gyrus and is distinguishable by the polygonal darker spots corresponding to the islands of layer 2 [24]. In terms of connectivity, the EC projects largely toward the dentate gyrus of the different parts of the hippocampal formation [21–23]. The subfields of the EC [24] have specific patterns of projections; the more mesial subfields have more rostral projections and the more lateral subfields have more posterior projections. The more lateral subfields tend to project more on gyrus dentatus and the more mesial more on cornu ammoni [54]. As demonstrated by retrograde tracing in nonhuman primate afferents of the EC include several paralimbic areas (cingulate, orbitofrontal, insular, parahippocampal cortex) olfactory bulb and superior temporal sulcus cortex [22, 23]. The EC is supposed to play also a major role in the contralateral propagation of the commissural connections of the hippocampal formation as it is restricted to the caudal EC and uncal portion of the hippocampus [1]. Several experimental studies have demonstrated the important role of the EC [12, 25], but the more convincing evidence came from the clinical experience [47]. The systematic analysis of the involvement of each of the structures from the hippocampal formation and its correlation with seizure cessation rate demonstrated in both microsurgical [53] and radiosurgical [19] experience the predominant role of EC resection or treatment for a high probability of seizure cessation. Kawai et al. [27] demonstrated the inefficacy of radiosurgery when only the amygdala and hippocampus are targeted. One of the first patients treated in Marseille was treated a similar way with a small volume confined to the amygdaloid complex and the hippocampus with high doses and a necrotizing effect inside the target volume. However, in spite of the destruction of the amygdala and hippocampus, the typical semiology of MTLE continued quite unchanged. An SEEG investigation allowed us to demonstrate that this epilepsy was essentially organized in the remaining anterior parahippocampal cortex. A cortectomy cured the patient. This demonstrated that all the different kinds of temporal lobe epilepsy cannot be cured by highly selective radiosurgery [42].

The present time is a period of reappraisal of neurosurgery for functional disorders. The enhanced level of care and the higher level of education of patients have led to higher expectations of those suffering from functional disorders like Parkinson disease, pain or epilepsy.

Concomitantly, some limits of drug strategies have been reached and minimally invasive neurosurgical techniques have demonstrated their safety and efficacy. Stereotactic minimally invasive procedures for functional neurosurgery include quite a large spectrum of techniques like thermocoagulation, deep brain stimulation, grafting or radiosurgery. Neurosciences have now entered into a very productive period where every day new discoveries are opening a new understanding of brain functioning and new future directions for innovative therapies. As our understanding of the role of each brain structure increases, we will be able to make new more precise therapeutic proposals intended to act precisely with more subtlety in this complex anatomy. Conversely, the idea to develop therapeutic strategies respecting the functioning of the normal brain sounds more and more realistic. Thus, the capacity of high-precision radiosurgery to tailor its action in the complex 3-D anatomy of the brain while sparing the surrounding critical structures make it very appealing for modern functional neurosurgery.

Epilepsy surgery is certainly one of the most challenging fields in functional disorders. The variability of the organization of the epileptic network from one patient to another, the very close relationship between these networks and normal neuronal networks underlying important neuropsychological functions, the necessity to operate the majority of these patients in young age make the requirement for development of new versatile high-precision minimally invasive methods more acute.

Today, there is no doubt that radiations can improve or cure epilepsy. This positive effect was first suspected in patients treated for a brain lesion associated with epilepsy as well as demonstrated in a series of experimental studies in animals [9, 29, 32, 33, 36, 49] and now demonstrated in several prospective clinical trials in MTLE and hypothalamic hamartoma patients.

Conclusion

Thanks to experimental studies and the last 12 years of clinical evaluation, a series of facts have been established:

1 Radiosurgery can provide seizure reduction or seizure cessation in epilepsies related to space-occupying lesions like arteriovenous malformations or tumors, epilepsies of mesial temporal lobe, epilepsies without space-occupying lesions and specific epileptic syndromes like hypothalamic hamartomas.
2 The antiepileptic effect of radiosurgery can be mediated by nondestructive tissue changes and has been demonstrated to induce very low rate of functional complications in MTLE and hypothalamic hamartomas.
3 Radiosurgery can lead to a real reversal of the epileptic encephalopathy in young patients presenting with hypothalamic hamartomas (with an improvement in cognitive abilities and a reduction in hyperkinetic and/or aggressive behavior associated with seizure cessation or reduction).
4 Radiosurgery in MTLE is associated with the persistence of the sudden unexpected death in epilepsy risk during the months preceding the seizure cessation which can be delayed by 1–36 months.

A series of issues need further clinical and experimental work for a better management of these patients:
1 The detailed mechanism of the nondestructive antiepileptic effect of radiosurgery.
2 The precise optimum target and dose selection in MTLE.
3 Several decades are required to confirm the prolonged safety and efficacy of radiosurgery in epilepsy.
4 Role of radiosurgery in epilepsies associated with dysplasia or heterotopia.
5 Role of radiosurgery in highly functional EC.
6 Role of radiosurgery in pathway disruption in complex epileptic networks.
7 Potential role of combined strategies with microsurgery and radiosurgery.

However, based on the extensive data available today, we expect a major role of radiosurgery in epilepsy surgery provided the rules of good practice in terms of patient selection, dose planning and patient clinical postoperative management are respected.

References

1 Amaral DG, Insausti R, Cowan WM: The commissural connections of the monkey hippocampal formation. J Comp Neurol 1984;224:307–336.
2 Barbaro N: Standard versus Selective Resection versus Radiosurgery, What Have We Learned from Comparative Trials? San Francisco, 2004.
3 Barcia Salorio JL, Garcia JA, Hernandez G, et al: Radiosurgery of epilepsy: long-term results. Eur Soc Stereotact Funct Neurosurg 1993.
4 Barcia Salorio JL, Roldan P, Hernandez G, et al: Radiosurgery treatment of epilepsy. J Appl Neurophysiol 1985;48:400–403.
5 Bartolomei F, Khalil M, Wendling F, et al: Entorhinal cortex involvement in human mesial temporal lobe epilepsy: an electrophysiological and volumetric study. Epilepsia 2005;46:677–687.

6 Bartolomei F, Wendling F, Bellanger JJ, et al: Neural networks involving the medial temporal structures in temporal lobe epilepsy. Clin Neurophysiol 2001;112:1746–1760.
7 Bartolomei F, Wendling F, Regis J, et al: Pre-ictal synchronicity in limbic networks of mesial temporal lobe epilepsy. Epilepsy Res 2004;61:89–104.
8 Bernasconi N, Bernasconi A, Caramanos Z, et al: Mesial temporal damage in temporal lobe epilepsy: a volumetric MRI study of the hippocampus, amygdala and parahippocampal region. Brain 2003;126:462–469.
9 Chen ZF, Kamiryo T, Henson SL, et al: Anticonvulsant effects of gamma surgery in a model of chronic spontaneous limbic epilepsy in rats. J Neurosurg 2001;94:270–280.
10 Clusmann H, Schramm J, Kral T, et al: Prognostic factors and outcome after different types of resection for temporal lobe epilepsy. J Neurosurg 2002;97:1131–1141.
11 Cmelak AJ, Abou-Khalil B, Konrad PE, et al: Low-dose stereotactic radiosurgery is inadequate for medically intractable mesial temporal lobe epilepsy: a case report. Seizure 2001;10:442–446.
12 Cohen I, Navarro V, Clemenceau S, et al: On the origin of interictal activity in human temporal lobe epilepsy in vitro. Science 2002;298:1418–1421.
13 Eisenschenk S, Gilmore RL, Friedman WA, et al: The effect of LINAC stereotactic radiosurgery on epilepsy associated with arteriovenous malformations. Stereotact Funct Neurosurg 1998;71: 51–61.
14 Elomaa E: Focal irradiation of the brain: an alternative to temporal lobe resection in intractable focal epilepsy? Med Hypotheses 1980;6:501–503.
15 Gaffey C, Monotoya V, Lyman J, et al: Restriction of the spread of epileptic discharges in cats by mean of Bragg Peak intracranial irradiation. Int J Appl Radiat Isot 1981;32:779–787.
16 Ghossoub M, Nataf F, Merienne L, et al: Evolution of epileptic seizures associated with cerebral arteriovenous malformations after radiosurgery. Neurochirurgie 2001;47:344–349.
17 Gleissner U, Helmstaedter C, Schramm J, et al: Memory outcome after selective amygdalohippocampectomy: a study in 140 patients with temporal lobe epilepsy. Epilepsia 2002;43:87–95.
18 Gleissner U, Sassen R, Lendt M, et al: Pre- and postoperative verbal memory in pediatric patients with temporal lobe epilepsy. Epilepsy Res 2002;51:287–296.
19 Hayashi M, Bartolomei F, Rey M, et al: MR changes after Gamma knife radiosurgery for Mesial Temporal Lobe Epilepsy: an evidence for the efficacy of subnecrotic doses; in Kondziolka D (ed): Radiosurgery. Basel, Karger, 2002, vol 4, pp 192–202.
20 Helmstaedter C, Reuber M, Elger CC: Interaction of cognitive aging and memory deficits related to epilepsy surgery. Ann Neurol 2002;52:89–94.
21 Insausti R: Comparative anatomy of the entorhinal cortex and hippocampus in mammals. Hippocampus 1993;3:19–26.
22 Insausti R, Amaral DG, Cowan WM: The entorhinal cortex of the monkey: II. Cortical afferents. J Comp Neurol 1987;264:356–395.
23 Insausti R, Amaral DG, Cowan WM: The entorhinal cortex of the monkey: III. Subcortical afferents. J Comp Neurol 1987;264:396–408.
24 Insausti R, Tunon T, Sobreviela T, et al: The human entorhinal cortex: a cytoarchitectonic analysis. J Comp Neurol 1995;355:171–198.
25 Jones R, Heinemann U, Lambert J: The entorhinal cortex and generation of seizure activity: studies of normal synaptic transmission and epileptogenesis in vitro; in Avanzini G, Engel J, Fariello R, et al. (eds): Neurotransmitters in Epilepsy. Elsevier Science, 1992, pp 173–180.
26 Jutila L, Ylinen A, Partanen K, et al: MR volumetry of the entorhinal, perirhinal, and temporopolar cortices in drug-refractory temporal lobe epilepsy. AJNR Am J Neuroradiol 2001;22: 1490–1501.
27 Kawai K, Suzuki I, Kurita H, et al: Failure of low-dose radiosurgery to control temporal lobe epilepsy. J Neurosurg 2001;95:883–887.
28 Kida Y, Kobayashi T, Tanaka T, et al: Seizure control after radiosurgery on cerebral arteriovenous malformations. J Clin Neurosci 2000;7:6–9.
29 Kitchen N: Experimental and clinical studies on the putative therapeutic efficacy of cerebral irradiation (radiotherapy) in epilepsy. Epilepsy Res 1995;20:1–10.

30 Lindquist C, Kihlstrom L, Hellstrand E: Functional neurosurgery – a future for the gamma knife? Stereotact Funct Neurosurg 1991;57:72–81.
31 Lopez E, Regis J, Bartolomei F, et al: Metabolic changes after selective temporo-mesial radiosurgery versus amygdalo-hippocampectomy in mesio-temporal lobe epilepsy. Epilepsia 2004; 45:113.
32 Maesawa S, Kondziolka D, Balzer J, et al: The behavioral and electroencephalographic effects of stereotactic radiosurgery for the treatment of epilepsy evaluated in the rat kainic acid model. Stereotact Funct Neurosurg 1999;73:115.
33 Maesawa S, Kondziolka D, Dixon C, et al: Subnecrotic stereotactic radiosurgery controlling epilepsy produced by kainic acid injection in rats. J Neurosurg 2000;93:1033–1040.
34 Maillard L, Vignal JP, Gavaret M, et al: Semiologic and electrophysiologic correlations in temporal lobe seizure subtypes. Epilepsia 2004;45:1590–1599.
35 Monnier M, Krupp P: Action of gamma radiation on electrical brain activity; in Haley TJ, Snider RS (eds): Response of the Nervous Systeme to Ionizing Radiation. New York, Academic Press, 1962, pp 359–368.
36 Mori Y, Kondziolka D, Balzer J, et al: Effects of stereotactic radiosurgery on an animal model of hippocampal epilepsy. Neurosurgery 2000;46:157–165; discussion 165–168.
37 Regis J, Bartolomei F, Hayashi M, et al: Gamma Knife surgery, a neuromodulation therapy in epilepsy surgery! Acta Neurochir Suppl 2002;84:37–47.
38 Régis j, Bartolomei F, Kida Y, et al: Radiosurgery of epilepsy associated with cavernous malformation: retrospective study in 49 patients. Neurosurgery 2000;47:1091–1097.
39 Régis J, Bartolomei F, Rey M, et al: Gamma knife surgery for mesial temporal lobe epilepsy. Epilepsia 1999;40:1551–1556.
40 Regis J, Bartolomei F, Rey M, et al: Gamma knife surgery for mesial temporal lobe epilepsy. J Neurosurg 2000;93(suppl 3):141–146.
41 Régis J, Hayashi M, Perez Eupierre L, et al: Gamma knife surgery for epilepsy related to hypothalamic hamartomas. Acta Neurochir 2004;91:33–50.
42 Regis J, Levivier M, Motohiro H: Radiosurgery for intractable epilepsy. Tech Neurosurg 2003;9:191–203.
43 Régis J, Peragut JC, Rey M, et al: First selective amygdalohippocampic radiosurgery for mesial temporal lobe epilepsy. Stereotact Funct Neurosurg 1994;64:191–201.
44 Regis J, Rey M, Bartolomei F, et al: Gamma knife surgery in mesial temporal lobe epilepsy: a prospective multicenter study. Epilepsia 2004;45:504–515.
45 Regis J, Semah F, Bryan R, et al: Early and delayed MR and PET changes after selective temporomesial radiosurgery in mesial temporal lobe epilepsy. AJNR Am J Neuroradiol 1999;20: 213–216.
46 Schrottner O, Eder HG, Unger F, et al: Radiosurgery in lesional epilepsy: brain tumors. Stereotact Funct Neurosurg 1998;70:50–56.
47 Spencer S, Spencer D: Entorhinal-hippocampal interactions in medial temporal lobe epilepsy. Epilepsia 1994;35:721–727.
48 Srikijvilaikul T, Najm I, Foldvary-Schaefer N, et al: Failure of gamma knife radiosurgery for mesial temporal lobe epilepsy: report of five cases. Neurosurgery 2004;54:1395–1402; discussion 1402–1404.
49 Sun B, DeSalles AA, Medin PM, et al: Reduction of hippocampal-kindled seizure activity in rats by stereotactic radiosurgery. Exp Neurol 1998;154:691–695.
50 Talairach J, Bancaud J, G.Szikla, et al: Approche nouvelle de la neurochirurgie de l'epilepsie. Méthodologie stéréotaxique et résultats thérapeutiques; in Neurochirurgie (ed): Congrés Annuel de la Société de Langue Française. Marseille 25–28 Juin 1974:Masson, 1974, Vol 20, suppl 1, pp 205–213.
51 Tracy S: High-frequency high potential currents, and X-radiations in the treatement of epilepsy. N Y Med J 1905;81:422–424.
52 Velasco A, Wilson C, Babb T, et al: Functional and anatomic correlates of two frequently observed temporal lobe seizure-onset patterns. Neural Plast 2000;7:49–63.

53 Wieser HG, Siegel AM, Yasargil GM: The Zurich amygdalo-hippocampectomy series: a short up-date. Acta Neurochir Suppl (Wien) 1990;50:122–127.
54 Witter MP, Amaral DG: Entorhinal cortex of the monkey: V. Projections to the dentate gyrus, hippocampus, and subicular complex. J Comp Neurol 1991;307:437–459.

Prof. Jean Régis
Service de Neurochirurgie Fonctionnelle et Stéréotaxique
264 Bvd St Pierre
FR–13385 Marseille Cedex 05 (France)
Tel. +33 4 91 38 70 58, Fax +33 4 91 38 70 56, E-Mail jregis@ap-hm.fr

Szeifert GT, Kondziolka D, Levivier M, Lunsford LD (eds): Radiosurgery and Pathological Fundamentals. Prog Neurol Surg. Basel, Karger, 2007, vol 20, pp 279–288

11.3.2. Radiosurgery in Epilepsy – Pathological Considerations

Paul A. House[a], *Jung H. Kim*[b], *Nihal De Lanerolle*[b], *Nicholas M. Barbaro*[c]

[a]Department of Neurosurgery, University of Utah, Salt Lake City, Utah, [b]Department of Pathology, Yale University School of Medicine, New Haven, Conn., [c]Department of Neurosurgery, University of California San Francisco, San Francisco, Calif., USA

Abstract

Radiosurgery is being investigated as an alternative to open surgical resection for patients with medial temporal lobe epilepsy. Additionally, the biological effects of mesial temporal radiosurgery are being evaluated using several animal models. The mechanisms through which radiosurgery exerts antiepileptic effects have not yet been proven, but time and dose dependency have been repeatedly demonstrated. Thus, there is a need to carefully examine the histological changes in patients who have undergone radiosurgical treatment of epilepsy.

Medial temporal lobe epilepsy (MTLE) is perhaps the epilepsy syndrome most responsive to surgical intervention. When MTLE is due to underlying mesial temporal sclerosis (MTS), surgical cure can be expected in approximately 65% of patients [1, 2]. Current studies indicate that freedom from seizures after withdrawal of medication can be expected in at least 30% of patients [3]. Recently, radiosurgery has been explored as an alternative to open resective surgery. A prospective European study demonstrated rates of epilepsy cure similar to those obtained from resective surgery [4]. The early results of a multicenter study in the United States similarly suggest a clear biological effect of radiosurgery on seizures, and seizure cessation rates similar to those seen with open resection [unpubl. obs.].

As the interest in radiosurgery as therapy for temporal lobe epilepsy increases, there is a need to evaluate what is known about the biological effects of radiosurgery in the setting of MTS. An early study of radiosurgery for epilepsy suggested that radiation has an antiepileptic effect, even when administered in subnecrotic doses [5]. However, it is unclear if the antiepileptic effects are caused by tissue necrosis (i.e. neuronal death) or if the radiation eliminates seizure activity in still functional brain tissue through some heretofore undiscovered mechanism. To date, histological examination of irradiated mesial temporal tissue has been very limited. This review evaluates histological specimens from patients with MTS who have undergone radiosurgery, and discusses the histological effects of radiosurgery on animal models of epilepsy.

Materials and Methods

A Medline search of the relevant English literature regarding radiosurgery for control of epilepsy was performed. From this review, we identified 6 patients who underwent surgical resection of the mesial temporal structures following radiosurgery. In addition, 2 patients enrolled in an ongoing multicenter trial (Radiosurgical Treatment of Temporal Lobe Epilepsy, Barbaro N.M., Principal Investigator) have required resection following radiosurgery. Histological analysis of the tissue from these 2 patients was performed at a single center. The UCSF Committee on Human Research approved the clinical trial.

Results

In total, histological examinations of tissue from 8 patients with temporal lobe epilepsy who had undergone radiosurgery were available (table 1). The patients from the ongoing multicenter trial have not been previously described.

The first patient from the clinical trial was a 30-year-old female with medically refractory epilepsy beginning at the age of 20. She was identified as having right MTLE based on semiology and video electroencephalography (EEG). Findings consistent with right hippocampal sclerosis were found on MRI. She was originally treated with radiosurgery; 24 Gy was delivered to the 50% isodose line, with a target volume of 6.8 cm^3. At 11 months following treatment, the patient experienced a decrease in her seizures but had troubling headaches and decreased vision. Papilledema and increased visual blind spots persisted despite administration of corticosteroids. Based on these clinical findings, the patient underwent resection of the amygdala, hippocampus, and 5 cm of the temporal neocortex 14 months after radiosurgery. Her papilledema resolved. Histological analysis revealed extensive necrosis and radiation-induced changes consisting of thickened, hyalinized vessels and early calcification (figs. 1 and 2).

The second patient from the clinical trial was a 29-year-old male who developed medically refractory MTLE at the age of 23. Video EEG demonstrated a left

Table 1. Summary of data from histological examinations of tissue from 8 patients with temporal lobe epilepsy who underwent radiosurgery

Patient	Age years	Sex	Radiation dose, Gy	Isodose line, %	Radiated volume cm^3	Time until resection months	Histology	Reference
1	30	f	24	50	6.8	14	extensive tissue necrosis and radiation changes	unpublished
2	29	m	20	50	6.9	>24	hippocampal sclerosis, small necrotic foci	unpublished
3	36	m	15	57	2.4	~12	sclerosis, no radiation induced changes seen	Cmelak et al. [6]
4	31	f	18	50	6.2	30	sclerosis, 5-mm necrotic focus, vascular wall thickening	Kawai et al. [7]
5	22	m	18	–	8.7	16	sclerosis, no necrosis or vascular changes, reactive astrocytes and scattered degenerated neurons	Kawai et al. [7]
6	19	f	20	50	6.1	20	hippocampal sclerosis and radiation effect, including necrosis	Srikijvilaikul et al. [8]
7	22	m	20	50	8.7	22	hippocampal sclerosis and radiation effect, including necrosis	Srikijvilaikul et al. [8]
8	50	f	20	50	7.2	18	hippocampal sclerosis and radiation effect, including necrosis	Srikijvilaikul et al. [8]

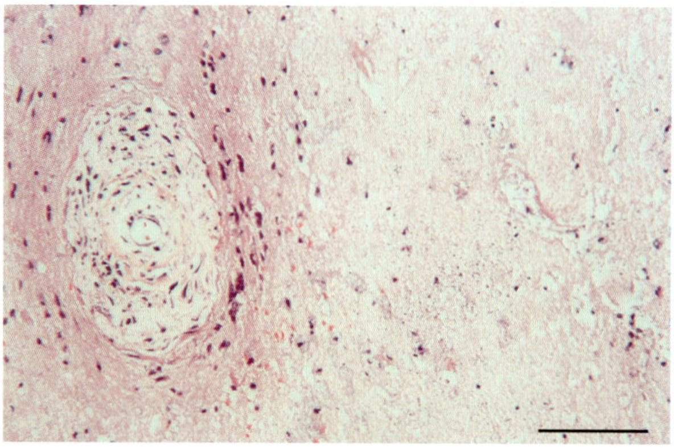

Fig. 1. An anomalous vessel with a thickened vascular wall (left) is seen in an area adjacent to necrosis (right). HE (bar = 100 μm).

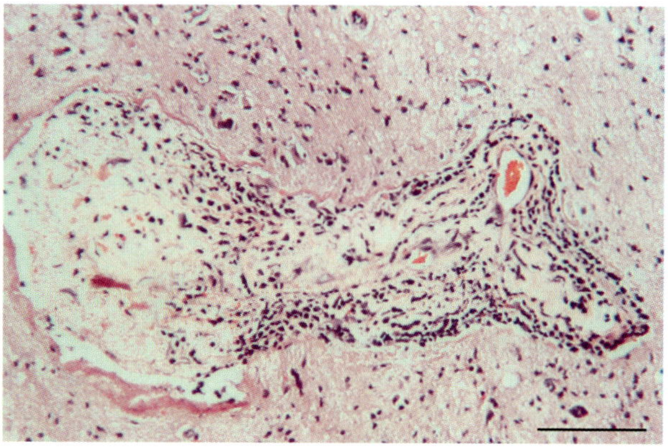

Fig. 2. An abnormal vessel with a thickened partially hyalinized wall infiltrated by mononuclear inflammatory cells. HE (bar = 100 μm).

temporal onset consistent with his MRI diagnosis of left MTS. He underwent radiosurgery to the medial temporal structures using a dose of 20 Gy at the 50% isodose line. Six isocenters were used to cover the 6.9-cm^3 target volume. The patient experienced no change in his seizure frequency and underwent resection 24 months after radiosurgery. Histological examination showed clear hippocampal sclerosis with extensive loss of CA1 neurons. The remaining neurons in the hippocampus had eosinophilic cytoplasm and dark nuclei, representing degenerative changes secondary to radiation. Also observed were isolated vessels with a

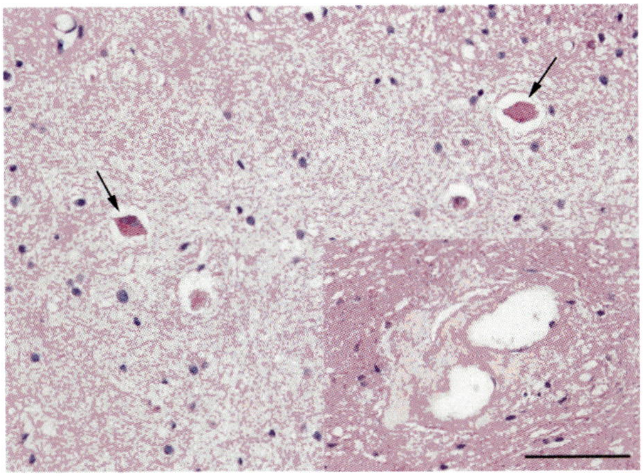

Fig. 3. CA2 of the hippocampal pyramidal layer showing a marked neuronal loss. The remaining neurons (arrows) are shrunken, displaying dark nuclei and eosinophilic cytoplasm. Inset: a vessel in the white matter with a thickened hyalinized wall. Main image and inset: HE (bar = 100 μm).

thickened hyalinized wall, a typical radiation-induced alteration (fig. 3). There was a vacuolar change in the hippocampal hilar region. Small foci of necrosis were identified in the subependymal layer of the floor of the temporal horn.

Three patients reported in 2001 (table 1) underwent resection due to lack of seizure control [6–8]. Patient 3 was a 36-year-old male who developed complex partial seizures at the age of 18. His seizures temporarily decreased after radiosurgery, but returned to baseline by 1 year. He therefore underwent resection of the amygdala, 2.5 cm of hippocampus and 5.5 cm of lateral neocortex. Histological evaluation of the tissue obtained at the time of surgery revealed hippocampal sclerosis with fibrillary astrocytosis. No radiation-induced histopathologic changes were seen [6].

Patient 4 was a 31-year-old female who had experienced refractory temporal lobe epilepsy since the age of 6. Due to persistent seizures, the patient underwent resection of the amygdala, hippocampus, and 5 cm of lateral neocortex 30 months after radiosurgery. Histological examination revealed hippocampal sclerosis with a single 5-mm necrotic focus in the posterior hippocampal head. Prominent vascular changes consisting of vessel wall thickening, fibrinoid and hyaline degeneration were seen in the area of necrosis [7].

Patient 5 was a 22-year-old male with a 13-year history of seizures. Seizures continued and no MRI changes were noted up to 15 months following radiosurgery. Temporal lobectomy was performed 16 months after radiosurgery and resulted in seizure cessation. Histological evaluation showed typical hippocampal sclerosis with additional gemistocytic astrocytes and scattered degenerated neurons. No necrotic focus or vascular changes were identified [7].

Srikijvilaikul et al. [8] from the Cleveland Clinic reported 5 patients in whom radiosurgical treatment failed to provide seizure control. Two patients died, likely due to seizure events, less than 14 months after radiosurgery. The remaining patients underwent resection at 18, 20, and 22 months following radiosurgery, respectively. Histological analysis revealed findings consistent with hippocampal sclerosis and radiation effects. Perivascular sclerosis, macrophage infiltration and necrosis were noted in all patients.

Discussion

The efficacy of radiosurgery for treating various forms of epilepsy is reviewed in an accompanying chapter in this volume. While radiosurgery has been shown to reduce seizures in both lesional and nonlesional epilepsy, the mechanism by which this abatement occurs is not clear. Insights into the mechanism of action and the biological effects of radiosurgery are currently being gleaned through both human and animal investigations. Due to the scarcity of histological samples from patients who have undergone radiosurgery for the treatment of epilepsy, animal models have been important in this field of study.

Experiments undertaken at the University of Virginia were designed to evaluate the effects of radiosurgery on a chronic spontaneous limbic epilepsy model in rats. In this model, hippocampal electrodes are implanted and a single 90-min period of stimulation is used to produce a spontaneous limbic epileptic state. The animals underwent Gamma Knife radiosurgery 10 weeks later at doses of 10–40 Gy, using a 4-mm collimator. The lowest dose group (10 Gy) showed no decrease in seizures. The 20 Gy group showed a gradual and continuous reduction in seizure occurrence from 2 to 6 months after irradiation. The 40 Gy group had a dramatic reduction is seizures by the second month. No radiation necrosis was noted on histological samples from any group. In a parallel study, hippocampal slices taken from animals more than 6 days after 40-Gy radiosurgery were significantly more resistant to penicillin-induced epileptiform bursting than nonirradiated specimens. Synaptically driven neuronal firing was found to be intact in these slices, suggesting that neuronal death was not responsible for the identified seizure resistance [9].

An initial evaluation to determine what dose of radiosurgery was necessary to eliminate seizures in a kainic acid rat model was undertaken by Mori et al. [4] from the University of Pittsburgh. In this study, rats underwent stereotactic injection of 8 μg of kainic acid into the right hippocampus to induce seizures.

Ten days after injection, the animals underwent unilateral Gamma Knife radiosurgery. Radiosurgery was performed using a 4-mm collimator and a range of doses between 20 and 100 Gy. The animals given 20 Gy showed a significant reduction in the number of daily seizures during each successive week of observation. Indeed, all radiation groups – 20, 40, 60 and 100 Gy – showed a significant reduction in the number of seizures observed during the last half of this 6-week study. These results were confirmed with EEG evaluations. The authors concluded that no radiation-induced necrosis was observed in any animals except for the 100 Gy cohort. However, as the injection of kainic acid induced a loss of CA3 neurons in all animals, interpretation of histological findings may have been confounded. For example, small areas of necrosis were seen in 2/20 control animals and in 14/37 irradiated animals. Only in the 100 Gy group did the necrosis noted match the collimator size. Furthermore, animals were evaluated only 6 weeks after radiosurgery.

A second study by the same group was undertaken to evaluate the pathological and behavioral effects of 'subnecrotic' radiosurgery doses in the same kainic acid rat epilepsy model [10]. Stereotactic hippocampal kainic acid injections were followed by single isocenter radiosurgery using a 4-mm collimated Gamma Knife. Groups of animals were irradiated with doses of 30 or 60 Gy. A significant reduction in seizures was noted in all animals that underwent radiosurgery. This effect was seen earlier in the 60 Gy than in the 30 Gy group (weeks 5–9 compared to weeks 7–9). Water maze testing did not reveal any deficit in new memory attainment tasks in irradiated animals compared with nonirradiated animals who underwent kainic acid injection, though both groups showed impairment compared to controls. Two blinded, experienced observers rated the histological specimens from all animals 13 weeks after irradiation. Changes typical for kainic acid injections were seen in all animals, including a loss of pyramidal cells in CA3–4. In 25/46 injected animals, unilateral hippocampal atrophy with cell loss extending into CA1 and CA2 was noted. Necrosis matching the target volume of radiosurgery was not observed in any animals. The authors again conclude that cessation of seizures following radiosurgery does not require concomitant loss of neurons.

Unfortunately, the relationship between radiosurgery dose and structural damage to the hippocampus has not been precisely defined. Two recent studies from the radiosurgery group in Prague are helping to clarify what should be considered a 'subnecrotic' dose [11, 12]. The investigators studied doses of 25, 50, 75, or 100 Gy to the 70% isodose line delivered bilaterally to the rat hippocampus. Memory function tests, MRI, and histological examination were performed at 1, 3, 6, and 12 months after radiosurgery. A time- and dose-dependent effect was noted on memory function testing, T_2 edema, and necrotic histopathology. Animals treated with 100 Gy died by 6 months following radiation and had necrotic lesions. All animals treated with 75 Gy displayed memory impairment at 6 and 12 months, edema on MRI, and necrotic lesions. In 1 of the animals treated with 50 Gy, edema and necrosis were noted. Otherwise, animals treated with 25 or 50 Gy did not show functional or structural impairment at any time up to 1 year after radiosurgery. This finding of potentially subnecrotic radiosurgery dose parameters prompted a second phase to this study where a 35-Gy radiosurgery dose was used and the animals were evaluated over 16 months. By 6 months after irradiation, T_2 edema was evident on MRI, but the edema peaked at 9 months after irradiation. By 16 months after irradiation, 2 of 6 animals had postnecrotic cavities. The 4 animals without frankly necrotic cavities had severe atrophy of the corpus callosum, loss of thickness of somatosensory cortex, and damage to the striatum oriens hippocampi. While the number of animals used for this study was small, the results are highly suggestive that the full histological effects of radiosurgery require observation for an adequate period of time to become apparent.

It has been suggested that radiation has a direct antiseizure effect. This effect has been purported to operate through several mechanisms. As glial cells are more radiosensitive than neurons, Barcia-Salorio [13] proposed that low-dose radiosurgery may reduce glial scar formation, allowing increased dendritic sprouting, improved cortical reorganization, and fewer seizures. Elomaa [14] proposed that the antiepileptic effect of radiation is mediated through effects of somatostatin. The results of the most recent human studies suggest that the therapeutic efficacy of radiosurgery is linked to necrosis of mesial temporal structures. Proof for this concept would require direct observation of tissue samples in patients where radiosurgery has controlled seizures, something that is unlikely to occur, as only patients with persistent seizures are likely to undergo further surgery. Surrogate markers of radiation effects, such as MRI, have thus far shown mixed results. Radiation-induced edema becomes evident in most patients 9–15 months following radiosurgery. While these changes usually reverse with time, they are often followed by focal atrophy. Perhaps, as in surgical resection, there is a critical volume of tissue that must be functionally ablated to obtain seizure control.

As with the first animal trials, results from 2 early human trials suggested that control of seizures might be possible with doses of radiosurgery that were lower than those typically applied to tumors [5, 15]. These early results have been somewhat tempered by recent case reports describing the failure of low-dose radiosurgery to control seizures [6–8]. While failure of seizure control is easy to identify, it is a much more difficult task to determine that this is due to an insufficient radiosurgery dose. There is a lack of consensus among treating centers as to when one can determine if radiosurgery has 'failed' [16]. Prospective results suggest that radiosurgery may have results very similar to resection, and that approximately 30% of patients will continue to have seizures [17]. The reported failures of low-dose radiosurgery are case reports, and as yet do not demonstrate a failure rate of ≥30%. Having said this, it is important to note that 7 out of the 8 patients described in this paper whose seizures were not controlled by radiosurgery became seizure-free following resection. The 8th patient continued to have auras only. It is also interesting to note that 5 of the 6 patients described in this paper who had radiosurgery and did not show adequate seizure reduction received radiation doses of 20 Gy or less. None of these patients showed evidence of radiation-induced necrosis in their histological specimens. The 1 patient who did have evidence of radiation-induced necrosis was treated with 24 Gy and was later operated upon to relieve increased intracranial pressure. In this patient, findings were typical of radiation necrosis. Thus, the best evidence to date from human studies suggests that there is a steep dose-response effect for seizure reduction, that some neuronal damage is required to produce seizure abatement, and that the dose required to eliminate seizures is very close to the maximum dose tolerated by human brain tissue.

Conclusions

Recent data suggest that radiosurgery is effective at reducing epileptiform activity and seizures in several rat models of epilepsy. The doses of radiation used have not been shown to cause histological changes, disruption of normal neuronal firing patterns, or significant learning deficits. When multiple isocenters are employed, and animals are observed over longer time periods, the patterns of changes seen on MRI closely mimic those observed in human trials, and histological analysis indicates that structural lesions are created. Animal studies have not yet proven if the antiepileptic effects of radiosurgery are due to tissue damage sufficient to cause functional ablation, or if seizure activity has been eliminated in still functional parenchyma. However, the available data suggest that it is necessary to produce changes on MRI consistent with tissue necrosis in order to eliminate seizures in humans. There is a need for further evaluation of tissue obtained from patients treated with radiosurgery to answer these questions.

References

1 Wiebe S, Blume WT, Girvin JP, Eliasziw M: A randomized, controlled trial of surgery for temporal-lobe epilepsy. N Engl J Med 2001;345:311–318.

2 Spencer SS, Berg AT, Vickrey BG, Sperling MR, Bazil CW, Shinnar S, Langfitt JT, Walczak TS, Pacia SV, Ebrahimi N, Frobish D: Initial outcomes in the multicenter study of epilepsy surgery. Neurology 2003;61:1680–1685.

3 Schmidt D, Baumgartner C, Loscher W: The chance of cure following surgery for drug-resistant temporal lobe epilepsy. What do we know and do we need to revise our expectations? Epilepsy Res 2004;60:187–201.
4 Mori Y, Kondziolka D, Balzer J, Fellows W, Flickinger JC, Lunsford LD, Thulborn KR: Effects of stereotactic radiosurgery on an animal model of hippocampal epilepsy. Neurosurgery 2000;46:157–165; discussion 165–168.
5 Barcia-Salorio JL, Barcia JA, Hernandez G, Lopez-Gomez L: Radiosurgery of epilepsy. Long-term results. Acta Neurochir Suppl 1994;62:111–113.
6 Cmelak AJ, Abou-Khalil B, Konrad PE, Duggan D, Maciunas RJ: Low-dose stereotactic radiosurgery is inadequate for medically intractable mesial temporal lobe epilepsy: a case report. Seizure 2001;10:442–446.
7 Kawai K, Suzuki I, Kurita H, Shin M, Arai N, Kirino T: Failure of low-dose radiosurgery to control temporal lobe epilepsy. J Neurosurg 2001;95:883–887.
8 Srikijvilaikul T, Najm I, Foldvary-Schaefer N, Lineweaver T, Suh JH, Bingaman WE: Failure of gamma knife radiosurgery for mesial temporal lobe epilepsy: report of five cases. Neurosurgery 2004;54:1395–1402; discussion 1402–1404.
9 Chen ZF, Kamiryo T, Henson SL, Yamamoto H, Bertram EH, Schottler F, Patel F, Steiner L, Prasad D, Kassell NF, Shareghis S, Lee KS: Anticonvulsant effects of gamma surgery in a model of chronic spontaneous limbic epilepsy in rats. J Neurosurg 2001;94:270–280.
10 Maesawa S, Kondziolka D, Dixon CE, Balzer J, Fellows W, Lunsford LD: Subnecrotic stereotactic radiosurgery controlling epilepsy produced by kainic acid injection in rats. J Neurosurg 2000;93:1033–1040.
11 Liscak R, Vladyka V, Novotny J Jr, Brozek G, Namestkova K, Mares V, Herynek V, Jirak D, Hajek M, Sykova E: Leksell gamma knife lesioning of the rat hippocampus: the relationship between radiation dose and functional and structural damage. J Neurosurg 2002;97:666–673.
12 Herynek V, Burian M, Jirak D, Liscak R, Namestkova K, Hajek M, Sykova E: Metabolite and diffusion changes in the rat brain after Leksell Gamma Knife irradiation. Magn Reson Med 2004;52:397–402.
13 Barcia-Salorio JL: Radiosurgery in epilepsy and neuronal plasticity. Adv Neurol 1999;81:299–305.
14 Elomaa E: Focal irradiation of the brain: an alternative to temporal lobe resection in intractable focal epilepsy? Med Hypotheses 1980;6:501–503.
15 Heikkinen ER, Heikkinen MI, Sotaniemi K: Stereotactic radiotherapy instead of conventional epilepsy surgery. A case report. Acta Neurochir (Wien) 1992;119:159–160.
16 Regis J, Bartolomei F: Comment on: failure of gamma knife radiosurgery for mesial temporal lobe epilepsy: report of five cases. Neurosurgery 2004;54:1404.
17 Regis J, Rey M, Bartolomei F, Vladyka V, Liscak R, Schrottner O, Pendl G: Gamma knife surgery in mesial temporal lobe epilepsy: a prospective multicenter study. Epilepsia 2004;45:504–515.

Nicholas M. Barbaro, MD
Box 0112, Department of Neurological Surgery
University of California at San Francisco
San Francisco, CA 94143 (USA)
Tel. +1 415 353 3557, Fax +1 415 353 3907, E-Mail barbaron@neurosurg.ucsf.edu

Szeifert GT, Kondziolka D, Levivier M, Lunsford LD (eds): Radiosurgery and Pathological Fundamentals. Prog Neurol Surg. Basel, Karger, 2007, vol 20, pp 289–296

12.1.1. Stereotactic Intracavitary Irradiation of Cystic Craniopharyngiomas with Yttrium-90 Isotope

Jenö Julow[a,b], *Ferenc Lányi*[b], *Márta Hajda*[b], *György T. Szeifert*[b], *Árpád Viola*[a], *Katalin Bálint*[b], *István Nyáry*[b]

[a]Department of Neurosurgery, St. John's Hospital, [b]National Institute of Neurosurgery and Department of Neurological Surgery, Semmelweis University, Budapest, Hungary

Abstract

The authors analyzed data from nearly 30-year follow-up period to assess the value of intracavitary irradiation with stereotactically implanted beta-emitting radioisotope yttrium-90 (^{90}Y) silicate colloid for the treatment of cystic craniopharyngiomas. Seventy-three cysts in 60 patients were selected for retrospective analysis. The cumulative dose aimed at the inner surface of the cyst wall was 300 Gy. An average of 79% (mean 88.3%) shrinkage of the initial cyst volume was observed. In 47 cysts, the reduction was more than 80%, and the cyst disappeared totally in 29 out of those 47 cases, usually within a year. Mean survival duration after intracavitary irradiation was 9.4 years. Neuroophthalmological prognosis was only favorable when the optic disc was normal or nearly normal at the time of the treatment. In the presence of preexisting optic atrophy, visual damage proved to be irreversible. The long-term results support the view that intracavitary ^{90}Y irradiation is a noninvasive and effective method for the treatment of craniopharyngioma cysts. Because of the mean penetration pathway of beta irradiation is 3.6 mm in the soft tissues (maximum 11 mm) it cannot influence the solid part of the tumor; therefore, the best result can be expected in solitary cysts.

Results with intracavitary implantation of yttrium-90 (^{90}Y) silicate colloid (Amersham, UK) and ^{90}Y citrate colloid (CIS, France) into cystic craniopharyngiomas were analyzed following partial tumor resection, usually through a frontotemporal craniotomy. Stereotactic insertion of beta-emitting isotopes into a craniopharyngioma cyst had already been performed by Leksell [1] and especially by Backlund [2], who formulated a protocol for complex stereotactic management (^{90}Y + Gamma Knife) of craniopharyngiomas as well.

The aim of the present study was to follow volume changes in craniopharyngioma cysts to study time course of volume reduction (VR), and to assess ophthalmological signs following ^{90}Y isotope intracavitary treatment.

Materials and Methods

^{90}Y implantations were performed in 89 craniopharyngioma cysts in 63 patients between December 1975 and February 2004. There were 27 female and 36 male patients (3 patients were excluded from the study). Fifty-seven patients had direct operations prior to ^{90}Y implantation, whereas in 3 cases ^{90}Y implantation was the primary treatment. Mostly recurrent cysts were treated, following one or more surgical procedures, and follow-up data of 73 procedures in 60 patients were available. Median age of patients was 27.7 years (range 2.9–67.5 years).

Following routine neuroradiological and neurosurgical examination, cyst volume has been determined by CT since 1980 (in the early period of the treatment by cystography or isotope dilution methods) [3, 4]. The volume was used for the calculation of radioactivity to be injected. A technique, including dosimetry comparable with Backlund's method was introduced into our practice [1, 2, 5, 6, 7, 8, 23, 24]. Implantation of ^{90}Y into the cyst was carried out through a frontal burr hole or by transsphenoidal puncture. At the beginning, a freehand technique had been used; however, since 1989 stereotactic techniques were integrated using the Leksell and Riechert-Mundinger frames. Since 1996, the BrainLab PatXfer 4.21 and Target 1.9 software has been applied for 3D planning of the cyst puncture. To avoid vessel injury, Ultravist 300 contrast (2.5 ml/kg)-enhanced 2.5-mm slices were used. Both planning of irradiation and follow-up of cyst shrinkage were based on CT/MR fused images. The mean dose delivered to the cyst wall was 302 Gy (range 150–320 Gy). To exclude possible leakage of the inserted isotope, gamma camera examinations were carried out in all cases following implantation [5]. To simplify representation, the original cyst volume (OCV) was normalized to 100% in all cases.

Results

Results of the stereotactically applied intracavitary irradiation (STAIR) using the ^{90}Y isotope were available on 73 craniopharyngioma cyst treatments in 60 patients. Preliminary data with the technique have been published previously [9–11]. Additional treatments were performed before and/or after the ^{90}Y-STAIR, including resection, aspiration, and shunt placement (table 1). Leakage of ^{90}Y was not detected by gamma camera examination in any case.

Neuroophthalmological Results

Neuroophthalmological data of available 55 cases before and after ^{90}Y treatment are summarized in table 2, (excluding the 3 cases with normal pre- and postoperative examinations). Visual field defects or impairment of visual acuity were observed preoperatively in 52 out of 55 patients. A unilateral optic nerve lesion

Table 1. Additional treatments before and after the first ^{90}Y-STAIR treatment in 60 patients with craniopharyngioma

Procedure	Before 1st ^{90}Y implant	After 1st ^{90}Y implant
Resection	57 (1 resection) 12 (2 resections) 3 (3 resections)	14
Aspiration	33	9
Shunt	16	7

Seventeen patients received second and third ^{90}Y implants.

Table 2. Neuroophtalmological data before and after ^{90}Y-STAIR treatment in patients with craniopharyngioma

Signs	Before treatment	After treatment			
		complete recovery	improved	unchanged	Progression
Visual acuity					
5/5–5/12	15	2	1	11	1
5/10–5/50	15	3	4	7	1
<5/50	12	1	2	8	1
Blind	10	0	0	10	0
Total	52	6	7	36	3
Optic disc					
Normal	7	2	2	2	1
Temporal pallor	15	3	5	7	0
Severe pallor or atrophy	30	0	2	26	2
Total	52	5	9	35	3
Visual field lesions					
Unilateral optic nerve	8	3	2	2	1
Chiasmal	36	2	5	27	2
Optic tract	8	0	0	8	0
Total	52	5	7	37	3

was present in 8 cases, chiasmal damage in 36, and optic tract lesion in 8. Only 7 patients had a normal optic disc. Temporal pallor was found in 15 cases, and optic atrophy was documented in 30 patients preoperatively. The ophthalmological status improved in 12 patients and did not change in 37 cases following

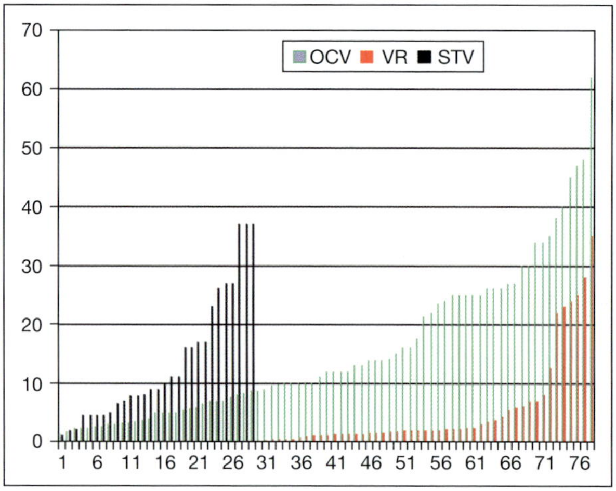

Fig. 1. Bar graph showing frequency distribution of original cyst volume (OCV), VR and solid tumor volume (STV).

^{90}Y irradiation. Visual deterioration occurred in 3 patients: radiation damage was suspected in 2, and compression of the optic nerve by the solid part of the tumor in the other case. Five patients had transient oculomotor nerve palsy: one occurred at the time of the puncture due to direct injury of the oculomotor nerve, and in the remaining 4 patients neuropathy developed during the follow-up period.

Cyst Volume Changes

Shrinkage occurred following ^{90}Y implantation procedures in 73 cysts. The cumulative volume of all cysts diminished from 1,061 to 180.9 ml, and the mean OCV was reduced from 10.6 to 1.0 ml after ^{90}Y-STAIR. VR of all cysts is demonstrated in figure 1. VR of the cystic part of craniopharyngiomas was more than 80% in 47 cases (among them the cyst disappeared totally in 29 cases), 40–80% VR occurred in 20 cases, and less than 40% in 6. The mean VR in all 73 cysts was 88.3%. An illustrative case is shown in figure 2.

Survival Periods

The mean survival time during the 30-year follow-up period (1975–2004) was 9.4 years (range 0.7–28.8 years). The mean survival time of 34 patients still alive is 12.1 years. The mean survival period of 26 deceased patients was 3.9 years. Actuarial survival rates at 5, 10, 15, 20, 25 and 29 years were 80, 61, 42, 18 and 2%, respectively. Figure 3 shows the Kaplan-Meier survival analysis of our patients.

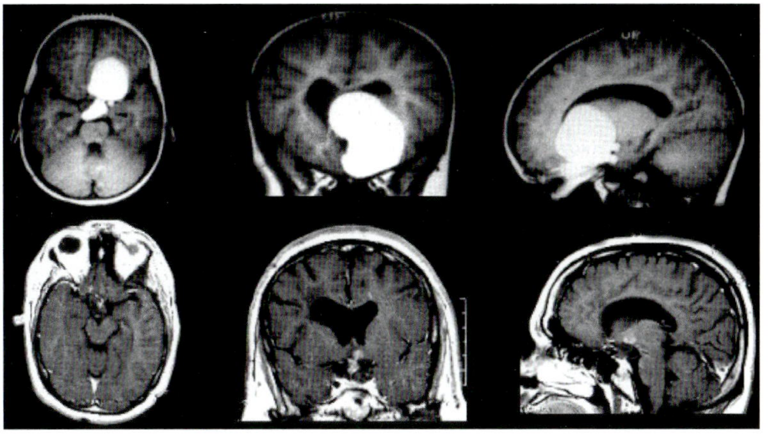

Fig. 2. A male patient born in 1983. He underwent partial removal of cystic CRF in 1987, ^{90}Y-STAIR of successive cysts at four occasions between 1988 and 1991, and Gamma Knife irradiation (Prof. Backlund) in 1990. In 2004, CT and MRI scans revealed suprasellar calcified remnant tumor. The patient attended high school.

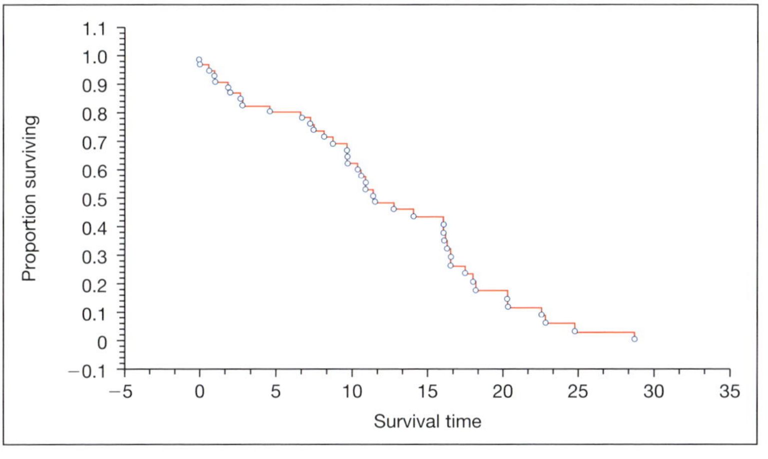

Fig. 3. Kaplan-Meier actuarial survival rates at 5, 10, 15, 20, 25 and 29 years were 80, 61, 42, 18 and 2%.

The ^{90}Y-STAIR did not produce significant changes in neurological symptoms of our patients. There was one perioperative death from meningo ventriculitis 1.5 months after a transnasal puncture. We have lost 2 patients with huge retrosellar cysts probably because of late injury of the basal perforating arteries. Twelve patients died due to unrelated causes several years following treatment (pulmonary embolism, cardiac and renal insufficiency, other causes). Ten more patients died due to progression of the solid part of the craniopharyngioma several years after ^{90}Y-STAIR, before the LINAC radiosurgery or iodine-125 irradiation era.

It seems obvious that our clinical results were impeded by the volume of the solid tumor, which occurred in 50% of our patients. The mean size of the solid part was 12.8 ml (median 9, range 1–37 ml).

Discussion

Possibilities and limitations of intracavitary radioisotope implantation into craniopharyngioma cysts have been documented in the last 2 decades [2, 4, 6]. Radioisotopes emitting short-range beta radiation with a short half-life time, like P^{32} ($Na^{32}PO_4$, $Cr^{32}PO_4$ and $Bi^{32}PO_4$) [1, 11–16], ^{198}Au colloid [17, 18], ^{90}Y silicate colloid [2, 4, 7, 9, 19–21], ^{186}rhenium [7, 21] have been used.

Our results presenting 88.3% mean OCV reduction are in accordance with previously reported data of 74–100% volume decrease following beta irradiation of cystic craniopharyngiomas [4, 7, 12, 14, 15, 20, 21].

Cyst shrinkage usually starts several months following ^{90}Y-STAIR and becomes stable in a period of 6–12 months [4, 12, 14, 16, 20, 21]. This process was accompanied by an improvement in ophthalmological signs in 23% of the treated patients. Subsequent surgery in 23%, shunting procedures in 12% of the patients were necessary following ^{90}Y-STAIR. A new cyst or cysts developed later in 28% of the cases. Such successive cysts could be treated with successive ^{90}Y implantations. However, we believe that multicystic craniopharyngiomas (when at least two or more cysts are present) require separate cyst puncture and dose calculation.

Radiation cyst wall doses that had been reported in previous series ranged from 50 to 1,000 Gy, and the generally accepted dose is about 200 Gy [2]. A 302-Gy mean radiation dose was applied to the cyst wall in the presented series. Our purpose is to decrease the radiation dose to 200 Gy or even less in cases with cysts adherent to the optic pathways or hypothalamic structures. Experience from Gamma Knife radiosurgery practice, that doses over 8 Gy may damage optic pathways, should be considered in dose planning of intracavitary craniopharyngioma treatments. The third, fourth, and fifth cranial nerves exposed to a dose from 4.5 to 30 Gy did not develop signs of neuropathy [22].

Ophthalmological prognosis was reported favorable in those cases where an intact optic disc or just slight temporal pallor was noticed before intracavitary treatment [17]. Visual acuity improved in 11 out of our 18 patients with intact optic discs or slight temporal pallor of the disc at the time of the treatment.

Changes in visual function usually occurred between 2 weeks and 6 months following ^{90}Y implantation. The lack of the ophthalmological improvement could be attributed to the fact that the treatment was carried out at a late stage of the disease. The optic disc in these patients was pale or clearly atrophic. When preoperative visual impairment exists for less than 1 year, improvement is still possible [16].

Our results are in accordance with data from the literature, and demonstrate that ^{90}Y-STAIR is a minimally invasive effective treatment modality of the cystic part in the complex management of craniopharyngiomas.

Conclusions

Stereotactic intracavitary irradiation of craniopharyngioma cysts with ^{90}Y colloid solution proved to be effective, with a low risk of complications, for reduction, annihilation or at least control of cysts, but not for the solid tumor components.

Acknowledgment

This work was supported by the Hungarian Ministry of Health and Welfare (ETT 028/2004).

References

1 Leksell L, Backlund EO, Johansson L: Treatment of craniopharyngiomas. Acta Chir Scand 1967;133:345–350.

2 Backlund EO: Stereotaktik behandling av kraniopharyngeom med intracystiskt ^{90}Y extern ^{60}Co Bestraling; thesis, Stockholm, 1972.

3 Kobayashi T, Negoro M, Asano Y, et al: Conray cystography and volumetry of the cysts using computed tomography (in Japanese). Progr Comput Tomogr 1980;2:101–105.

4 Sturm V, Rommel Th, Strauss L, Georgi P, Scheer KE, Steude U, Stock G, Penzholz H, Backlund EO: Preliminary results of intracavitary irradiation of cystic craniopharyngiomas by means of stereotactically applied ^{90}yttrium. Adv Neurosurg 1981;9:401–404.

5 Balachandran S, McGuire L, Flanigan S, Shah H, Boyd CM: Bremsstrahlung imaging after ^{32}P treatment for residual suprasellar cyst. Int J Nucl Med Biol 1985;12:215–221.

6 McGuire EL, Balachandran S, Boyd CM: Radiation dosimetry considerations in the treatment of cystic suprasellar neoplasms. Br J Radiol 1986;59:779–785.

7 Musolino A, Munari P, Blond S, Betti O, Lajat Y, Schaub C, Askienazy S, Chodkewicz JP: Traitment stereotaxique des kystes expansifs de cranio-pharyngiomes par irradiation endocavitaire Beta (^{186}Re, ^{198}Au, ^{90}Y). Neurochirurgie 1985;31:169–178.

8 van den Berge JH, Blaauw G, Breeman WAP, Rahmy A, Wlingaarde R: Intracavitary brachytherapy of cystic craniopharyngiomas. J Neurosurg 1992;77:545–550.

9 Huk WJ, Mahlstedt J: Intracystic radiotherapy (^{90}Y) of craniopharyngiomas. CT-guided stereotaxic implantation of indwelling drainage system. AJNR 1983;4:803–806.
10 Julow J, Lányi F, Hajda M, Seifert GT, Bálint K, Drasnyi G, Pásztor E, Fedorcsák I, Borbély K, Nyáry I: Treatment of cystic craniopharyngiomas yttrium-90 silicate colloid solution. Neurosurg Focus 1997;3:1–9.
11 Strauss L, Sturm V, Georgi P, Schlegel W, Ostertag H, Clorius JH, Kaick G: Radioisotope therapy of cystic craniopharyngeomas. Int J Radiat Oncol Biol Phys 1982;8:1581–1585.
12 Hasegawa T, Kondziolka D, Hadjipanayis CG, Lunsford LD: Management of cystic craniopharyngiomas with phosphorus-32 intracavitary irradiation. Neurosurgery 2004;54:813–820; discussion 820–822.
13 Pan DH, Lee LS, Huang CI, Wong TT: Stereotactic internal irradiation for cystic craniopharyngiomas: a 6-year experience. Stereotact Funct Neurosurg 1990;54/55:525–530.
14 Pollock BE, Natt N, Schomberg PJ: Stereotactic management of craniopharyngiomas. Stereotact Funct Neurosurg 2002;79:25–32.
15 Úlfarsson E, Lindquist Ch, Roberts M, Rahn T, Lindquist M, Thorén M, Lippitz B: Gamma knife radiosurgery for craniopharyngiomas: long term results in the first Swedish Patients. J Neurosurg 2002;97(suppl):613–622.
16 Voges J, Sturm V, Lehrke R, et al: Cystic craniopharyngioma: long-term results after intracavitary irradiation with stereotactically applied colloidal β-emitting radioactive sources. Neurosurgery 1997;40:263–270.
17 Gonzales-Feria L, Pedraza Muriel V, Ginoves-Sierra M: Treatment of recurrence of cystic craniopharyngioma with stereotaxic injection of Au 198 (in Spanish). Rev Esp Otoneurooftalmol 1976;34:83–88.
18 Kodama T, Matsukado Y, Uemura S: Intracapsular irradiation therapy of craniopharyngiomas with radioactive gold: indication and follow-up results. Neurol Med Chir 1981;21:49–58.
19 Blackburn TP, Doughty D, Plowman PN: Stereotactic intracavitary therapy of recurrent cystic craniopharyngioma by instillation of 90yttrium. Br J Neurosurg 1999;13:359–365.
20 Lange M, Kirsch CM, Steude U, Oeckler R: Intracavitary treatment of intrasellar cystic craniopharyngiomas with 90-yttrium by trans-sphenoidal approach – a technical note. Acta Neurochir 1995;135:206–209.
21 Munari C, Landre E, Musolino A, Turak B, Habert Mo, Chodkiewicz JP: Long-term results of stereotactic endocavitary beta irradiation of craniopharyngioma cysts. J Neurosurg Sci 1989;33: 99–105.
22 Rähn T: Gamma knife radiosurgery and intracystic colloidal isotope treatment of craniopharyngiomas; in Broggi G (ed): Craniopharyngiomas. Surgical Treatment. New York, Springer, 1995, pp 120–125.
23 Leber KA, Berglöff J, Langmann G, Mokry M, Schrottner O, Pendl G: Radiation sensitivity of visual and oculomotor pathways. Stereotact Funct Neurosurg 1995;64(suppl 1):233.
24 Lunsford LD, Levine G, Gumerman LW: Comparison of computerized tomographic and radionuclide methods in determining intracranial cystic tumor volumes. J Neurosurg 1985;63:740–744.

Dr. Jenö Julow
Department of Neurosurgery, St. John's Hospital
Diósárok út 1
HU–1125 Budapest (Hungary)
Tel. +36 458 4538, Fax +36 458 4560, E-Mail h12494jul@t-online.hu

Szeifert GT, Kondziolka D, Levivier M, Lunsford LD (eds): Radiosurgery and Pathological Fundamentals. Prog Neurol Surg. Basel, Karger, 2007, vol 20, pp 297–302

12.1.2. Pathological Findings in Cystic Craniopharyngiomas after Stereotactic Intracavitary Irradiation with Yttrium-90 Isotope

György T. Szeifert[a], *Katalin Bálint*[a], *László Sipos*[a], *Mainul H. Sarker*[a,c], *Sándor Czirják*[a], *Jenö Julow*[b]

[a]National Institute of Neurosurgery and Department of Neurological Surgery, Semmelweis University, [b]Department of Neurosurgery, St. John's Hospital, Budapest, Hungary; [c]Department of Neurosurgery, Dhaka Medical College, Dhaka, Bangladesh

Abstract

Histopathological, ultrastructural and polyacrylamide gel electrophoretic examinations were carried out on biopsy, cyst fluid, surgical pathology and autopsy specimens obtained from 7 cystic craniopharyngioma cases before and after yttrium-90 silicate colloid (^{90}Y) irradiation. Light microscopy revealed that the lining epithelial tumor cell layer of the cyst wall was destroyed, and scar tissue containing large amount of hyaline degenerated collagen bundles replaced it. Proliferative postirradiation vasculopathy was also demonstrated in the cyst wall following ^{90}Y installation. Electrophoretic property of cyst fluid was similar to the normal human serum. Considering that scar tissue has a certain propensity to shrink, the fibrosis in the cyst wall together with destruction of neoplastic epithelium and vascular changes might explain diminished fluid production and cyst volume reduction after ^{90}Y treatment.

Craniopharyngiomas represent histologically benign tumors of the sellar region with a suggested maldevelopmental origin either from ectopic cell rests of the enemal organ or from remnants of Rathke's pouch [1]. They account for 1.2–4.6% of all intracranial tumors and are the most common nonneuroepithelial intracerebral neoplasms in childhood [2]. Their macroscopic appearance might be solid, cystic or mixed [3]. Histopathologically two basic types, i.e. squamous papillary and adamantinomatous, are differentiated (fig. 1a–c).

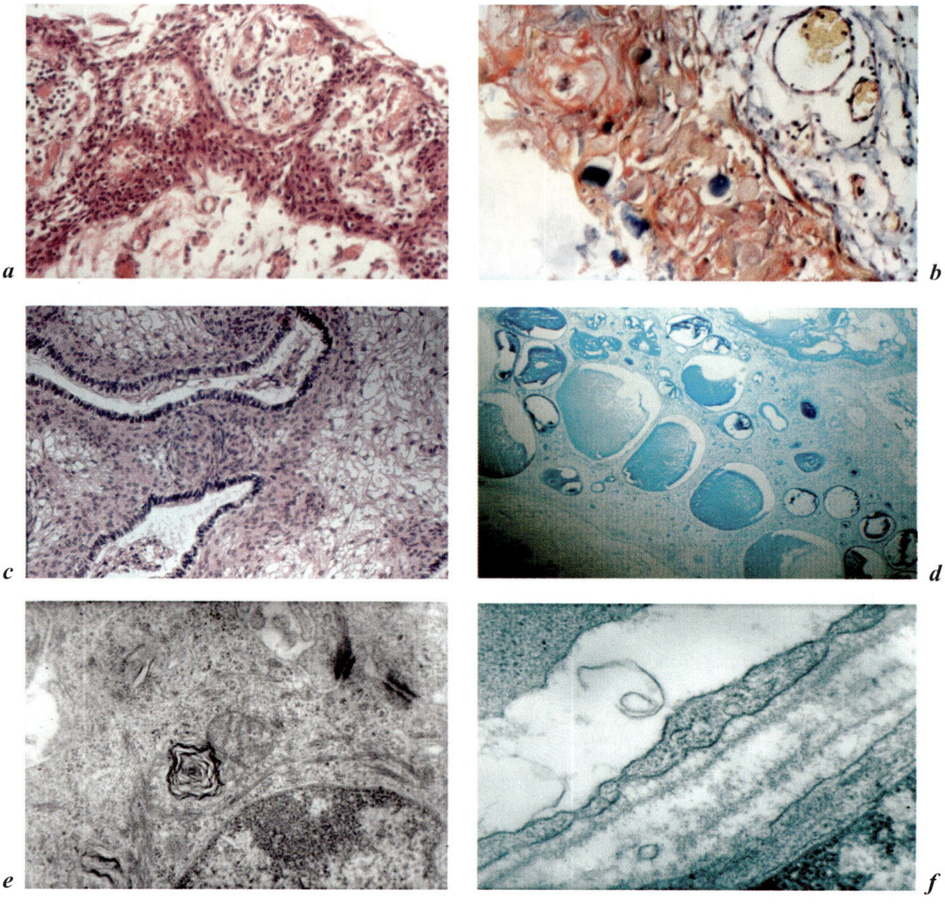

Fig. 1. Morphological characteristics of nontreated cystic craniopharyngiomas. ***a*** Lining squamous epithelial layer of the cyst. The loose connective tissue stroma contains numerous thin-walled small vessels (HE, ×300). ***b*** Keratinization and exfoliation into the cyst lumen (Lendrum's trichrom, ×300). ***c*** Adamantinomatous biphasic histological appearance with stellate cells and columnar epithelium (HE, ×300). ***d*** Fluid secretion in a micro-multicystic region (Alcian-blue, ×150). ***e*** Epithelial cell from the cyst wall rich in cytoplasmic organelles (EM, ×20,000). ***f*** Fenestrated endothelial lining in a stromal channel (EM, ×20,000).

Tumor recurrence following total resection usually occurs in adamantinomatous craniopharyngiomas. Light microscopic and electron microscopic investigations revealed that expanding cysts could be attributed to a 'motor-oil'-like fluid production. This results partly from a secretory activity of tumor cells (fig. 1d, e), combined with a fenestrated endothelial structure of stromal vessels (fig. 1f), and desquamation of neoplastic cells into the cyst cavity [4–8].

Pathological classification can influence the selected treatment modality, has a prognostic value and reflects in the clinical course [9, 10]. The aim of the present study was to investigate histopathological changes, and to explain the pathophysiological mechanism of volume reduction in craniopharyngioma cysts following intracavitary irradiation with yttrium-90 silicate colloid isotope (^{90}Y).

Materials and Methods

Histopathological investigations were carried out in 7 cystic craniopharyngioma cases treated with ^{90}Y intracavitary irradiation. Biopsy specimens were obtained from cyst walls in all cases before ^{90}Y implantation. Surgical pathology specimens were obtained from 4 cases, and 3 additional autopsy specimens were also studied in an 8- to 36-month interval after isotope treatment. In addition to hematoxylin and eosin, the 5-μm paraffin sections were stained with PAS, elastic van Gieson, Endes' and Lendrum's trichrom methods. Collagen production in the cyst wall was sensitively and specifically demonstrated by picrosirius-red F3BA topo-optical reaction in polarized light.

Protein composition of cyst fluid aspirated prior to isotope installation was investigated by polyacrylamide gel electrophoresis.

Results

Biopsy samples taken from the cyst wall before ^{90}Y treatment were composed by nests or trabeculae of epithelial tumor parenchyma surrounded by a loose connective tissue stroma (fig. 1a). Besides solid islands and a network of squamous neoplastic cells, there was stratified keratinization through maturation in the lining squamous epithelium of the cyst wall (fig. 1b). The connective tissue stroma contained thin-walled capillaries and small vessels as well. Cellular debris, sloughed off squamous cells intermingled with foreign body giant cells and an amorph eosinophilic proteinacous material accumulated in the cyst lumen.

The protein composition and electrophoretic distribution of cyst fluid taken at the time of isotope installation were similar to those of normal human serum controls (fig. 2a, b).

Histopathological investigation following ^{90}Y treatment revealed that the lining epithelial cell layer of the cyst cavity was destroyed, and a large amount of massive collagen bundles with hyaline degeneration accumulated in the wall (fig. 2c–e). Vascular proliferative and degenerative changes were also apparent

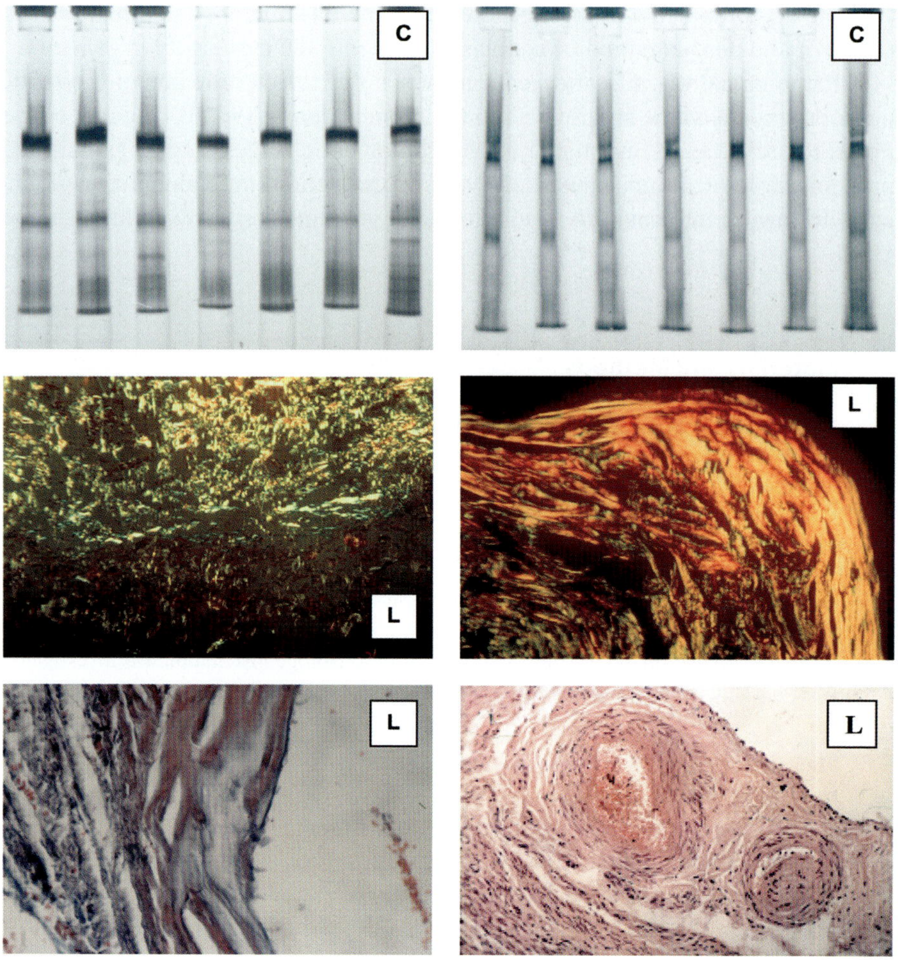

a b c d e f

Fig. 2. ***a*** Electrophoretic distribution of cyst fluid proteins (c = normal serum control). ***b*** Reaction with polyvalent human serum similar to that of normal control. ***c*** Loose connective tissue material of the pretreatment cyst wall sample demonstrating birefringence in polarized light (picrosirius-red F3BA reaction, ×300; courtesy of Prof. L. Módis). ***d*** Considerably enhanced birefringence 11 months following ^{90}Y treatment suggesting strong irradiation fibrosis in the cyst wall (×300). ***e*** Hyaline degeneration of thick collagen bundles in the irradiated cyst wall (Endes' trichrom, ×300). ***f*** Intimal spindle cell proliferation narrowing vessels' lumina in the fibrotic cyst wall 8 months after ^{90}Y irradiation (HE, ×300).

following irradiation. These included thickening of the vessel wall, cell proliferation and fibrous sclerosis in the intimal region of small arteries and arterioles narrowing the lumen (fig. 2f). Subendothelial deposition of hyaline-like substance and dystrophic calcification were also observed in the channels.

Discussion

Since 1950, when Leksell and Lidén introduced stereotactic inracavitary irradiation of cystic craniopharyngiomas with ^{32}P isotope [11], several studies have demonstrated the therapeutic effectiveness of the method [10, 12–15]. In the majority of cases, the symptoms are due to the expanding cyst, and obliteration of the cystic part with radioisotope injection solves most of the clinical problems. Solid tumors were effectively treated by radiosurgery [16]. A recent systematic protocol has been suggested to assess the role of the Gamma Knife treatment for tumors with cystic or multicystic component [17]. Present pathological observations indicate that the ionizing energy of ^{90}Y radioisotope produces biologic response both in the neoplastic squamous cell parenchyma, and in the connective tissue vascular stroma of cystic craniopharyngiomas. The short distance penetration capability of β-rays emitted by the ^{90}Y isotope can protect normal neural structures beyond the irradiated cyst wall from undesired side effects. Destruction of the lining tumorous epithelium, together with vascular changes and irradiation fibrosis generated in the cyst wall, might explain decreased fluid production and volume reduction following ^{90}Y intracavitary irradiation [18].

Conclusion

Light microscopic, ultrastructural and electrophoretic investigations provide pathological background to the radiobiological effect, and support the clinical benefit of stereotactic intracavitary ^{90}Y radioisotope irradiation in the management of cystic craniopharyngiomas.

References

1 Szeifert GT, Pásztor E: Could craniopharyngiomas produce pituitary hormones? Neurol Res 1993;15:68–69.

2 Janzer RC, Burger PC, Giangaspero F, Paulus W: Craniopharyngioma; in Kleihues P, Cavenee WK (eds): Pathology and Genetics of Tumours of the Nervous System. WHO Classification of Tumours. Lyon, IARC Press, 2000, pp 244–246.

3 Konovalov AN: Operative management of craniopharyngiomas; in Symon L (ed): Advances and Technical Standards in Neurosurgery. New York, Springer, vol 8, 1981.

4 Hirano A, Ghatak NR, Zimmerman HH: Fenestrated blood vessels in craniopharyngioma. Acta Neuropathol (Berlin) 1973;26:171–177.

5 Petito CK, de Girolami U, Earle KM: Craniopharyngiomas. A clinical and pathological review. Cancer 1976;37:1944–1952.

6 Adamson TE, Wiestler OD, Kleihues P, Yasargil MG: Correlation of clinical and pathological features in surgically treated craniopharyngiomas. J Neurosurg 1990;73:12–17.

7 Szeifert GT, Julow J, Szabolcs M, Slowik F, Bálint K, Pásztor E: Secretory component of cystic craniopharyngiomas: a mucino-histochemical and electron-microscopic study. Surg Neurol 1991;36:286–293.
8 Szeifert GT, Sipos L, Horváth M, Sarker MH, Major O, Salomvary B, Czirják S, Bálint K, Slowik F, Kolonics L, Pásztor E: Pathological characteristics of surgically removed craniopharyngiomas: analysis of 131 cases. Acta Neurochir (Wien) 1993;124:139–143.
9 Kobayashi T, Kageyama N, Yoshida J, Shibuya N, Yonezawa T: Pathological and clinical basis of the indication for treatment of craniopharyngiomas. Neurol Med Chir 1981;21:39–47.
10 Kobayashi T, Kageyama N, Ohara K: Internal irradiation for cystic craniopharyngioma. J Neurosurg 1981;55:896–903.
11 Leksell L, Lidén K: A therapeutic trial with radioactive isotopes in cystic brain tumor; in Radioisotope techniques: Medical and Physiological Applications. London, HM Stationery Office, vol 1, 1951.
12 Leksell L, Backlund EO, Johansson L: Treatment of craniopharyngiomas. Acta Chir Scand 1967;133: 345–350.
13 Backlund EO: Colloidal radioisotopes as part of a multi-modality treatment of craniopharyngiomas. J Neurosurg Sci 1989;33:95–97.
14 Julow J, Lányi F, Hajda M, et al: The radiotherapy of cystic craniopharyngioma with intracystic installation of ^{90}Y silicate colloid. Acta Neurochir (Wien) 1985;74:94–99.
15 Pollock BE, Lunsford LD, Kondziolka D, et al: Phosphorous-32 intracavitary irradiation of cystic craniopharyngiomas: current technique and long-term results. Int J Radiat Oncol Biol Phys 1995;33:437–446.
16 Leksell L: Stereotactic radiosurgery. J Neurol Neurosurg Psychiatry 1983;46:797–803.
17 Reda WA, Hay AA, Ganz JC: A planned combined stereotactic approach for cystic intracranial tumors. Report of two cases. J Neurosurg 2002;97(suppl 5):610–612.
18 Szeifert GT, Julow J, Slowik F, Bálint K, Lányi F, Pásztor E: Pathological changes in cystic craniopharyngiomas following intracavital ^{90}yttrium treatment. Acta Neurochir (Wien) 1990;102:14–18.

György T. Szeifert, MD, PhD
National Institute of Neurosurgery, Department of Neurological Surgery
Semmelweis University, Amerikai út 57
HU–1145 Budapest (Hungary)
Tel. +36 1 2512 999, Fax +36 1 2515 678, E-Mail gyorgyszeifert@yahoo.com

Szeifert GT, Kondziolka D, Levivier M, Lunsford LD (eds): Radiosurgery and Pathological Fundamentals. Prog Neurol Surg. Basel, Karger, 2007, vol 20, pp 303–311

12.2.1. Image Fusion-Guided Stereotactic Iodine-125 Interstitial Irradiation of Inoperable and Recurrent Gliomas

Jenö Julow[a], Árpád Viola[a], Katalin Bálint[b], György T. Szeifert[b]

[a]Department of Neurosurgery, St. John's Hospital, [b]National Institute of Neurosurgery and Department of Neurological Surgery, Semmelweis University, Budapest, Hungary

Abstract

Between 1996 and 2004, 27 patients with low grade gliomas (WHO grade I–II), 10 patients with WHO grade III gliomas and 6 patients with glioblastoma multiforme (WHO grade IV) were treated with stereotactic brachytherapy using low-dose rate iodine-125 (^{125}I) isotope seeds at the Department of Neurosurgery, St. John's Hospital, Budapest, Hungary. In all 43 cases, brachytherapy was used for surgically inoperable gliomas: in 32 cases for recurrent gliomas and in 11 cases as a primary treatment. Results of this study suggest that ^{125}I brachytherapy for inoperable and recurrent gliomas is an effective method and offers a chance for longer-term survival.

Survival rates of patients with anaplastic astrocytoma and glioblastoma multiforme (GBM) are discouraging. The majority of these patients die of local recurrence following surgery [1]. The Brain Tumor Cooperative Group (BTCG) trials demonstrated significant increase in the survival of patients with malignant gliomas when surgery was followed by radiotherapy (total dose of 60 Gy at 170–200 cGy daily) compared to surgery alone [2, 3]. The BTCG study has also demonstrated an increased survival rate using higher total irradiation doses from 50 to 60 Gy. Further increase in the dose of external irradiation is limited by the normal brain tolerance [4].

Because of the unifocal presentation of most malignant gliomas and the improvement in the local control with higher doses of radiation [5], brachytherapy has generated considerable interest as an alternative treatment modality

Table 1. Main characteristics of ^{125}I interstitial irradiation

	Mean	Median	Min.	Max.
Age, years	39.6	42	9	67
Tumor volume, cm^3	13.7	12.5	2.9	32
Catheters	1.8	2	1	5
Seeds	5.5	5	2	10
Activity, mCi	66.6	57.5	12.3	155.2
Length of irradiation, days	18	14	4	90
DVH, %	92.3	93.8	67	99.7
NTTV, %	80.5	77	21.8	190
Treatment dose, Gy	61.2	60	40	200
Dose rate, cGy/h	23.3	20.6	0.9	82.7

DVH = Dose volume histogram; NTTV = (irradiated) normal tissue in the % of tumor volume.

[6, 21, 22]. Stereotactic interstitial irradiation can deliver a large dose to the tumor volume while sparing surrounding normal tissue [4]. Gutin et al. [7] in 1987 first demonstrated the effectiveness of stereotactic brachytherapy for the treatment of recurrent glioblastomas. Conventional radiotherapy results in 80% local recurrence rate (within 2 cm of the primary site), but only 35% of patients receiving brachytherapy had local recurrences, whereas 65% of patients had marginal or distant recurrences [1, 8].

More promising results of the iodine-125 (^{125}I) interstitial irradiation of nearly 500 low grade gliomas (LGG) were analyzed by the classical papers of the Freiburg school [9, 10].

The integration of CT with modern stereotactic systems has made it possible to implant radioactive sources into selected brain tumor targets safely and accurately, eliminating the need for craniotomy [7, 11]. The application of the interstitial irradiation with CT control, including image fusions (CT-MRI, CT-PET, MRI-PET), discloses potential flaws of the operation. Hence, conformity of dose delivery becomes more accurate and reliable [12].

Methods

The effect of brachytherapy on brain tumors is achieved using low-energy gamma radiating radioactive ^{125}I isotope seeds (Iodine-125 Seeds IMC6702, Medi-Physics Inc., Arlington Heights, Ill., USA). The method has been described in previous publications [12, 13]. Between 1996 and 2004, 27 patients with LGG (WHO grade I–II), 10 patients with WHO grade III gliomas (HGG) and 6 patients with GBM (WHO grade IV) were treated at the Department of Neurosurgery, St. John's Hospital Budapest, Hungary (table 1). In all

Table 2. Additional treatments before and after the first ^{125}I implant in 43 patients with glioma

Procedure	Before 1st ^{125}I implant	After 1st ^{125}I implant
Resection	32	13
	19 (1 resection)	8
	5 (2 resections)	1
	1 (3 resections)	1
Shunt	2	13
Aspiration	2	3
Chemotherapy	11	1
WBRT	2	2
Stereotactic biopsy	7	1

Four patients received a second, 1 patient third and 1 patient fourth ^{125}I implant. In 8 cases, the reason for the resections following ^{125}I interstitial irradiation were recurrence (and edema) around radionecrosis. In 2 cases, only radionecrosis and edema were found and proved histologically. WBRT = Whole brain radiotherapy.

43 cases, brachytherapy was used for surgically inoperable gliomas: in 32 cases for recurrent gliomas and in 11 cases as a primary treatment (table 2). Tumors' locations were as follows: frontocentral region in 15, insular in 9, thalamic in 6, hypothalamic in 3, corpus callosum in 5 and brainstem in 5 cases. Patients' Karnofsky scale scores ranged from 70 to 100 (median 80).

Resection of radiation necrosis, stereotactic aspiration of cystic tumor compartment, stereotactic biopsy for differentiation of radionecrosis from tumor, whole brain radiotherapy and chemotherapy were used as additional treatments before and after brachytherapy (tables 2–4). Four patients underwent second, 1 patient third and 1 fourth brachytherapy operations (table 1).

We investigated the CT/MRI images for the 'triple ring' (tumor necrosis, reactive zone and edema) on average 14.5 months following the low-dose rate ^{125}I interstitial irradiation of 19 inoperable LGG. The images with the triple ring were fused with the planning images, and the isodose curves were superimposed on them. The volumes of the three regions were measured. The average dose at the necrosis border was determined by the isodose distribution [14].

Results

The median survival rate for LGG, HGG and GBM were 35.8, 16.2 and 7.6 months, respectively. Overall survival rate for LGG, HGG and GBM were 93,

Table 3. Additional treatments before and after the first ^{125}I implant in 16 patients with HGG and GBM

Procedure	Before 1st ^{125}I implant	After 1st ^{125}I implant
Resection	13	7
	9 (1 resection)	4
	2 (2 resections)	0
	0 (3 resections)	1
Shunt	0	1
Aspiration	2	0
Chemotherapy	3	1
WBRT	6	0
Stereotactic biopsy	3	0

One patient received a second ^{125}I implant. In 4 cases, the reason for the resections following ^{125}I interstitial irradiation were recurrence (and edema) around radionecrosis.

Table 4. Additional treatments before and after the first ^{125}I implant in 27 patients with LGG

Procedure	Before 1st ^{125}I implant	After 1st ^{125}I implant
Resection	19	6
	10 (1 resection)	4
	3 (2 resections)	1
	1 (3 resections)	0
Shunt	2	8
Aspiration	1	3
Chemotherapy	1	1
WBRT	4	1
Stereotactic biopsy	5	0

Three patients received a second, 1 patient third and 1 patient fourth implant. In 2 cases, the reason for the resections following ^{125}I interstitial irradiation were recurrence (and edema) around radionecrosis. In 2 cases, only radionecrosis and edema were found and proved histologically.

48, 17% at 1 year, 61, 19, 0% at 3 years and 40, 0, 0% at 5 years, respectively (fig. 1). Fifty-three percent of patients had toxicity or transient subacute or chronic side effects. Their edemas were manageable using mannitol-steroid infusions. Eighteen percent of patients with glioma underwent reoperation following ^{125}I implantation.

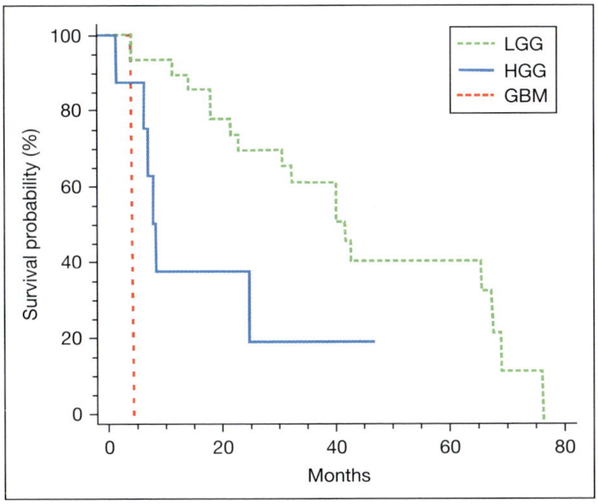

Fig. 1. Survival probability of 43 inoperable and recurrent LLG, HGG and GBM following ^{125}I irradiation.

The relative volumes of the different parts of the triple-ring after the interstitial irradiation compared to the reference dose volume were as follows: necrosis 54.9%, reactive zone 59.7%, and edema 445.3%. Tumor necrosis developed at 71.9-Gy dose, on average (fig. 2).

Discussion

Patients with GBM treated by surgery combined with or without chemotherapy at the time of recurrence have a median survival of 5–9 months [15, 16]. For patients with GBM, median survival times after brachytherapy at initial diagnosis range between 13.8–19 months [17–19].

The role of brachytherapy in the primary management of malignant gliomas has historically been controversial. Retrospective studies had suggested an improvement in the median survival of malignant glioma patients treated with brachytherapy [1, 20]. These results have been criticized by the presumed highly selected patient population receiving implants [19, 20]. Studies have suggested either a positive [4, 17, 23, 24] or no survival benefit [18, 25] for malignant glioma patients treated with brachytherapy. Some authors found that the extent of initial surgical resection did not influence the benefit of successive brachytherapy [17, 26–28].

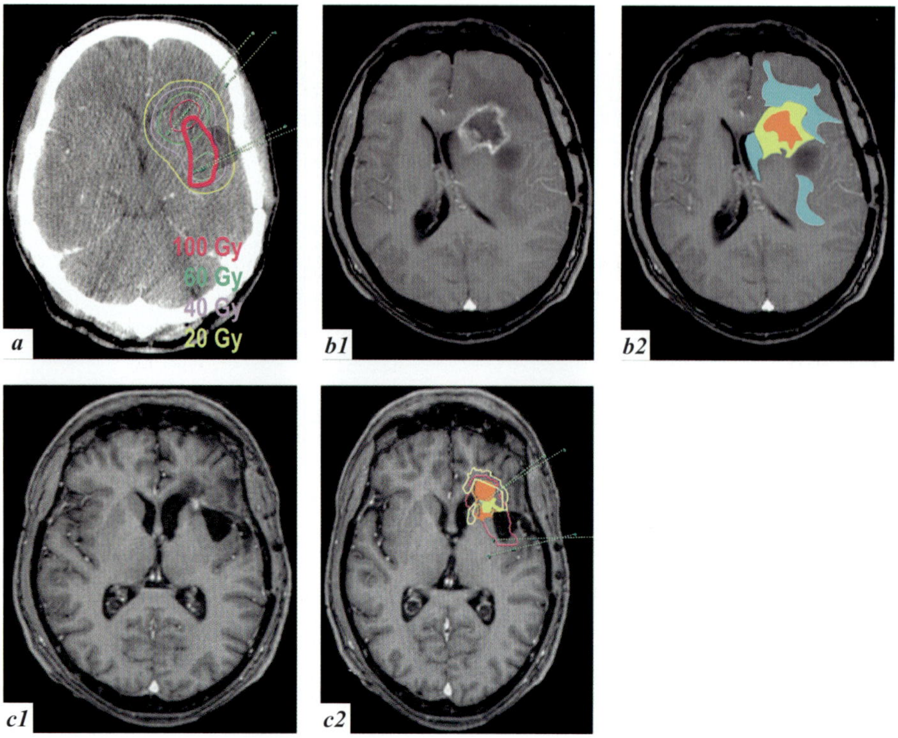

Fig. 2. The formation and change of the triple ring following ^{125}I interstitial irradiation (U.G. male, born in 1955). ***a*** In March 1998, a right insular space-occupying lesion was proved by CT after GM seizures. It was partially removed by right frontotemporal craniotomy using trans-Sylvian approach. In July 1998, the 2.6-cm^3 residual tumor marked by red line, was irradiated with 4 catheters and 8 102-mCi activity ^{125}I seeds through 13 days, by 60-Gy dose. The resection hollow is marked by grey line. ***b1, b2*** The MR images taken 14 months after the irradiation show the triple ring. The necrosis is ochre, the reactive zone yellow, the edema light blue. MRI (***c1***) and MRI/CT/MRI fusion (***c2***) images were taken 3–4 months after the irradiation. The edema disappeared; the reactive zone and the necrosis significantly shrank. ***c2*** The 14-month necrosis was marked with ochre, the reactive zone with yellow, and the tumor prior to irradiation with red line. The 4-year- and 3-month-old necrosis and reactive zone from (***c1***) are projected to (***c2***) filled with ochre and yellow colors. Recurrence cannot be seen on the images. The methionin PET examination made parallel with the MRI did not show any recurrence either. Today, the patient works as an electronic mechanic.

Age is a highly significant prognostic variable in patients with focal GBMs treated with external beam radiotherapy and brachytherapy boost. Sneed et al. [17] reported unusually good survival in the series of patients with GBM implant boost: patients aged between 18–29.9 years had a 3-year survival probability of 78%, and patients aged between 30–49.9 years had a 3-year survival probability of 29%, indicating that an aggressive approach to the treatment of GBM in young patients is justified.

The BTCG made a randomized study for a comparison of surgery, external beam radiotherapy, and carmustine versus surgery, external beam therapy, ^{125}I interstitial radiotherapy boost, and carmustine in newly diagnosed malignant gliomas [25]. The median survival for patients receiving additional therapy of ^{125}I was 68.1 weeks, and median survival for those receiving only external beam radiation and carmustine was 58.8 weeks without statistically significant difference between two survival rates.

In the study of Ostertag and Kreth [9], the 5-year survival rates were 77% for pilocytic astrocytomas, 65% for grade II astrocytomas, 80% for oligoastrocytomas, and 58% for oligodendrogliomas. The 2-year survival rates were 36% for anaplastic gliomas and 16% for glioblastomas. Kreth et al. [10] found the 5- and 10-year survival rates in patients with pilocytic astrocytomas (97 patients) were 84.9 and 83%, and in patients with WHO grade II astrocytomas (250 patients) 61 and 51%, respectively. Five-year survival rates for patients with oligoastrocytomas (60 patients), oligodendrogliomas (27 patients), and gemistocytic astrocytomas (21 patients) were 49, 50, and 32%, respectively.

Our results are comparable with the results of other brachytherapy centers. Brachytherapy with temporarily implanted ^{125}I sources for inoperable and recurrent gliomas is effective and offers a chance for longer-term survival even though edema surrounding the focal radiation necrosis might somewhat degrade the quality of survival in a minority of patients.

In ^{125}I brachytherapy of gliomas, the image fusion is a novel and important method for postoperative follow-up of effectiveness. The fusion of postirradiation CT/MRI images with the treatment images, including the isodose distribution, helps analyze the quantitative changes of necrosis, the reactive zone and edema (triple ring). This technique might also promote recognition of tumor recurrence, and altogether gives more information than measurement of volume changes alone.

Conclusion

Brachytherapy with temporarily implanted ^{125}I sources for inoperable and recurrent gliomas is an effective method and offers a chance for longer-term survival even though edema surrounding the focal radiation necrosis might degrade the quality of survival in a minority of patients. The image fusion technique proved to be useful to follow postirradiation changes. Fusion of posttreatment CT/MRI images with planning images, including the isodose distribution, helps analyze postirradiation quantitative changes of necrosis, the reactive zone and edema (triple ring), or even tumor recurrence.

References

1 Wallner KE, Galicich JH, Krol G, Arbit E, Malkin MG: Patterns of failure following treatment for glioblastoma multiforme and anaplastic astrocytoma. Int J Radiat Oncol Biol Phys 1989;16: 1405–1409.
2 Walker MD, Alexander E Jr, Hunt WE: Evaluation of BCNU and/or radiotherapy in the treatment of anaplastic gliomas. J Neurosurg 1978;49:333–343.
3 Walker MD, Green SB, Byar DP: Randomized comparisons of radiotherapy and nitrosoureas for malignant gliomas after surgery. N Engl J Med 1980;303:1323–1329.
4 Scharfen CO, Sneed PK, Wara WM, Larson DL, Phillips TL, Prados MD, Weawer KA, Malec M, Acord P, Lamborn KR, Lamb SA, Ham B, Gutin PH: High activity iodine-125 interstitial implant for gliomas. Int J Radiat Oncol Biol Phys 1992;24:583–591.
5 Walker MD, Strike TA, Sheline GE: An analysis of dose-effect relationship in the radiotherapy of malignant gliomas. Int J Radiat Oncol Biol Phys 1979;5:1725–1731.
6 Leibel S, Gutin PH, Sneed D, Prados M, Levin K, Larson D, Wara W, Weaver K, Philips TH: Interstitial irradiation for the treatment of primary and metastatic brain tumors. PPO Update 1987;13:1–11.
7 Gutin PH, Leibel SA, Wara WM, Choucair A, Levin VA, Phillips TL: Recurrent malignant gliomas: survival following interstitial brachytherapy with high-activity iodine-125 sources. J Neurosurg 1987;67:864–873.
8 Hochberg FH, Pruitt A: Assumptions in the radiotherapy of glioblastomas. Neurology 1980;30: 907–911.
9 Ostertag CB, Kreth FW: Iodine-125 interstitial irradiation for cerebral gliomas. Acta Neurochir 1992;119:53–61.
10 Kreth FW, Faist M, Warnke PC, Rossner R, Volk B, Ostertag CB: Interstitial radiosurgery of low-grade gliomas. J Neurosurg 1995;82:418–429.
11 Boethius J, Bergstrom M, Greitz T, et al: CT localization in stereotactic surgery. Appl Neurophysiol 1980;43:164–169.
12 Viola A, Major T, Julow J: The importance of postoperative CT image fusion verification of stereotactic interstitial irradiation for brain tumors. Int J Radiat Oncol Biol Phys 2004;60:322–328.
13 Julow J, Major T, Emri M, et al: The advantages of image fusion in stereotactic brachytherapy of brain tumours. Acta Neurochir 2000;142:1253–1258.
14 Julow J, Viola A, Major T, et al: Volumetric changes following I-125 interstitial irradiation of low grade gliomas. Clin Neurosci 2005;58:120–132.
15 Ammirati M, Vick N, Liao Y, Ciric I, Mikhael M: Effect of the extent of surgical resection on survival and quality of life in patients with supratentorial glioblastomas and anaplastic astrocytomas. Neurosurgery 1987;21:201–206.
16 Dirks P, Bernstein M, Muller PJ, Tucker WS: The value of reoperation for recurrent glioblastoma. Can J Surg 1993;36:271–275.
17 Sneed PK, Prados MD, McDermot MW, Larson DA, Malec MK, Lamborn KR, Davis RL, Weaver KA, Wara WM, Phillips TL, Gutin PH: Large effect of age on the survival of patients with glioblastoma treated with radiotherapy and brachytherapy boost. Neurosurgery 1995;36:898–904.

18 Laperriere NJ, Leung PMK, McKenzie S, Milosevic M, Wong S, Glen J, Pintilie M, Bernstein M: Randomized study of brachytherapy in the initial management of patients with malignant astrocytoma. Int J Radiat Oncol Biol Phys 1998;41:1005–1011.
19 Wen PY, Alexander E III, Black PM, Fine HA, Riese N, Levin JM, Coleman CN, Loeffler JS: Long term results of stereotactic brachytherapy used in the initial treatment of patients with glioblastomas. Cancer 1994;73:3029–3036.
20 Fernandez PM, Zamorano L, Yakar D, Gaspar L, Warmelink C: Permanent Iodine-125 implants in the up-front treatment of malignant gliomas. Neurosurgery 1995;36:467–473.
21 Voges J, Treuer H, Schlegel W, Pastyr O, Sturm V: Combined radiotherapy of high-grade gliomas with stereotactic implants iodine-125 seeds and fractionated low-dose rate beam irradiation: preliminary results. Adv Neurosurg 1992;20:298–303.
22 Zamorano L, Yakar D, Dujovny M, Sheehan M, Kim J: Permanent iodine-125 implant and external beam radiotherapy for the treatment of malignant brain tumors. Stereotact Funct Neurosurg 1992;59:183–192.
23 Selker RG, Shapiro WR, Green S: A randomized trial of interstitial radiotherapy (IRT) boost for the treatment of newly diagnosed malignant glioma: BTCG Study 87-01. Congr Neurol Surg 45 Annu Meet Prog, San Francisco, October 1995, pp 94–95.
24 Videtic GMM, Gaspar LE, Zamorano L, Stitt LW, Fontanesi J, Levin KJ: Implant volume as a prognostic variable in brachytherapy decision-making for malignant gliomas stratified by the RTOG recursive partitioning analysis. Int J Radiat Oncol Biol Phys 2001;51:963–968.
25 Selker RG, Shapiro WR, et al: The Brain Tumor Cooperative Group NIH Trial 87-01: a randomized comparison of surgery, external radiotherapy, and carmustine versus surgery, interstitial radiotherapy boost, external radiation therapy and carmustine. Neurosurgery 2002;51:343–357.
26 Nazzaro JM, Neuwelt EA: The role of surgery in the management of supratentorial intermediate and high-grade astrocytomas in adults. J Neurosurg 1990;73:331–344.
27 Hess KR: Extent of resection as a prognostic variable in the treatment of gliomas. J Neurooncol 1999;42:227–231.
28 Bampoe J, Glen J, Mackenzie I, Porter P, Bernstein M: Effect of implant dose/volume and surgical resection on survival in a rat glioma brachytherapy model: implications for brain tumor therapy. Neurosurgery 1997;41:1374–1383.

Jenö Julow, MD, PhD
Department of Neurosurgery, St. John's Hospital
Diósárok út 1
HU–1125 Budapest (Hungary)
Tel. +36 458 4538, Fax +36 458 4650, E-Mail h12494jul@t-online.hu

Szeifert GT, Kondziolka D, Levivier M, Lunsford LD (eds): Radiosurgery and Pathological Fundamentals. Prog Neurol Surg. Basel, Karger, 2007, vol 20, pp 312–323

12.2.2. Tissue Response to Iodine-125 Interstitial Brachytherapy of Cerebral Gliomas

Jenö Julow[a], *György T. Szeifert*[b], *Katalin Bálint*[b], *István Nyáry*[b], *Zoltán Nemes*[c]

[a]Department of Neurosurgery, St. John's Hospital, [b]National Institute of Neurosurgery and Department of Neurological Surgery, Semmelweis University, Budapest, [c]Department of Pathology, University Medical School of Debrecen, Debrecen, Hungary

Abstract

The purpose of this study was to investigate histopathological changes and the role of the microglia/macrophage cell system in the therapeutic effect of iodine-125 (^{125}I) interstitial brachytherapy on cerebral gliomas. Out of a series of 60 cases harboring cerebral astrocytomas and other brain tumors treated with ^{125}I interstitial brachytherapy, autopsy material was available in 10 cases between 0.75 and 60 months after irradiation. The patients were treated with 60-Gy maximum doses at the tumor periphery. Besides the routine HE and Mallory's PTAH trichrome staining, immunohistochemical reactions were carried out for CD15, CD31, CD34, CD45, CD68 (PG-M1), CPM, HAM 56 and HLA-DR antigens to study immunological characteristics of the reactive cell population around gliomas after ^{125}I treatment. The present immunohistochemical study demonstrated that the early lesions following ^{125}I interstitial brachytherapy of gliomas are characterized by migrating macrophages apparently concerned with the removal of necrotic debris. The established phase of reactive zone around the necrotic center disclosed a narrow inner rim of microglial accumulation, and a broad outer area consisting of astrocytic gliosis, vascular proliferation, activated microglia and infiltration by macrophages. In the burned-out phase, the necrosis undergoes liquefaction, the microglial rim is replaced by end-stage macrophages, and the reactive zone is transformed into astrocytic gliosis, which can be considered as equivalent to scar tissue formed around necrosis outside of the central nervous system.

There has been a considerable increase in the interest for the use of interstitial brachytherapy in the treatment of brain tumors during the last 20 years. The benefit

Table 1. The main characteristics of the therapy employed

Mean age, years	47.1
Females/males	33/27
Tumor volume, cm^3	11.9 (1.2–32)
Catheters	1.7 (1–5)
Seeds	4.7 (1–8)
Total activity, mCi	57.3 (8–155)
Irradiation time, days	16 (4–90)
DVH, %	91.6 (64–100)
NT of TV, %	78 (32.7–166)
Treatment dose, Gy	62.3 (45–120)
AV dose rate, cGy/h	23.9 (0.9–82.7)
Mean follow-up, months (49 cases)	25.4 (0.6–67.0)

Table 2. Primary antibodies employed in this study

Antigen	Clone	Source	Dilution	Specificity
CD68	PGM-1	DAKO	1:50	monocyte-derived cells only
HAM56		DAKO	1:50	macrophages, and some other cells
CD34	QBEND	DAKO	1:100	endothelial and progenitor cells
CD31	JC70A	DAKO	1:40	endothelial cells and some macrophages
CD45	2B11, PD7/26	DAKO	1:50	lymphoid cells
CD15	C3D1	DAKO	1:50	neutrophil granulocytes
HLA-DR	CR3-43	DAKO	1:100	MHC class 2
S100	polyclonal	DAKO	1:400	myeloid antigen presenting cells
Factor XIIIa	polyclonal	Calbiochem	1:400	mesenchymal dendritic cells
CPM	1C2	Novocastra	1:40	epithelioid cells, endstage macrophages

Calbiochem, La Jolla, Calif., USA; DAKO, Copenhagen, Denmark; Novocastra, Newcastle upon Tyne, UK.

of this procedure compared to traditional external-beam radiotherapy is the capacity to save normal brain tissue surrounding the tumor, thus improving the therapeutic ratio [1]. As the irradiation sources are placed inside the tumor, dose distribution can be confirmed to the shape of the tumor with a high dose gradient fall-off towards the normal neural tissue. The goal of interstitial brachytherapy is to produce well-defined, small volume tissue necrosis that develops centrifugally from the implant and is subsequently removed by macrophage activity [22].

Despite of the widespread application of brachytherapy in the complex management of cerebral gliomas, only sparse human pathological data are available in the literature explaining histopathological changes following interstitial irradiation [12]. Relatively little is known about the cellular mechanism underlying the induction of 'triple ring' phenomenon, that is necrosis-reactive zone edema as a consequence of glioma irradiation. Ostertag [20] has demonstrated that after ^{192}Ir, ^{198}Au and iodine-125 (^{125}I), interstitial irradiation of dog brain necrosis develops and is later eliminated by macrophages, and such a treatment can be regarded as a radiosurgical procedure.

Following radiosurgical interventions performed by the Gamma Knife or by a linear accelerator, similar pathological changes appear (i.e. necrosis, cellular zone, edema). However, literature regarding these treatment modalities is far more prevalent than literature on interstitial irradiation [10, 13, 14]. Therefore, the goal of the present study was to characterize pathological changes, and the role of the microglia/macrophage cell system following interstitial irradiation of cerebral gliomas.

Patients and Methods

We have performed interstitial brachytherapy on 25 low grade, 10 high grade gliomas and 25 other brain tumors (pinealomas, meningiomas, craniopharyngiomas and schwannomas) using radioactive ^{125}I seeds between 1996 and 2003. The main characteristics of this method are summarized in table 1.

The seeds were placed in Teflon catheters into the tumor under local anesthesia, with stereotactic operation using determined geometrical parameters. The delivered dose was 50–60 Gy at the periphery of the tumor. The placement of the catheters was temporary, and they were removed after the expiration of the irradiation period (usually 1–5 weeks). Treatment planning was based on CT/MR/PET image fusion. Three-dimensional examinations revealed the conformity of isodose distribution on the target volume, as well as outcomes of the irradiation changes. Image fusion was performed with Target 1.19 (BrainLab, Germany) planning system used for planning of brachytherapy before, and during the operation [11].

Out of the brachytherapy-treated 35 glioma cases, 15 patients died until now. Postmortem examinations were carried out in 10 cases. Brain tumors representing the necrotic area, the reactive ring and outer edematous zone were routinely fixed in 10% buffered formaldehyde, embedded in paraffin, and cut at 4–5 μm. Paraffin sections were used for both histological staining and immunohistochemical methods. Histological stain included HE and Mallory techniques. Immunohistochemical reactions were carried out with the avidin-biotin-peroxidase technique. Prior to immunohistochemistry antigen, unmasking was performed by heating the slides in citrate buffer (10 mM, pH 6.0) for 3 min using a pressure cooker. Endogenous peroxidase was blocked with 30 min incubation in 0.5% hydrogen peroxide at room temperature. Primary antibodies employed are listed in table 2. Biotinylated goat antimouse antisera (1:200) and avidin-biotin pereoxidase complex (1:100) were the second and third steps of the immunohistochemical technique (DAKO, Copenhagen, Denmark). In control sections, the primary

Table 3. Immunohistochemical results of postirradiation tissue alterations

Case	Migration of phagocytes	Vascular proliferation	Astrocytic proliferation	Microglial proliferations	End-stage macrophages	Tumor type	Postirradiation period, months
1	++	–	–	–	–	A3	0.75
2	–	++	++	++	–	Gb1	5
3	–	–	+	+/–	++	A2	54
4	–	+	++	+	–	Gb1	12
5	–	–	+	–	+	A2	57
6	–	+	+	+	–	A3	15
7	–	++	++	++	–	A3	15
8	–	–	+	–	+	03	60
9	–	+	++	++	–	03	10
10	–	–	++	–	+	Gb1	23

antibody was either omitted or substituted with an irrelevant monoclonal antibody of the same isotype. Peroxidase was detected using Vector VIP SK-4600 chromogene (Vector Laboratories, Burlingame, Calif., USA) and 0.01% H_2O_2. Slides were counterstained with methyl green.

Results

The immunohistochemical results of all ten postmortem examinations are summarized in table 3. Findings in typical illustrative cases are detailed below:

Case 1 (1 month following brachytherapy): a recent hemorrhagic necrosis was seen in the central area. No nuclear material was stained in this necrotic region. The central area was surrounded by small focal hemorrhages. The formation of a reactive zone was not apparent with HE. Immunohistochemistry revealed no glial cell response around the necrotic tumor. However, the reactive zone was evidenced by immunohistochemical staining for macrophages: a diffuse scattered and a dense focal perivascular accumulation of PGM-1-positive cells were demonstrated (fig. 1). There was no inflammatory reaction and no vascular proliferation around the necrotic area.

Case 2 (6 months following irradiation): coagulation necrosis was seen in the innermost zone of the tumor. Cell contours were lost and fragmented nuclear material was stained as basophilic stippling in the necrotic area. The necrosis had no hemorrhagic character. The necrotic tumor showed no apparent demarcation zone with HE staining: cellular density was not increased, and no orderly arrangement of nuclei (pseudopalisading) was seen in the viable tissue immediately surrounding the necrotic area (fig. 2). However, immunohistochemical reaction with macrophage-specific antibody (PGM-1) revealed a rim formed by

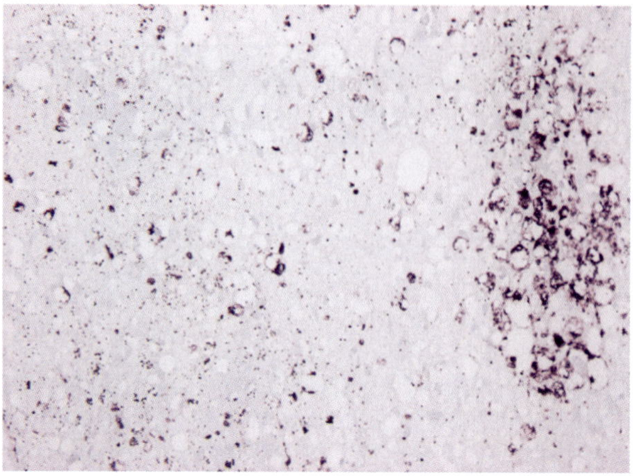

Fig. 1. Case 1. Tissue area around a recent postirradiation necrosis (1 month after ^{125}I brachytherapy). Scattered macrophages and a perivascular accumulation of macrophages. Phagocytosis of lipids is indicated by rounded clear spaces in their cytoplasm. Immunoperoxidase technique for PGM-1, ×400.

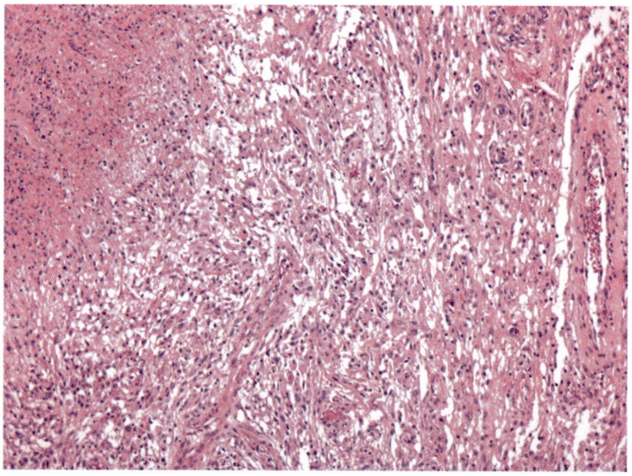

Fig. 2. Case 2. Reactive zone formed after 6 months around postirradiation necrosis (top, left). HE staining, ×200.

the dense accumulation of small stellate cells. Activated macrophages scattered throughout the broad reactive zone around the necrotic area were larger and disclosed more intense immunohistochemical reaction with PGM-1 (fig. 3) or HAM56. The reactive zone contained an accumulation of GFAP-positive glial

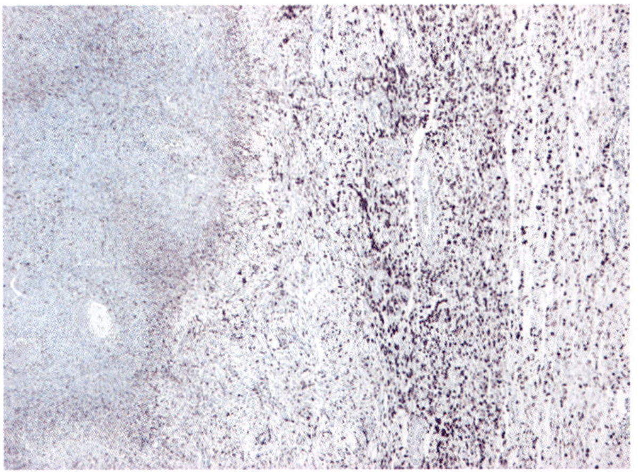

Fig. 3. Case 2. Adjacent section to that seen in figure 2. There is an inner ring formed by small stellate microglial cells (left) and an outer area of activated macrophages (right). Immunoperoxidase technique for PGM-1, ×200.

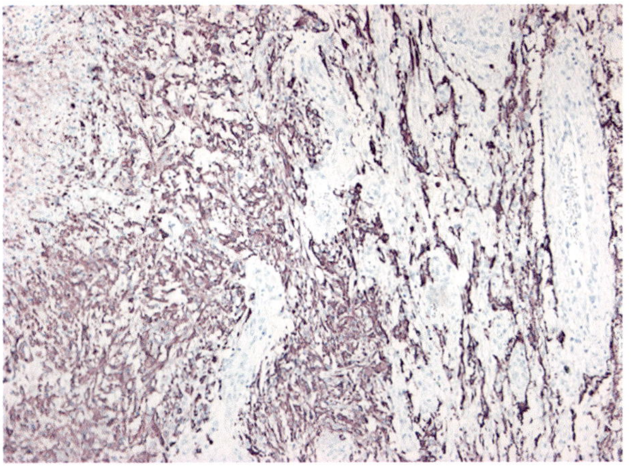

Fig. 4. Case 2. Adjacent section to that seen in figure 3. Dense accumulation of astrocytes around the necrotic zone. Immunoperoxidase for GFAP, ×200.

cells (fig. 4) and a vascular proliferation (fig. 5). The reactive zone contained only an insignificant amount of lymphocytes and no granulocytes. The outermost zone was formed by a broad area of edematous brain tissue. End-stage macrophages were not seen in the reactive or outermost zones.

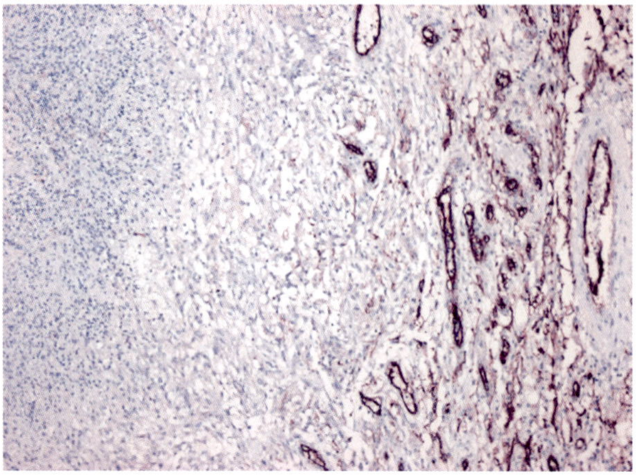

Fig. 5. Case 2. Adjacent reaction to that seen in figure 4. Endothelial lining of proliferating vessels in the reactive zone is strongly stained. Immunoperoxidase technique for CD34, ×200.

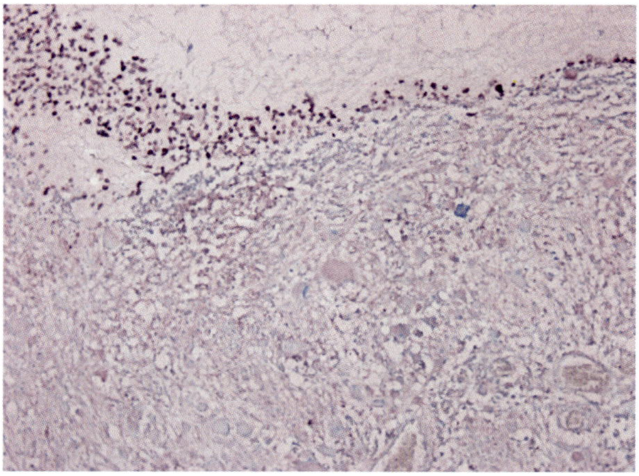

Fig. 6. Case 3. Reactive zone formed after 54 months around the postirradiation necrosis (top). A layer of rounded end-stage macrophages is strongly stained around the necrosis. Immunoperoxidase technique for carboxypeptidase M, ×200.

Case 3 (54 months following brachytherapy): the central necrotic zone was colliquative and cystic. The necrosis was lined by a dense layer of rounded end-stage macrophages which were positive for PGM-1, HAM56 and also for carboxypeptidase M (fig. 6). The reactive zone was characterized by a prominent

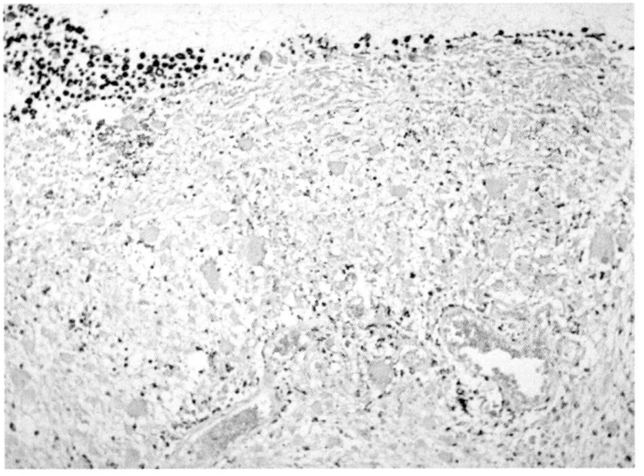

Fig. 7. Case 3. Adjacent section to that seen in figure 6. The end-stage macrophages (top) and a few scattered microglial cells are stained. Immunoperoxidase technique for PGM-1, ×200.

glial cell accumulation. Scattered microglial elements were also seen with PGM-1 (fig. 7). Vascular proliferation was lacking in the reactive zone.

Discussion

Brain tumors, especially gliomas examined by MRI, CT and PET imaging demonstrate characteristic changes several months after Gamma Knife [16], linear accelerator or interstitial irradiation, what we denominated as 'triple ring' phenomenon. The necrotized part of the tumor is situated innermost. The necrosis is surrounded by a layer called 'reactive zone', in our terminology. Edema, later demyelinization can encircle the reactive ring, especially in the white matter. These changes were studied by Higashi et al. [8] and Tada et al. [31]. Colliquation and coagulation necrosis can be seen around the implanted isotopes. Early lesions resulted from inflammatory phenomena and elimination of necrotic debris by phagocytes originating from the surrounding veins [9]. Kumar et al. [15] described contrast-enhancing CT ring lesions 2–6 months after ^{60}Co AL HDR treatment of glioblastomas (in 21 patients out of 41). Harisiadis et al. [6] also observed an 'enhancing rim' on CT images of irradiated gliomas. The 6- to 8-mm-thick 'contrast-enhancing CT ring', or 'contrast-medium enhanced ring', what we designated as 'reactive ring' is even easier to demonstrate with MRI. Even more striking on T_1-weighted images after administering gadolinium contrast material, than with CT. Numerous papers refer to the radiological lesions after Gamma Knife surgery or interstitial irradiation [2, 15, 18, 22, 24, 31]. The reactive ring is believed to consist of dilated and proliferating vessels. Macrophages are supposed to play a key role in angiogenesis [30]. The third part of triple ring phenomenon is tissue edema production that has great clinical importance. In our practice, it can be reduced by dehydration in about half of the cases. There are papers in the literature demonstrating the frequency of edema production after radiotherapy [7], and the development of edema time course was analyzed by Groothuis et al. [5] and Nakata et al. [19]. Perinecrotic edema is one of the most serious complications of interstitial irradiation of gliomas; however, the exact pathogenesis of this condition is still unknown. Macrophages are known to secrete various substances (including arachidonate metabolites) that may interfere with vascular permeability [29].

Both of our imaging techniques, i.e. image fusion and the histological examination of autopsy material, supported the existence of the triple ring theory. Distribution and characterization of the microglia/macrophage system in human brain tumors have previously been investigated by other authors [17, 24, 27, 28]. Our study was focused on the role of the microglia/macrophage cell system in the tissue reaction around postirradiation necrosis after brachytherapy of gliomas. We investigated 10 autopsy material 0.75–60 months following ^{125}I interstitial irradiation using immunohistochemical markers. Formation of the reactive zone around the early radiation-induced necrosis (1 month) was not evident with conventional histological staining techniques. There was no glial or vascular response in the brain tissue adjacent to the necrotic zone. The mobilization of macrophages, however, was obvious using macrophage-specific immunohistochemical reactions.

Phagocytes emigrating from the blood into the perinecrotic zone serve to remove tissue debris. Antibodies to CD68 are used as immunohistochemical markers for macrophages. CD68 is a highly glycosylated lysosomal membrane protein which belongs to a family of lysosomal glycoprotein/plasma membrane shuttling proteins that play a role in endocytosis and/or lysosomal trafficking. Unlike many other CD leukocyte antigens, the CD68 molecule is antigenically very heterogeneous, and different antibodies to CD68 show different cellular reactivities [3]. PGM-1 is regarded as the most macrophage selective because it fails to react with granulocytes like KP-1 [26], and some endothelial or lymphoid cells like HAM56 [4]. PGM-1 antibody detects only a fixative-resistant epitope on the macrophage-restricted form of the CD68 antigen [3]. The PGM-1-positive macrophages do not show zonal arrangement, they are diffusely scattered in a broad area around the necrosis with occasional perivascular accumulation.

A clear-cut microglial rim is seen immediately adjacent to the radiation-induced necrosis in the reactive zone after a few months. The rim is formed by a dense accumulation of PGM-1-positive stellate cells, which have only a limited amount of cytoplasm. Larger macrophages with rounded cytoplasm and more intense PGM-1 positivity are seen in the zone, which is characterized also by a proliferation of vessels and GFAP-positive astrocytic glial elements. After about 2 years, the reactive zone around the necrosis is characterized by astrocytic gliosis but microglial and vascular components disappear. The necrotic area is surrounded by rounded end-stage macrophages. They are positive for carboxypeptidase M, HLA-DR and CD31. These macrophages do not appear to be migratory cells and seem to be concerned with the storage of some phagocytosed material. Astrocytic gliosis in the burned-out phase of radiation-induced necrosis is an equivalent of scarring formed around necrosis in mesenchymal tissues.

Conclusion

The present immunohistochemical study demonstrated that the early lesions following ^{125}I interstitial brachytherapy of gliomas are characterized by migrating macrophages apparently concerned with the removal of necrotic debris. The established phase of the reactive zone around the necrotic center disclosed a narrow inner rim of microglial accumulation and a broad outer area consisting of astrocytic gliosis, vascular proliferation, activated microglia and infiltration by macrophages. In the burned-out phase, the necrosis undergoes liquefaction, the microglial rim is replaced by end-stage macrophages, and the reactive zone is transformed into astrocytic gliosis, which can be considered as equivalent to scar tissue formed around necrosis outside of the central nervous system.

References

1 Bellezza DM, Berner BM: Stereotactic interstitial brachytherapy; in Gildenberg PL, Tasker RR (eds): Textbook of Stereotactic and Functional Neurosurgery. New York, McGraw-Hill, 1998, pp 577–580.

2 Castel JC, Caille JM: Imaging of irradiated brain tumours. Value of magnetic resonance imaging. J Neuroradiol 1989;16:81–132.

3 Falini B, Flenghi L, Pileri S, Gambacorta M, Bigerna B, Durkop H, et al: PG-M1: a new monoclonal antibody directed against a fixative-resistant epitope on the macrophage-restricted form of the CD68 molecule. Am J Pathol 1993;142:1359–1372.

4 Gown AM, Tsukada T, Ross R: Human atherosclerosis. II. Immunocytochemical analysis of the cellular composition of human atherosclerotic lesions. Am J Pathol 1986;125:191–207.

5 Groothuis DR, Wright DC, Ostertag CB: The effect of 125 I interstitial radiotherapy on blood-brain barrier function in normal canine brain. J Neurosurg 1987;6:895–902.

6 Harisiadis L, Wechsler-Jentzsch K, Harisiadis S, Dina TS: Glioblastoma oncometry. Strahlenther Onkol 1990;166:808–817.

7 Helenowski TK, Pothiawala B: Role of Gamma Knife in the treatment of large lesions. Stereotact Funct Neurosurg 1993;6:103–115.

8 Higashi H, Matsumoto K, Ono Y: Patterns of recurrence in malignant gliomas after brachytherapy. No Shinkei Geka 1994;22:321–326.

9 Ishikawa S, Otsuki T, Kaneki M, Jokura H, Yoshimoto T: Dose-related Effects of Single Focal Irradiation in the medial Temporal Lobe Structures in Rats. MRI and Histological Study Neurol Med Chir 1999;39:1–7.

10 Julow J, Slowik F, Kelemen I, Gorácz I: Late post Irradiation necrosis of the Brain. Acta Neuriochirurgica 1979;46:135–150.

11 Julow J, Major T, Emri M, Valálik I, Sági S, Mangel L, et al: The advantages of Image Fusion in Stereotactic Brachytherapy of Brain Tumours. Acta neurochir 2000;142:1253–1258.

12 Kiessling M, Kleihues P, Gassega E, et al: Morphology of intracranial tumors and adjacent brain structures following interstitial iodine-125 radiotherapy. Acta Neurochir 1984;33(suppl):281–289.

13 Kondziolka D, Lunsford LD, Claassen D, Pandalai S, Maitz HA, Flickinger JC: Radiobiology of Radiosurgery. Part II. The Rat C6 Glioma Model. Neurosurgery 1992;31:280–287.

14 Kamiryo T, Kassel NF, Thai A, Lopes MBS, Lee KS, Steiner L: Histological changes in the Normal Rat Brain after Gamma Irradiation. Acta Neurochir 1996;138:451–459.

15 Kumar PP, Good RR, Jones EO, Skultety FM, Leibrock LG, McComb RD: Contrast-enhancing computer tomography ring in glioblastoma multiforme after intraoperative endocurietherapy. Cancer 1988;61:1795–1796.

16 Levivier M, Wikler D, Goldman S, Massager N, Van Houtte P, Brotchi J, et al: Integration of metabolic data of positron emission tomography in the dosimetry planning of radiosurgery with the Leksell Gamma Knife: early experience with brain tumors. J Neurosurg 2000;93(suppl 3): 233–238.

17 Morimura T, Neuchrist C, Kitz K, Budka H, Scheiner O, Kraft D, Lassmann H: Monocyte subpopulations in human gliomas: expression of Fc and complement receptors and correlation with tumor proliferation. Acta Neuropathol 1990;80:287–294.

18 Moringlane JR, Voges M, Huber G, Müller J, Letz H: Short-term CT and MR changes in brain tumours following 125 I interstitial irradiation. J Comput Assist Tomogr 1997;21:15–21.

19 Nakata H, Yoshimine T, Murasawa A, Kumura E, Harada K, Ushio Y, et al: Early blood-brain barrier disruption after high-dose single-fraction irradiation in rats. Acta Neurochir 1995;136: 82–87.

20 Ostertag CB: Brachytherapy-interstitial implant radiosurgery. Acta Neurochir 1993;58(suppl): 79–84.

21 Ostertag BC: Interstitial radiosurgery of brain tumors; in Gildenberg PL, Tasker RR (eds): Textbook of stereotactic and functional neurosurgery. New York, McGraw-Hill, 1998, pp 589–598.

22 Park YG, Kim EZ, Chang JW, Chung SS: Volume changes following gamma knife radiosurgery of intracranial tumors. Surg Neurol 1997;48:488–493.

23 Penfield W: Microglia and the process of phagocytosis in gliomas. Am J Pathol 1925;1:77–97.

24 Plowman PN: Stereotactic radiosurgery VIII. The classification of postirradiation reactions. Br J Neurosurg 1999;13:256–264.

25 Pulford KAF, Rigney EM, Micklem KJ, Jones M, Stross WP, Gatter KC, et al: KP1: a new monoclonal antibody that detects a monocyte/macrophage associated antigen in routinely processed tissue sections. J Clin Pathol 1989;42:414–421.

26 Roggendorf W, Strupp S, Paulus W: Distribution and characterisation of microglia/macrophages in human brain tumors. Acta Neuropathol 1996;92:288–293.

27 Rossi MI, Hughes JT, Esiri MM, Coakham HB, Brownell DB: Immunhistological study of mononuclear cell infiltrate in malignant gliomas. Acta Neuropathol 1987;74:269–277.

28 Shinonaga M, Chang Ch, Suzuki N, Sato M, Kuwabara T: Immunohystological evaluation of macrophage infiltrates in brain tumor. J Neurosurg 1988;68:259–265.

29 Sunderkötter C, Steinbrink K, Goeveler M, Bhardwaj R, Sorg C: Macrophages and angiogenesis. J Leukoc Biol 1994;55:410–422.

30 Tada E, Matsumoto K, Kinoshita K, Tamesa N, Maeda Y, Adachi H, et al: Combined brachytherapy and external beam radiotherapy in normal monkey brains. Experimental Radiation Necrosis Evaluated by Sequential Magnetic Resonance Imaging. Neurol Med Chir 1998;38:203–212.
31 Vuorinen V, Heikokken J, Brander A, Setala K, Sane T, Randell T, et al: Interstitial radiotherapy of 25 parasellar/clival meningiomas and 19 meningiomas in the elderly. Analysis of short-term tolerance and responses. Acta Neurochir 1996;138:495–508.

Jenö Julow, MD, PhD
Department of Neurosurgery, St. John's Hospital
Diósárok út 1
HU–1125 Budapest (Hungary)
Tel. +36 1 458 4538, Fax +36 1 458 4650, E-Mail h12494jul@t-online.hu

Szeifert GT, Kondziolka D, Levivier M, Lunsford LD (eds): Radiosurgery and Pathological Fundamentals. Prog Neurol Surg. Basel, Karger, 2007, vol 20, pp 324–339

13. Radiosurgery in Ocular Disorders: Clinical Applications

Roman Liščák, Vilibald Vladyka

Department of Stereotactic and Radiation Neurosurgery, Na Homolce Hospital, Prague, Czech Republic

Abstract

Radiosurgery using the Leksell Gamma Knife (LGK) applied to ophthalmologic indications is a specific area where the eye target has a very eccentric location, since the eye can move, its fixation is required and the patient is generally treated in a prone position. It was demonstrated that the LGK is sufficiently accurate to be used for ophthalmic radiosurgery. Current spectrum of treated indications includes uveal melanomas, eye metastases, advanced glaucoma, age-related macular degeneration (ARMD), hemangioblastoma, angioreticuloma, pseudotumors and vegetative pain. The results for uveal melanomas are recognized and the value of the LGK in the treatment of glaucoma and ARMD seems promising after initial studies. Gamma Knife radiosurgery of the ciliary body leads to a significant alleviation of pain and reduction in intraocular pressure in advanced glaucoma. The latency of the treatment effect is relatively short. In the majority of patients with ARMD, both ultrasonography and fluorescein angiography demonstrated a regression of the neovascular complex or stabilization after LGK radiosurgery. A number of rare ophthalmologic indications have also been treated by the Gamma Knife in our Center with more or less prominent therapeutic responses.

Due to its radiobiological principles, radiosurgery is limited to the treatment of small lesions, and it is logical from this point of view that the eye should attract deserved attention. During 2003, we treated 800 patients with the Leksell Gamma Knife (LGK) in our Center, and of these 75 (9.4%) had ophthalmologic indications. First experiences with ophthalmologic indications involved the treatment of patients suffering from uveal melanomas [1–6]. However, it would appear that the potential of radiosurgery to provide effective treatment for ophthalmologic indications is far greater and, besides uveal melanomas, the current spectrum of treated indications also includes eye

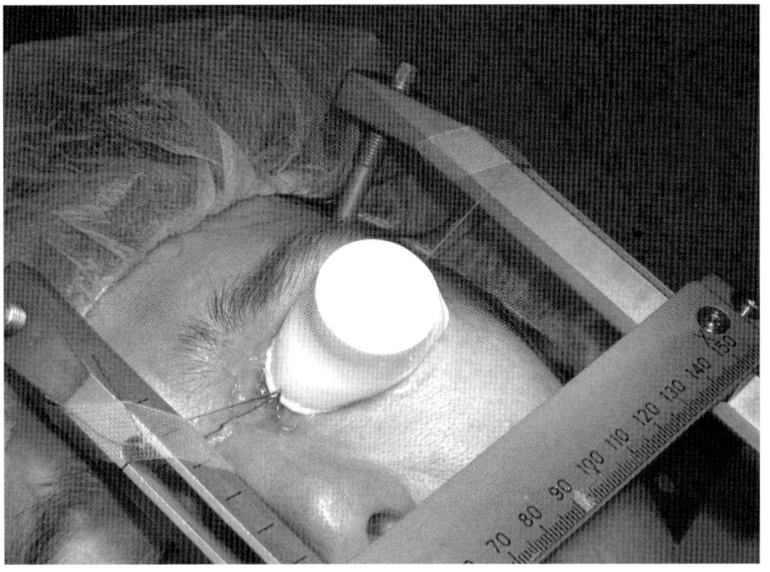

Fig. 1. Fixation of the eye.

metastases, advanced glaucoma, age-related macular degeneration (ARMD), hemangioblastoma, angioreticuloma, pseudotumors and vegetative pain.

The LGK was originally designed to treat brain targets with the skull rigidly fixed to the stereotactic coordinate frame. For this reason, radiosurgery using the LGK applied to ophthalmologic indications is a specific area where the eye target has a very eccentric location, since the eye can move, its fixation is required and the patient is generally treated in a prone position.

Method

Radiosurgery at our Center was performed using the LGK Model B, which was upgraded to Model C in 2002 (Elekta Instrument AB). The stereotactic frame must be fixed in a position relative to the marginal position of the eye. The eye to be treated must be close to the midline of the stereotactic system. The stereotactic frame has to be rotated accordingly and pushed as far forward as possible. The occipital panel of the MRI indicator box was in contact with the occipital bone. The treated eye was fixed under local anesthesia by suturing two rectus eye muscles to the stereotactic frame. Fixation of the eye was performed by the ophthalmologist. To assure the build-up and homogenous propagation of radiation between the tissues and the air, partial tarsorrhaphy was performed and a plastic cover filled with tissue-equivalent gel was used (fig. 1). This simultaneously acted as protection for the cornea. The stereotactic targeting was performed by MRI (Magnetom Expert 1 T, Siemens).

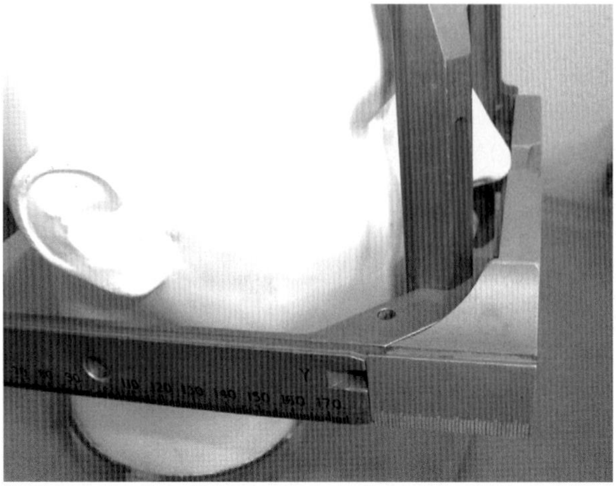

Fig. 2. Triangle adapter to enlarge the y coordinate.

Gradient echo T_1-weighted 3-D sequences and 1.3-mm slices were used for targeting. Treatment planning was performed using Leksell GammaPlan® (Elekta Instrument AB). The coordinates of eye targets are usually beyond the scale available to the automatic positioning system, and therefore the trunnion mode was used for the majority of patients. There is no problem setting the x and z coordinates, but the y coordinates frequently lie beyond the scale of the stereotactic coordinate frame ($y > 175$). Where this was the case, a special triangle adapter was used (fig. 2). Because of the marginal position of the eye, an extreme gamma angle has to be used to avoid collision of the skull with the collimator helmet. Usually, the gamma angle differs from the 90° standard position by 40°, which means 50° when patients are in a supine position, which they do not tolerate. Therefore the prone position is used in most cases. In this prone position, a gamma angle of up to 135–140° can be tolerated (fig. 3). The treatment could not be performed in a small number of patients suffering from rigid kyphosis or Bechterev disease. In our experience, the number of patients with ophthalmologic indications who could not be treated with the LGK for these technical reasons has not exceeded about 3%.

The accuracy of the MRI of the eye as an eccentric target was tested using phantoms. A special cylindrical phantom with two inserts (axial and coronal) was constructed to assess the accuracy of MRI. The phantom was fixed in the Leksell stereotactic frame and underwent stereotactic MRI under routine clinical conditions. Coronal MRI slices demonstrated higher image distortion and were not accepted for eye stereotactic localization. Consequently, only MRI axial slices were acquired, and reconstruction in the treatment planning system was performed. The standard imaging procedure for eye lesions was 3-D gradient echo image sequence with 1.3-mm slice thickness. Detailed phantom measurements are required for each MRI scanner employed and each individual sequence used for the imaging [7].

Because MRI is performed in a supine position, while the patient is treated in a prone position, the stability of the eye fixation was also tested. Two subsequent MRIs were performed on a patient with a fixed eye in different positions (supine and prone). To assess the

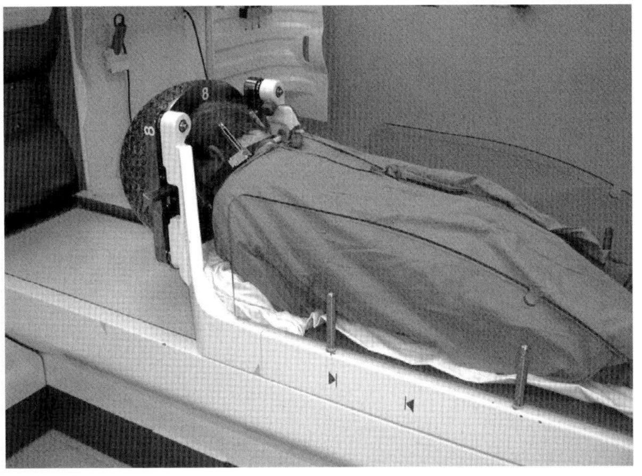

Fig. 3. Prone position of the patient.

stability of eye fixation as well, these two subsequent scans were done at least 2 h apart. Very good stability of eye fixation was observed for all 10 tested patients. No significant difference in stereotactic localization was observed when MRI was done in either the supine or the prone position. Consequently, no limitations were imposed on treating patients in a prone position, while MRI was performed in a supine position.

Leksell GammaPlan calculations and treatment delivery were also tested. To assess the accuracy of the treatment planning system, relative and absolute dose calculations and treatment delivery, a special head phantom was constructed. This phantom was filled with water and dosimeters employed in relative and absolute dosimetry were fixed in the correct position (eye of the head phantom). A PinPoint PTW Freiburg TW 31006 ion chamber (PTW Freiburg, Germany) and PTW UNIDOS electrometer (PTW Freiburg) were used for absolute dosimetry. For relative dosimetry, a polymer gel dosimeter was poured into spherically shaped glass test vessels and fixed in the head phantom. The composition, calibration and evaluation of this dosimeter have been described elsewhere [8, 9]. The phantom with the selected dosimeter was fixed to the Leksell stereotactic frame and underwent imaging, treatment planning and treatment following standard patient procedures. The polymerization that occurred in the polymer gel, together with the 3-D treatment plan can be seen in figure 4.

Absolute doses measured by pinpoint ion chamber at depths of 10 mm and deeper showed relatively close conformity with the treatment planning system-calculated data. Absolute doses delivered during head phantom irradiation were systematically lower than those calculated by Leksell GammaPlan, usually within 5%. Absolute doses measured by pinpoint ion chamber at depths of less than 10 mm showed relatively large deviations when compared to the treatment planning system-calculated data. In this situation, absolute doses delivered during phantom irradiation were systematically lower, usually between 15 and 20%. One should be aware of this, especially when reporting doses for structures such as the eyelid, eye lens, etc. A sufficient volume of a proper build-up material fixed to the patient's eye could probably reduce calculation errors. The application of tissue-equivalent build-up material on a treated eye was tested in this study to reduce inaccuracy in absolute dose

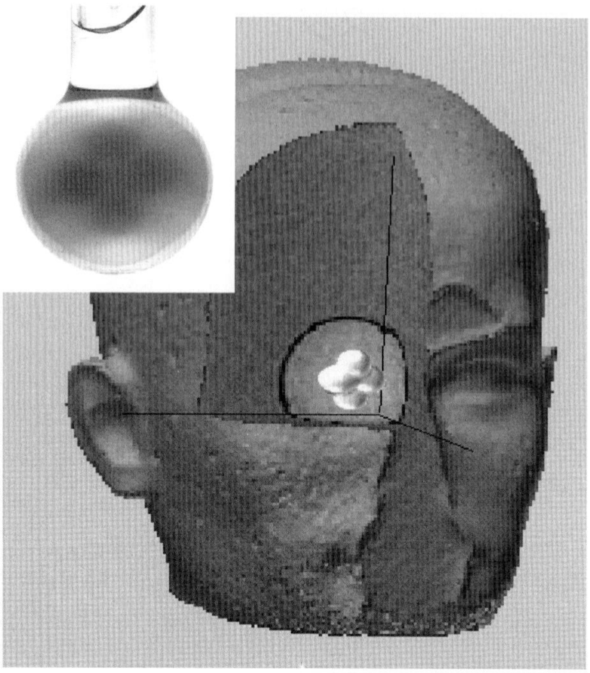

Fig. 4. Polymerization occurring in polymer gel together with the 3-D treatment plan used for the treatment of advanced glaucoma (four isocenters using an 8-mm collimator).

calculations. A gel used for ultrasound was poured into a special vessel and then fixed to the patient's eye and used as build-up material. Preliminary measurements taken using the above-mentioned head phantom demonstrated that calculation errors should probably not exceed 10% even in surface structures when build-up material is used. However, more measurements and analyses are needed to prove this hypothesis.

Relative dose distributions measured by polymer gel dosimeter were in close conformity with the Leksell GammaPlan-calculated data.

It was demonstrated that the LGK is sufficiently accurate to be used for ophthalmic radiosurgery.

Uveal Melanomas

Uveal melanoma represents the most common malignant primary tumor of the eye in adult patients. Several therapeutic options for this tumor are available: resection or enucleation, brachytherapy and stereotactic irradiation [1–6, 10–28]. It is typically resistant to standard fractionation radiotherapy and chemotherapy. Better results were noticed after application of a higher dose per fraction (hypofractionated scheme) and with immunotherapy. Wide variations in the grading of malignity can be observed, from relatively benign types with several years survival without dissemination, to other tumors with fast multi-organ dissemination, which lead to the patient's death within a few months.

We studied a group of 81 patients with uveal melanoma treated using the LGK over a period of 6 years [5]. The characteristics of this group of patients were as follows: a median age of 59 years (range 22–85 years), 45 males and 36 females, with 75 patients undergoing minimal follow-up 10 months after treatment. The LENT SOMA scoring system was used to measure radiation side effects [29]. The median target volume was 640 mm^3 and the median applied minimal dose was 31.4 Gy. All patients were examined by an ophthalmologist and MRI at regular intervals. The following ophthalmologic methods were employed for diagnostic investigation and patient follow-up at regular intervals after Gamma Knife surgery (GKS): ultrasonography, indocyanine and fluorescein angiography, optical coherence tomography, ultrabiomicroscopy (for tumors located anterior to the equator), visual function and biomicroscopy. Factors influencing patient survival and side effects after treatment were statistically analyzed.

In our group, 57 out of 81 patients were still alive with a median survival period of 15 months (6–74 months), 16 patients died (other organ dissemination) with a median survival period of 35 months (14–70 months).

Local tumor control in the 75 patients who underwent minimal follow-up after 10 months was achieved in 63 patients (84%; fig. 5), while progression was observed in 12 patients (16%), 10 of whom were enucleated. The most frequent side effect was secondary glaucoma, which was detected in 18 patients (25%). This side effect was observed to have a significantly higher incidence when the total volume of peripheral isodose was greater than 1 cm^3. There was also a significantly higher toxicity recorded in the optic nerve when the maximal dose to this structure was higher than 9 Gy, in the cornea when the maximal dose to this structure was higher than 15 Gy, and in the lens when the maximal dose was higher than 10 Gy. Statistically significant positive prognostic factors may identify the characteristics of patients with longer life expectancy (patients younger than 50 years old, lesions located posterior to the equator, a minimal applied dose 40 Gy and higher, and no dissemination to other organs).

All the eyes in this group of patients that required secondary enucleation had an initial tumor height exceeding 9 mm, and the secondary reason for their enucleation was the presence of ciliary body tumors. Zehetmayer et al. [6] reported that 13% of eyes enucleated as a result of this complication. A proton beam irradiation study found ciliary body involvement, a tumor height greater than 8 mm and the proximity of the tumor to the fovea to be the leading risk factors for enucleation [19].

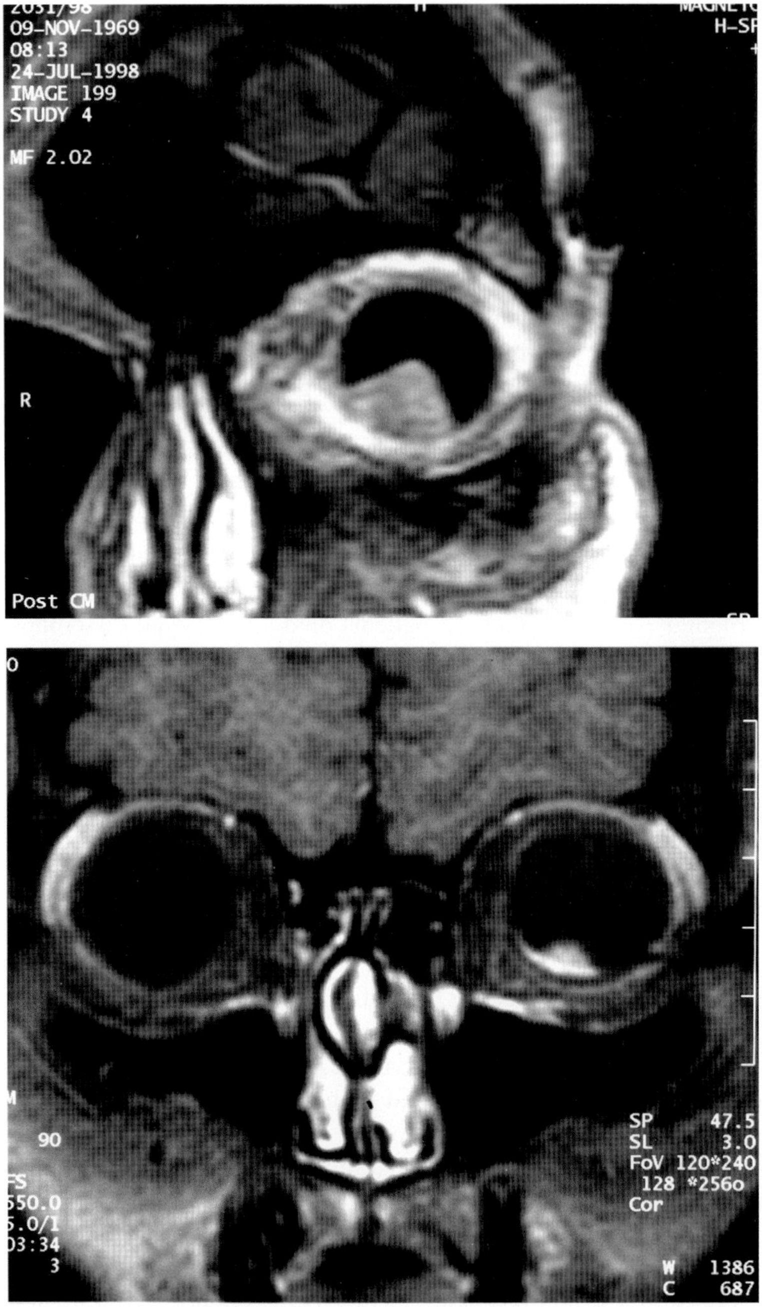

Fig. 5. A 29-year-old woman with uveal melanoma before and 18 months after Gamma Knife radiosurgery.

The occurrence of secondary glaucoma as a typically late side effect mainly depends on the time interval of the follow-up and on different radiation techniques. Because of this, the rate of enucleation ranges from 6% at a 2-year follow-up to 19% at 8 years after the treatment [11, 12, 14, 19, 28].

Radiosurgery represents a treatment modality for patients with uveal melanoma and fulfils the primary objective of protecting the majority of patients from enucleation. The choice of treatment modality depends in particular on the location of the tumor within the eye, the tumor volume and its dissemination into other organs.

Glaucoma

Glaucoma is a chronic, slowly progressive, usually bilateral neuropathy of the optic nerve. Untreated glaucoma eventually leads to complete loss of vision. About 10% of patients with glaucoma become uni- or bilaterally blind [30, 31]. We currently understand the pathophysiology of glaucoma to be a progressive loss of ganglion cells resulting in visual field damage related to the intraocular pressure (IOP) [32]. Although many clinicians now feel that there are several factors involved in the pathogenesis of glaucoma, the only rigorously proven treatment method is the lowering of IOP [33].

The conventional antiglaucomatous treatment – local and systemic pharmacotherapy, laser and cryotherapy and incisional surgery – sometimes fails and progressive optic nerve head neuropathy is manifested. We are then faced with a difficult situation of advanced and sometimes painful glaucoma with major defects in visual functions and, in the final stages of the disease, enucleation of the painful blind eye must be considered. Therefore, a new effective method of treatment has to be sought [30, 31, 34].

During treatment of patients with different tumoral and vascular ocular lesions using the LGK at our Center in the past years [2, 35], some of these lesions were located near the ciliary body, and we observed that the radiation exerted a positive influence on secondary glaucoma, which was sometimes present. The ciliary body, as the source of intraocular aqueous production, had been simultaneously irradiated.

As there was no previous experience of the radiosurgical treatment of glaucoma to refer to, we started to elaborate an effective and safe irradiation of the corpus ciliare as the source of intraocular aqueous humor [36]. The goal of the radiosurgical treatment is determined by the stage of the disease. When vision has been totally or partially lost, the main aim is to abolish the elevated IOP and to eliminate severe pain. In the early stages of the disease, when conventional therapy has failed and visual acuity is still preserved, the treatment has

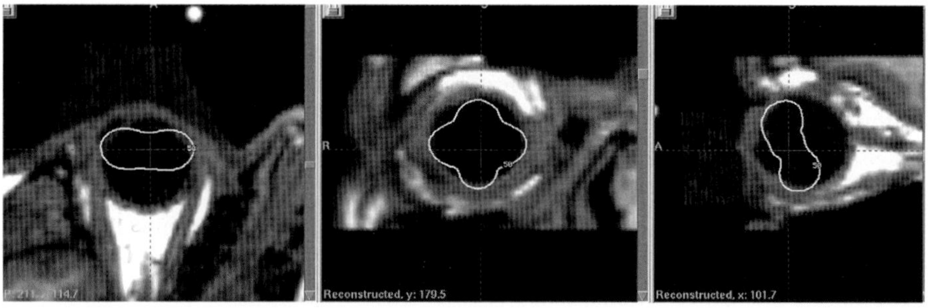

Fig. 6. A plan of irradiation of the ciliary body using four 8-mm collimators (50% isodose displayed); the eye bulb with aphakia.

the more difficult task of preventing any further progress of the pathogenic mechanisms.

The radiation pattern was elaborated in successive steps [36, 37] and finally four isocenters of an 8-mm collimator were displaced in a cruciform manner (fig. 4 and 6). A total of 90 eyes in 88 patients were irradiated in this way. All the patients had a long history of the disease, had exhausted all kinds of conventional therapy, had remained refractory to all kinds of treatment and had progressively suffered severe damage of their visual functions. We delivered 20 Gy at 50% isodose, but for patients with some preserved vision, the dose was lowered to 15 Gy at 50% isodose. The patients were followed ophthalmologically for a median period of 20 months (range 2–54 months) at regular 3-month intervals during the 1st year after the irradiation and then twice yearly to assess the irradiation influence on pain, IOP and neovascularization. Any eventual side effects were recorded.

In 89% of cases, severe pain in patients with secondary glaucoma was substantially ameliorated by the irradiation. In primary open angle glaucoma the pain was less frequent and of a low grade. In more than half of the patients it disappeared. The median latency was 6 weeks, ranging from 2 to 32 weeks. Similarly, the IOP was lowered in patients with secondary glaucoma from the median of 51.3 to 27 mm Hg after the irradiation. The same values for primary open angle glaucoma were 25.3 and 16.1 mm Hg, respectively, after a median latency of 12 weeks. Forty patients were suffering from neovascular glaucoma, and there was a marked reduction in neovascularization in 27 patients after a median latency of 18 weeks. Treatment complications were not significant – short-term postoperative lacrimation in 61% of those treated, postirradiation cataracts in 2 patients and noninfectious keratitis in another 2 patients. During the follow-up period, pharmacotherapy could be reduced in all patients and was interrupted in about one third of them. Meanwhile, no recurrence of the initial symptoms was observed and there was no worsening of visual acuity.

Gamma knife radiosurgery of the ciliary body leads to a significant alleviation of pain and a reduction in IOP in advanced glaucoma. It is effective in secondary glaucoma, especially in terms of neovascularization [36, 37]. The latency of the treatment effect is relatively short. Patients with primary open-angle glaucoma suffer less pain, their IOP is less elevated and their disease is mainly expressed by visual loss as a manifestation of the optic neuropathy. Even in the early stages of glaucoma, this can be detected by confocal laser scanning tomography and nerve fiber layer testing and analysis [38–42]. The treatment effect on optic neuropathy can be evaluated after a longer follow-up by registering visual function and performing other tests for glaucoma neuropathy. We assume that GKS can help achieve 'the target IOP' and thus prevent further progression of optic neuropathy.

A long follow-up is needed to evaluate whether progressive optic neuropathy will be stabilized by GKS. Special ophthalmologic examinations have to be performed in order to make this evaluation. A prospective 5-year clinical study to halt progressive optic neuropathy in the early stages of glaucoma is underway.

Age-Related Macular Degeneration

ARMD is the most common cause of blindness in older people in the western world. The most severe form of this degeneration is characterized by the development of the so-called choroidal neovascularization membrane (CNVM) – an exudative form of ARMD. Currently, there is no effective treatment for this serious illness. Laser coagulation, photodynamic therapy, transpupillary thermotherapy, and subretinal surgical techniques are successful in small numbers of strictly indicated cases. The effect of those methods – the destruction or reduction of the neovascular complex – is better in well-defined CNVMs. In severe cases of ARMD with 'malignant destroying CNVMs', these treatments are ineffective. These advanced forms of CNVMs are characterized by the fast growth of subfoveal neovascular tissue with strong exudation, covered with blood and lipid, which cause damage of the neurosensory retina overlying the CNVMs.

CNVMs, which are composed of endothelial cells and proliferate more rapidly than the endothelial cells of the retina, may be more sensitive than the retinal vasculature. Consequently, radiation therapy has been suggested as a treatment for subfoveal CNVMs [43–49]. Clinical experience with conventional fractionated irradiation for head and neck malignancies has demonstrated

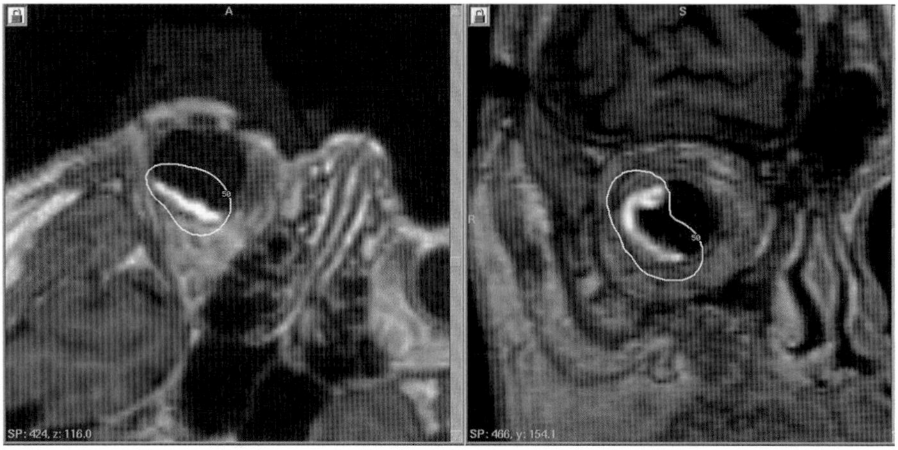

Fig. 7. An 80-year-old woman with ARMD, 15 Gy on 50% isodose.

that cumulative doses (multiple fractions) of up to 25 Gy cause no damage to the retina or optic nerve, and the susceptibility of retinal vasculature endothelial cells has been confirmed in other studies described by Archer et al. [50]. Many pilot studies for exudative ARMD show stabilization or regression of CNVM with different kinds of radiation therapy [51–53].

Initial results from patients treated with GKS for ARMD show that GKS is able to affect tissues beneath the retina (CNV in ARMD) without damaging the overlying retinal structures. Haas et al. [52] in their pilot study had investigated the effect of single-fraction (10 Gy at the 90% isodose) GKS in patients with classic subfoveal CNVM due to ARMD. Ten patients were followed up for a period of 12 months. Fluorescein angiography and indocyanine green chorioangiography demonstrated a regression of the neovascular complex in 1 patient and stabilization in 3 patients. Enlargement of the CNVM was found in 6 patients and was associated with a decrease in visual acuity in 4 patients. In our study, we treated 11 patients with occult forms of CNVM in ARMD with a dose of 15 Gy at a 50% isodose in a single fraction (fig. 7). Both ultrasonography and fluorescein angiography demonstrated a regression of the neovascular complex in 2 patients and stabilization in 8 patients. An enlargement of the CNVM was found in 1 patient. As in the study of Haas et al. [52], we did not observe a decrease in vision immediately after treatment, and no severe radiation-related side effects (retinopathy, optic neuropathy, cataract progression, or keratitis) have been detected. The fact that our results are relatively better is probably due to the more problematic indications in the study of Haas et al. [52] (classic

CNVM in ARMD) and their lower radiation dose (which is, on the other hand, understandable because of the level of visual acuity in their patients).

Our results show that radiosurgery could play a significant role in very advanced forms of CNVMs or large CNVMs, which are not treatable using other procedures. On this basis, we have constructed a new, prospective, non-randomized study, which is now underway.

Rare Indications for Ophthalmic Radiosurgery

A number of rare indications have been treated by Gamma Knife irradiation in our Center with more or less prominent therapeutic responses.

Four patients suffered from retinal or choroidal hemangiomas. One of them, with typical Von Hippel-Lindau disease, was treated radiosurgically and then followed up for 7 years. The irradiated lesion in one eye regressed in volume by 50% and stabilized even when several lesions in other organs progressed and had to be surgically treated. The other patient with Sturge-Weber syndrome similarly showed a 40% regression at follow-up after 6 years [35]. The remaining 2 patients had one eye radiosurgically irradiated for a solitary hemangioma, which markedly regressed 1–2 years after irradiation. Radiosurgery also prevented secondary glaucoma with possible refractory symptoms.

We also treated 2 patients with carcinomatous juxtabulbar infiltration. The primary lesion in 1 patient was bronchial carcinoma with multiple organ dissemination. The progression of the intraorbital metastasis was stopped by irradiation, but the patient died after several months due to the generalization of the disease. The other patient was operated on for a basalioma of the nasal orbital angle with subsequent invasion to the medial orbital wall. The lesion disappeared totally after irradiation and only partial stenosis of lacrimal pathways resulted.

Retinoblastoma represents the most common primary malignant tumor of the eye in small children (in the first 2 years of life). Over a period of 3 years, 4 patients were admitted for stereotactic irradiation using the Gamma Knife and they had vitreous seeding of malignant cells. All patients were pretreated according to the SIOP (Society International of Pediatric Oncology) protocol and relapsed after standard treatment. The only remaining possibility was enucleation. The whole vitreous body was irradiated using the Gamma Knife in a single session, with a collimator diameter of 14 mm. To avoid growth retardation of the irradiated eye and bony structures, the minimal dose did not exceed 15 Gy in all these patients. For this reason, and also bearing in mind the risk of complications of previous treatment, the applied doses were relatively low. Local progression was observed in 3 out of 4 patients and 3 patients were enucleated a median of 2 months after radiosurgery.

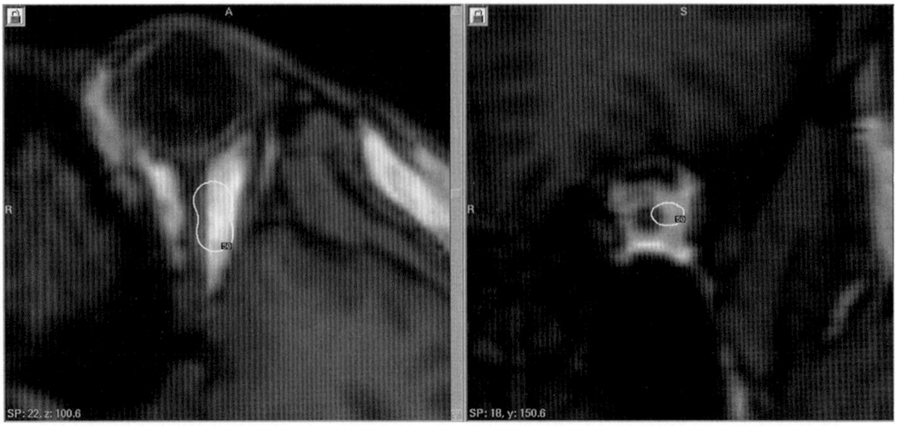

Fig. 8. A 32-year-old woman with a blind painful eye; irradiation of ganglion ciliare (two isocenters using a 4-mm collimator, 37.5 Gy on 50% isodose).

One patient with a blind eye was partially operated for a giant cell tumor of the orbital apex, and we irradiated the residual part of the tumor. Its volume had decreased by 60% at the 1-year follow-up.

We further treated a young woman with recurrent infections of the anterior orbital segment, followed by an orbital pseudotumor. Because of therapeutic resistance, the edematous suprabulbar and lateral orbital tissue was irradiated. A volume of 2.3 cm^3 was covered by 12 Gy to the periphery. The protrusion of the eye regressed.

Finally, a 32-year-old woman was suffering from severe vegetative orbital pain after a longer history of penetrating bulbar injury, 3 operations for retinal ablation and a cyclocryocoagulation for secondary glaucoma (fig. 8). The affected eye was blind. The intraocular hypertension normalized but the pharmacoresistant pain accompanied by the vegetative symptoms persisted. We irradiated the ciliary ganglion in the affected orbit by the Gamma Knife and the pain disappeared within a week. Two and a half years after treatment, still pain free, the patient could reassume her job abroad and after several years of continual suffering she fully appreciates the difference Gamma Knife radiosurgery has made to her life.

Conclusion

Ophthalmologic indications currently make up as much as 10% of all our annual Gamma Knife treatments. The results for uveal melanomas are recognized and the value of the LGK in the treatment of glaucoma and ARMD seems promising after initial studies. The number of treated patients can provide the inspiration for further technical innovations to make radiosurgical treatment of the eye easier and more comfortable for the patient.

Acknowledgements

We thank our colleagues from Department of Ophthalmology, 1st Medical Faculty, Charles University and Central Military Hospital, Prague (J. Pašta, MD, PhD; J. Pilbauer, MD; J. Vladyková, MD, DSc; J. Ernest, MD, PhD; P. Němec, MD; L. Nováček, MD; Y. Hejdkuová, MD; L. Rajmont, MD), as well as colleagues from our own Department (G. Šimonová, M.D, PhD, and J. Novotný, Jr, PhD) for their care for our patients and their assistance in the preparation of the manuscript.

References

1 Marchini G, Gerosa M, Piovan E, et al: Gamma Knife stereotactic radiosurgery for uveal melanoma: clinical results after 2 years. Stereotact Funct Neurosurg 1996;66(suppl 1):208–213.

2 Pochop P, Pilbauer J, Křepelková J, Vladyka V, Liščák R, Šimonová G: Two years of experience with therapy of uveal melanoma by using the Leksell gamma knife (in Czech). Cs Oftal 1998;54: 232–235.

3 Rand RW, Khonsary A, Brown WJ, et al: Leksell stereotactic radiosurgery in the treatment of eye melanoma. Neurol Res 1987;9:142–146.

4 Rennie I, Forster D, Kemeny A, Walton L, Kunkler I: The use of single fraction Leksell stereotactic radiosurgery in the treatment of uveal melanoma. Acta Ophthalmol Scand 1996;74:558–562.

5 Šimonová G, Novotný J. Jr, Liščák R, Pilbauer J: Leksell gamma knife treatment of uveal melanoma. J Neurosurg 2002;97(suppl 5):635–639.

6 Zehetmayer M, Kitz K, Menapace R, et al: Local tumor control and morbidity after one to three fractions stereotactic external beam irradiation for uveal melanoma. Radiother Oncol 2000;55: 135–144.

7 Novotný Jr J, Novotný J, Vymazal J, Liščák R, Vladyka V: Assessment of the accuracy of stereotactic target localization using magnetic resonance imaging: a phantom study. J Radiosurg 1998;1: 99–111.

8 Novotný Jr J, Dvořák P, Spěváček V, et al: Quality control of the stereotactic radiosurgery procedure with the polymer-gel dosimetry. Radiother Oncol 2002;63:223–230.

9 Novotný Jr J, Spěváček V, Hrbáček J, et al: Measurement of relative dose distributions in stereotactic radiosurgery by the polymer-gel dosimeter; in Kondziolka D (ed): Radiosurgery. Basel, Karger, 2004, vol 5, pp 225–235.

10 Brady LW, Markoe AM, Amendola BE, et al: The treatment of primary intraocular malignancy. Int J Radiat Oncol Biol Phys 1988;15:1355–1361.

11 Castro JR, Char D, Opetti P, et al: 15 years experience with helium ion radiotherapy for uveal melanoma. Int J Radiat Oncol Biol Phys 1997;39:989–996.

12 Char DH, Quivey JM, Castro JR, et al: Helium ion versus iodine-125 brachytherapy in the management of uveal melanoma. Arch Ophthalmol 1990;108:209–214.

13 Char DH, Kroll S, Quivey J, et al: Long term visual outcome of radiated uveal melanomas in eyes eligible for randomisation to enucleation versus brachytherapy. Br J Ophthalmol 1996;80:117–124.

14 Char DH, Castro JR, Kroll SM, et al: Five-year follow-up of helium ion therapy for uveal melanoma. Arch Ophthalmol 1990;108:209–214.

15 Char DH, Kroll SM, Castro J: Ten-year follow-up of helium ion therapy for uveal melanoma. Am J Ophtalmol 1998;125:81–89.
16 Courdi A, Caujolle JP, Grange JD, et al: Results of proton therapy of uveal melanoma treated in Nice. Int J Radiat Oncol Biol Phys 1999;45:5–11.
17 Damato BE, Paul J, Foulds WS: Risk factors for residual and recurrent uveal melanoma after trans-scleral local resection. Br J Ophthalmol 1996;80:102–108.
18 Dieckmann K, Bogner J, Georg D, Zehetmayer M, Kren G, Potter R: A linac-based stereotactic irradiation technique of uveal melanoma. Radiother Oncol 2001;61:49–56.
19 Egan KM, Gragoudas ES, Seddon JM, et al: The risk of enucleation after proton beam irradiation for uveal melanoma. Ophthalmology 1989;96:1377–1383.
20 Gragoudas ES, Egan KM, Walsh SM, et al: Intraocular recurrence of uveal melanoma after proton beam irradiation. Ophthalmology 1992;99:760–766.
21 Gradoudas ES, Seddon JM, Egan K, et al: Long-term results of proton beam irradiated uveal melanomas. Arch Ophthalmol 1987;94:349–353.
22 Gragoudas ES, Lane AM, Regan S, et al: A randomized controlled trial of varying radiation doses in the treatment of chorioidal melanoma. Arch Ophthalmol 2000;118:773–778.
23 Petrovich Z, Luxton G, Langohlz B, et al: Episcleral plaque radiotherapy in the treatment of uveal melanomas. Int J Radiat Oncol Biol Phys 1992;24:247–251.
24 Saunders WM, Char DH, Quivey JM, et al: Precision, high dose radiotherapy: Helium ion treatment of uveal melanoma. Int J Radiat Oncol Biol Phys 1985;11:227–233.
25 Seregard S, aft Trampe E, Lax I, Kock E, Lundell G: Results following episcleral ruthenium plaque radiotherapy for posterior uveal melanoma. Acta Ophtlamol Scand 1997;75:11–16.
26 Shields CL, Shields JA, Karlsson U, et al: Enucleation after plaque radiotherapy for posterior uveal melanoma. Ophthalmology 1990;97:1665–1670.
27 Tokuuye K, Aknine Z, Sumi M, et al: Fractionated stereotactic radiotherapy for chorioideal melanoma. Radiother Oncol 1997;43:87–91.
28 Wilson MW, Hungerford JL: Comparison of episcleral plaque and proton beam radiation therapy for the treatment of chorioidal melanoma. Ophthalmology 1999;106:1579–1587.
29 LENT SOMA Tables. Radiother Oncol 1995;35:25–26.
30 Alfonso A: Relationship of structural and functional measurements; in Weinreb RN, Kitazawa Y, Kriegelstein GK (eds): Glaucoma in the 21st Century. London, Mosby International Ltd., 2000, pp 57–65.
31 Fuchs HJ, Nissen KR, Goldschmidt E: Glaucoma blindness in Denmark. Acta Ophtalmol 1992;70: 73–78.
32 Harwerth RS, Carter-Dawson L, Shen F, Smith EL, Crawford ML: Ganglion cell losses underlying visual field defects from experimental glaucoma. Invest Ophtalmol Vis Sci 1999;40: 2242–2250.
33 Langham ME, Farrel R, Krakau T, Silver D: Ocular pulsatile blood flow, hypotensive drugs, and differential light sensitivity in glaucoma; in Krieglstein GK (ed): Glaucoma Update IV. Berlin, Springer-Verlag, 1991, pp 162–172.
34 Goldberg I: How common is glaucoma worldwide? in Weinreb RN, Kitazawa Y, Kriegelstein GK (eds): Glaucoma in the 21st Century. London, Mosby International Ltd., 2000, pp 3–8.
35 Pilbauer J, Hejduková I, Pašta J,Vladyka V, Liščák R, Šimonová G: Our experience with treatment of some ocular vascular diseases by using the Leksell Gamma Knife (in Czech). Cs Oftal 1998;54: 235–241.
36 Pilbauer J, Hejduková I, Němec P, Liščák R, Vladyka V: Treatment of advanced glaucomas using Leksell Gamma Knife – A pilot clinical study. J Radiosurg 2000;3:155–158.
37 Vladyka V, Liščák R, Šubrt O, et al: Initial experience with gamma knife radiosurgery for advanced glaucoma. J Neurosurg 2000;93:180–183.
38 Brigatti L, Caprioli J: Correlation of visual field with scanning confocal laser optic disc measurements in glaucoma. Arch Ophthalmol 1995;113:1191–1194.
39 Burk RO, Rohnrschneider K, Takamoto T, et al: Laser scanning tomography and stereophotogrammetry in three-dimensional optic disc analysis. Graefe's Arch Clin Exp Ophthalmol 1993;231: 193–198.

40 Cauchan BC, Blanchard JW, Hamilton DC: Technique for detecting serial topographic changes in the optic disc and peripapillary retina using scanning laser tomography. Invest Ophthalmol Vis Sci 2000;41:775–782.
41 Greenfield DS: Optic nerve and retinal nerve fiber layer analyzers in glaucoma. Curr Opin Ophthalmol 2002;13:68–76.
42 Mardin CY, Junemann AG: The diagnostic value of optic nerve imaging in early glaucoma. Curr Opin Ophthalmol 2001;12:100–104.
43 Bergink GJ, Deutman AF, van den Broek JF: Radiation therapy for subfoveal choroidal neovascular membranes in age-related macular degeneration. A pilot study. Graefes Arch Clin Exp Ophthalmol 1994;232:591–598.
44 Bergink GJ, Deutman AF, van den Broek JE, et al: Radiation therapy for age-related subfoveal choroidal neovascular membranes. A pilot study. Doc Ophthalmol 1995;90:67–74.
45 Berkow JW, Flower RW, Orth DH, Kelley JS: Fluorescein and Indocyanine Green Angiography, ed 2. San Francisco, American Academy of Ophthalmology, 1997, p 7.
46 Berson AM, Finger PT, Sherr DL: Radiotherapy for age-related macular degeneration: preliminary results of a potentially new treatment. Int J Radiat Oncol Biol Phys 1996;36:861–865.
47 Finger PT, Berson A, Sherr D, et al: Radiation therapy for subretinal neovascularisation. Ophthalmology 1996;103:878–889.
48 Finger PT, Berson A, Ng T: Ophthalmic plaque radiotherapy for age-related macular degeneration associated with subretinal neovascularization. Am J Ophthalmol 1999;127:170–177.
49 Weinberger AW, Wolf S, Kube T: Radiation therapy of occult choroidal neovascularisation (CNV) in age-related macular degeneration (AMD). Klin Monatsbl Augenheilkd 1999;214:96–99.
50 Archer DB, Amoaku WM, Gardiner TA: Radiation retinopathy-clinical, histopathological, ultrastructural and experimental correlations. Eye 1991;5:239–251.
51 Chakravarthy U, Houston RF, Archer DB: Treatment of age-related subfoveal neovascular membranes by teletherapy: a pilot study. Br J Ophthalmol 1993;77:265–273.
52 Haas A, Papaefthymiou G, Langmann G: Gamma knife treatment of subfoveal, classic neovascularization in age-related macular degeneration: a pilot study. J Neurosurg 2000;93(suppl 3): 172–176.
53 Spaide RF, Guyer DR, McCormick B, et al: External beam radiation therapy for choroidal neovascularization. Ophthalmology 1998;105:24–30.

Roman Liščák, MD, PhD
Na Homolce Hospital
Roentgenova 2
CZ–150 30 Prague 5 (Czech Republic)
Tel. +420 257 272 552, Fax +420 257 272 972, E-Mail roman.liscak@homolka.cz

Szeifert GT, Kondziolka D, Levivier M, Lunsford LD (eds): Radiosurgery and Pathological Fundamentals. Prog Neurol Surg. Basel, Karger, 2007, vol 20, pp 340–358

14. CyberKnife Radiosurgery for Spinal Neoplasms

Peter C. Gerszten, Steven A. Burton, Cihat Ozhasoglu

Departments of Neurological Surgery and Radiation Oncology, University of Pittsburgh Medical Center, Pittsburgh, Pa., USA

Abstract

The role of stereotactic radiosurgery for the treatment of intracranial lesions is well established. Its use for the treatment of spinal lesions has been limited by the availability of effective target immobilization and localization technologies. Conventional external beam radiotherapy lacks the precision to allow delivery of large doses of radiation near radiosensitive structures such as the spinal cord. The CyberKnife® (Accuray Inc., Sunnyvale, Calif., USA) is an image-guided frameless stereotactic radiosurgery system that allows for the radiosurgical treatment of spinal lesions. The system utilizes the coupling of an orthogonal pair of X-ray cameras to a dynamically manipulated robot-mounted lightweight linear accelerator which has 6 d.f. that guides the therapy beam to the intended target without the use of frame-based fixation. Real-time imaging tracking allows for patient movement tracking with 1 mm spatial accuracy. Cervical spine lesions are located and tracked relative to skull bony landmarks; lower spinal lesions are tracked relative to percutaneously placed gold fiducial bone markers. Spinal stereotactic radiosurgery using a frameless image-guided system is now both feasible and safe. The major potential benefits of radiosurgical ablation of spinal lesions are short treatment time in an outpatient setting with rapid recovery and good symptomatic response. This technique offers a successful therapeutic modality for the treatment of a variety of spinal lesions as a primary treatment or for lesions not amenable to open surgical techniques, in medically inoperable patients, lesions located in previously irradiated sites, or as an adjunct to surgery.

Radiotherapy for Spinal Lesions

Standard treatment options for spinal tumors include radiotherapy alone, radionuclide therapy, radiotherapy plus systemic chemotherapy, hormonal therapy, or surgical decompression and/or stabilization followed by radiotherapy [1]. If a spinal tumor causes compression of the spinal cord or other neural elements, surgical decompression is often necessary with or without spinal fixation based on the extent of spinal column destruction and instability of the spine. The role of radiation therapy in the treatment of tumors of the spine has been well established. The goals of local radiation therapy in the treatment of spinal tumors have been palliation of pain, prevention of pathologic fractures, and halting progression of or reversing neurological compromise.

A primary factor that limits radiation dose in this tumor control with conventional radiotherapy is the relatively low tolerance of the spinal cord to radiation. Conventional external beam radiotherapy lacks the precision to deliver large single-fraction doses of radiation to the spine near radiosensitive structures such as the spinal cord. It is the low tolerance of the spinal cord to radiation that often limits the treatment dose to a level that is far below the optimal therapeutic dose [2–4]. Precise confinement of the radiation dose to the treatment volume, as is the case for intracranial radiosurgery, should increase the likelihood of successful tumor control at the same time that the risk of spinal cord injury is minimized [5].

Spinal Radiosurgery

Lars Leksell introduced the term 'radiosurgery' in 1951 to refer to single-fraction, high-dose irradiation of a limited target volume of tissue [6]. Stereotactic radiosurgery was conceived to be more analogous to conventional surgery than to conventional radiotherapy [7]. Stereotactic radiosurgery offers a method for delivering a high dose of radiation in a single or limited number of fractions to a small volume encompassing the tumor while minimizing the dose to adjacent normal structures [8]. The use of multiple beams of radiation requires extremely precise control of position and movement of the linear accelerator. In the past, stereotactic radiosurgery was limited to intracranial disease because precise localization could be achieved only by neurosurgical frames fixed to the patient's skull. The frame acts as a fiducial reference system to provide accurate targeting and delivery of the radiation dose. As a corollary, treatment is typically limited to single-fraction treatments. Intracranial radiosurgery is practical because the lesions are fixed with respect to the cranium, which can be immobilized rigidly in a stereotactic frame. Spinal lesions also have a fixed relationship to the spine. However, stereotactic radiosurgery techniques developed for spinal lesions using standard linear accelerators require the placement of an invasive rigid external frame system directly to the spine and therefore have not been adopted for general use [9].

Since Hamilton et al. [9] first described the possibility of linear-accelerator-based spinal stereotactic radiosurgery in 1995, multiple centers have attempted to pursue large-fraction conformal radiation delivery to spinal lesions using a variety of technologies [10–16]. Treatment of spinal lesions by stereotactic conformal radiotherapy and intensity-modulated radiotherapy (IMRT) have shown promising clinical results [15]. Others have demonstrated the effectiveness of protons for spinal and paraspinal tumors [17]. Recent studies using hypofractionated or single-dose treatments for spinal metastases reported results that were comparable to conventional fractionation [12–14, 18]. With advances in conformal treatment techniques using multileaf collimators such as IMRT, Chang et al. [11–16] found that intensity-modulated, near-simultaneous, CT image-guided stereotactic radiotherapy is a feasible and highly precise technique for the noninvasive treatment of spinal metastases. Bilsky et al. [11–16] found successful tumor control in 13 of 15 patients with spinal metastases using an IMRT technique. Milker-Zabel et al. [11–16] achieved tumor control in 95% of patients. Nevertheless, conformal radiotherapy and intensity-modulated radiation therapy (IMRT) are limited by problems with target immobilization as well as localization. This limitation of IMRT precludes large single-fraction treatment to spinal lesions.

The image-guided frameless stereotactic radiosurgery delivery system known as the CyberKnife® Stereotactic Radiosurgery System (Accuray Inc., Sunnyvale, Calif., USA) was developed by Dr. John Adler, Jr., and colleagues at Stanford University. It was approved in 2001 by the United States Food and Drug Administration for use throughout the body [19]. The CyberKnife was first developed for treatment of brain tumors at Stanford University. Since 1994, the device has been used at a number of sites around the world to treat a variety of benign and malignant intracranial lesions [20, 21]. As expected, treatment outcome has closely mirrored the results of conventional frame-based radiosurgery [3]. With the ability to treat lesions outside of the skull using fiducial tracking, a growing interest in the treatment of spinal lesions using the CyberKnife has emerged [3, 22–24]. The CyberKnife technology is now being adopted worldwide as a feasible method to perform spinal radiosurgery. Our work with the CyberKnife at the University of Pittsburgh has demonstrated both the feasibility as well as the clinical efficacy of spinal radiosurgery for a variety of both benign and malignant lesions [5, 22, 24, 25].

The CyberKnife System

The CyberKnife is a frameless image-guided stereotactic radiosurgical system that uses X-ray radiographic imaging to locate and track the treatment site while controlling the alignment of radiation beams via a robot-mounted linear accelerator [19]. The CyberKnife system consists of a lightweight linear accelerator (weight, 120 kg) mounted on a robotic arm (fig. 1). Real-time imaging tracking

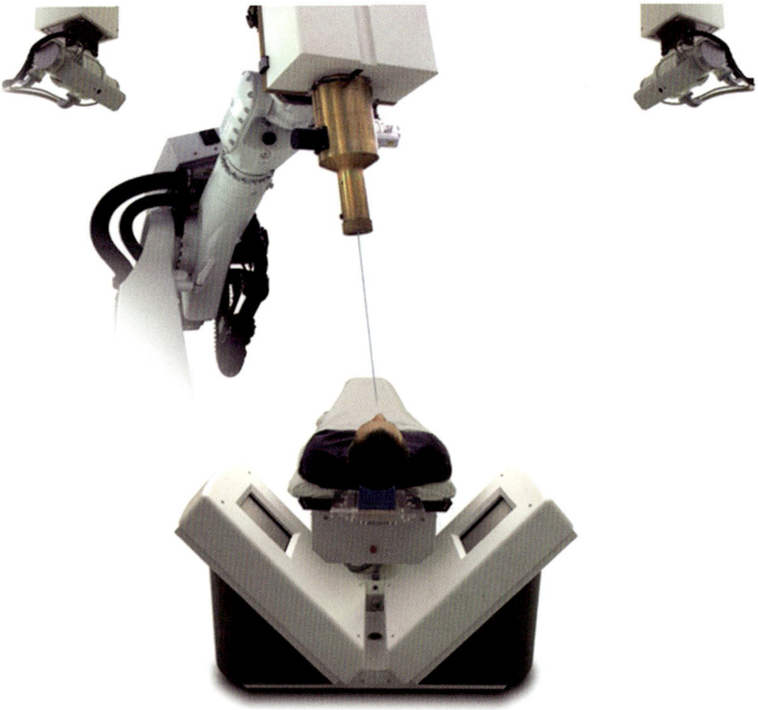

Fig. 1. The CyberKnife radiosurgical system. The X-ray tubes in the ceiling fire simultaneously to the amorphous silicone projectors mounted orthogonally under the table. The couch can be moved in 0.1-mm increments with 5 d.f. to position the fiducials in front of the cameras.

allows for patient movement tracking with 1 mm spatial accuracy [3, 21, 26]. Dosimetry compares favorably with other intracranial radiosurgery devices [27].

The CyberKnife was developed as a noninvasive means to precisely align treatment beams with targets. It differs from conventional frame-based radiosurgery in three fundamental ways [3]. First, it references the position of the treatment target to internal radiographic features such as the skull or implanted fiducials rather than a frame. Second, it uses real-time X-ray imaging to establish the position of the lesion during treatment and then dynamically brings the radiation beam into alignment with the observed position of the treatment target. Third, it aims each beam independently, without a fixed isocenter.

Changes in patient position during the treatment are compensated for by adaptive beam pointing rather than controlled through rigid immobilization. This allows the patient to be positioned comfortably in the treatment room without precise reproduction of the position in the treatment planning study. Because of the spatial precision with which the CyberKnife can administer

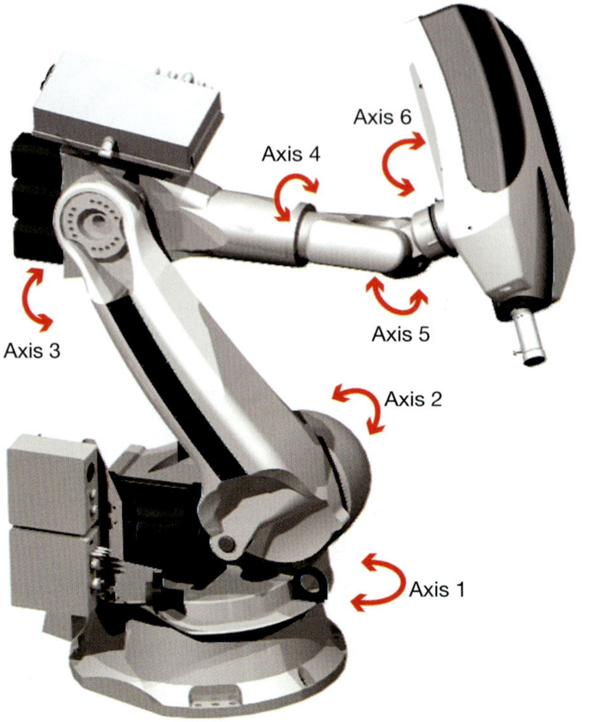

Fig. 2. The CyberKnife consists of a linear accelerator mounted on a six-axis robotic manipulator that permits a wide range of beam orientations.

radiation, it is theoretically feasible to administer a tumorcidal radiation dose in a single outpatient treatment. By minimizing the irradiation of surrounding healthy tissue, it should also be possible to decrease the rate of complications. The design of the CyberKnife makes it intrinsically capable of treating sites anywhere in the body in either a single-fraction or multifraction manner [28].

The CyberKnife consists of a computer controlled, compact 6-MV linear accelerator, that is smaller and lighter in weight than linear accelerators used in conventional radiotherapy [23, 29, 30]. The smaller size allows it to be mounted on a computer-controlled six-axis robotic manipulator that permits a much wider range of beam orientations than can be achieved with conventional radiotherapy devices (fig. 2). The CyberKnife system utilizes image-guided frameless robotic radiosurgery. Two ceiling-mounted diagnostic X-ray cameras are positioned orthogonally (90° offset) to acquire real-time images of the patient's internal anatomy during treatment. The images are gathered using two amorphous silicon X-ray screens capable of generating high-resolution digital

Table 1. Candidate lesions for CyberKnife spinal radiosurgery

Well-circumscribed lesions
Minimal spinal cord compromise
Radioresistant lesions that would benefit from a radiosurgical boost
Residual tumor after surgery
Previously irradiated lesions
Recurrent surgical lesions
Lesions requiring difficult surgical approaches
Relatively short life expectancy as an exclusion criteria for open surgical intervention
Significant medical comorbidities precluding open surgical intervention
No overt spinal instability

images [31]. The images are processed automatically to identify radiographic features and then registered to the treatment planning study to measure the position of the treatment site. The measured position is communicated through a real-time control loop to a robotic manipulator that aims the linear accelerator.

The system can adapt to changes in patient position during treatment by acquiring targeting images repeatedly and then adjusting the direction of the treatment beam. If the patient moves during treatment, the change is detected during the next imaging cycle and the beam is adjusted and realigned with the target [28]. The target to be treated is identified prior to treatment on planning images. Between 100 and 200 beams are commonly used to irradiate the target in a stereotactic fashion. The treatment beam can be maneuvered and pointed nearly anywhere in space. Treatment beams are also not confined to isocentric geometry, so they can be arranged in complex overlapping patterns that conform irregularly shaped tumor volumes [3]. An analysis of the accuracy of the CyberKnife radiosurgery system found that the machine has a clinically relevant accuracy of 1.1 ± 0.3 mm using a 1.25-mm CT slice thickness. Hence, the CyberKnife precision is comparable to published localization errors of other current frame-based radiosurgical systems [31].

Indications for Spinal Radiosurgery

The indications for spine radiosurgery using the CyberKnife are currently evolving and will continue to evolve as clinical experience increases. This is similar to the evolution of indications for intracranial radiosurgery which occurred in the past. Table 1 summarizes the candidate lesions for CyberKnife spinal radiosurgery. Similar to intracranial radiosurgery, candidate lesions may be of either benign or malignant histology. Spinal vascular malformations are also amenable to spinal radiosurgery [3].

This new technique is an important treatment modality whose clinical role has not yet been fully defined. The most frequent indication for the treatment of spinal tumors is pain, and spinal radiosurgery is most often used to treat tumor pain. Radiation is well known to be effective as a treatment for pain associated with spinal malignancies. Our clinical experience has found a 92% improvement in pain after CyberKnife therapy. We have found CyberKnife spinal radiosurgery to be highly effective at decreasing pain in this difficult patient population. Spinal radiosurgery was also found to successfully alleviate radicular pain caused by tumor compression of adjacent nerve roots.

Another indication for spinal radiosurgery might be to halt tumor progression that could lead to spinal instability or neural compromise. The ideal lesion should be well circumscribed such that the lesion can be easily outlined (contoured) for treatment planning. Our initial experience has found that many of our cases have already received irradiation with significant spinal cord doses or have lesions that recurred after open surgical removal. Currently, it appears that CyberKnife radiosurgery is often being used as a 'salvage' technique for those cases in which further conventional irradiation or surgery are not appropriate.

Other candidate lesions are those that would require difficult surgical approaches for adequate resection. Spinal radiosurgery can delivery radiation to anywhere along the spine. Candidate patients may have significant medical comorbidities precluding open surgical intervention or a relatively short life-expectancy that would deem them inappropriate for open surgical intervention. We have treated several radioresistant tumors (e.g. renal cell carcinoma, melanoma, sarcoma) that have completed external beam irradiation with or without IMRT, and we have used CyberKnife radiosurgery for a boost treatment. Other lesions have been treated with CyberKnife radiosurgery as their sole radiation treatment. The benefits for this treatment option include a single treatment with minimal radiation dose to adjacent normal tissue. In addition, a much larger radiobiologic dose can often be delivered compared to external beam irradiation. With greater clinical experience, upfront radiosurgery perhaps will become more commonly used in certain cases such as patients with a single symptomatic spine tumor of a radioresistant histology.

If a tumor is only partially resected during an open surgery, fiducials can be left in place to allow for radiosurgery treatment to the residual tumor at a later date. Given the steep falloff gradient of the CyberKnife target dose, such treatments can be given early in the postoperative period as opposed to the usual significant delay before standard external beam irradiation is permitted by the surgeon. With the ability to effectively perform spinal radiosurgery, the current surgical approach to these lesions might change. Open surgery for

Table 2. Overview of CyberKnife spinal radiosurgery treatment

Fiducials placed (lower spinal lesions only) or facemask molded (cervical lesions)
CT image-guided simulation performed using 1.25-mm slices
Treatment plan designed
Patient returns for outpatient treatment
Treatments may be fractionated if necessary
Patient has the opportunity to stop and rest at any point during the treatment
No recovery time

spinal metastases will likely evolve in a similar manner in which malignant intracranial lesions are debulked in such a way as to avoid neurological deficits and minimize surgical morbidity. The spinal tumors can be removed away from neural structures allowing for immediate decompression, the spine can be instrumented if necessary, and the residual tumor can be safely treated at a later date with radiosurgery, thus further decreasing surgical morbidity. We have found that anterior corpectomy procedures in certain cases can be successfully avoided by posterior decompression and instrumentation alone followed by radiosurgery to the remaining anterior lesion.

There are several relative contraindications for CyberKnife spinal radiosurgery. These include: (1) evidence of overt spinal instability (2) neurologic deficit resulting from bony compression of neural structures, or (3) previous radiation treatment to spinal cord tolerance dose. With time and further clinical experience, these contraindications will be better understood and defined.

Overview of the CyberKnife Treatment

The CyberKnife spinal radiosurgery treatment consists of three distinct components: (1) CT image acquisition based upon skull bony landmarks or implanted bone fiducials, (2) treatment planning, and (3) the treatment itself (table 2). Intracranial and cervical lesions are tracked relative to skull bony landmarks. All other lesions are tracked relative to fiducials placed adjacent to the lesion. Because these implanted fiducials have a fixed relationship with the bone in which they are implanted, any movement in the tumor in or adjacent to the vertebrae would be detected as movement in the fiducials, and this movement is detected and compensated for by the CyberKnife.

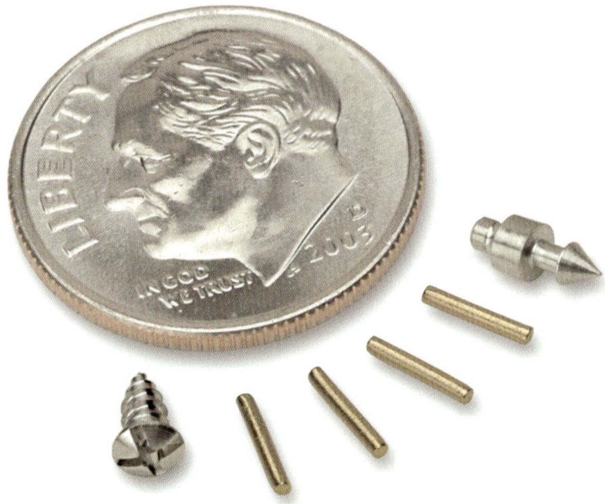

Fig. 3. Gold seed fiducials, stainless steel screws, or tacks may be used for image tracking.

Face Mask and Fiducial Placement

All patients with cervical lesions are first fitted with a noninvasive molded Aquaplast facemask (WRF/Aquaplast Corp., Wyckoff, N.J., USA) that stabilizes the head and neck on a radiographically transparent headrest [24]. The patient then proceeds directly with imaging. CT images are acquired using 1.25-mm-thick slices from the top of the skull to the bottom of the cervical spine. Images may be acquired using the addition of intravenous contrast enhancement. However, contrast is often not necessary for lesions that are completely within the bony elements. In fact, bony windowing is often more helpful for lesion localization and treatment planning than soft tissue windowing for many spinal lesions. For patients with allergies to intravenous contrast or renal function that precludes contrast, nonenhanced CT imaging is performed with little difficulty in determining precise lesion anatomy.

The CyberKnife is able to detect and track either straight gold fiducials (Alpha-Omega Services Inc., Bellflower, Calif., USA) or stainless steel screws (Accuray) (fig. 3). These fiducials are placed using fluoroscopic guidance using a percutaneous technique (fig. 4). The fiducial placement procedure is performed in the operating room in an outpatient setting. The gold fiducial markers are placed into the pedicles immediately adjacent to the lesion to be treated using a standard Jamshidi Bone Marrow Biopsy Needle (Allegiance Healthcare Corporation, McGraw Park, Ill., USA). The stainless steel screws are screwed directly into the posterior bony elements via a specially designed

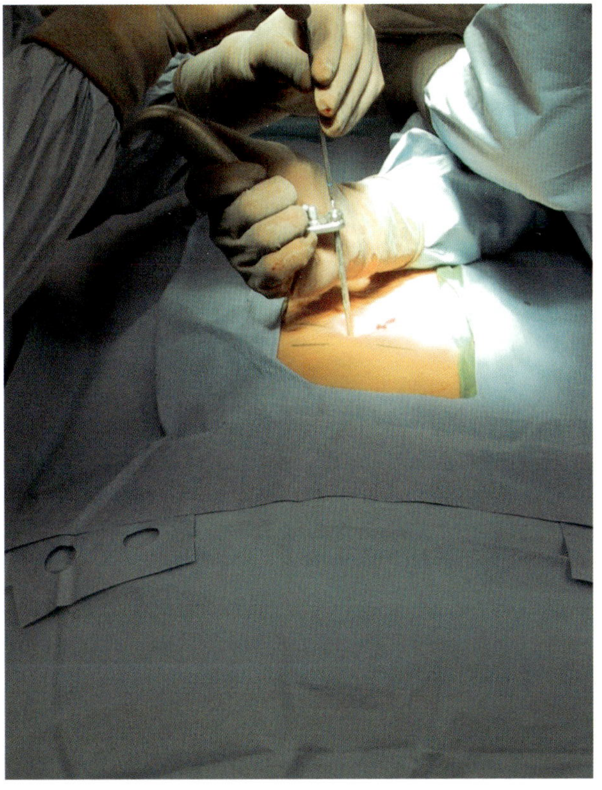

Fig. 4. Fiducials are placed percutaneously around the lesion in the bony structures using fluoroscopic guidance.

cannula. If fiducials are placed in conjunction with an open surgical procedure, the stainless steal screws are easily screwed into any adjacent exposed bone.

Four to five fiducial markers are usually placed, two in the vertebrae above, two in the vertebrae below, and one or two in the vertebrae at the level of the lesion. The reason for this number is that four fiducials are usually tracked during treatment to allow for maximum accuracy. Tracking more than four fiducials adds little to target accuracy. Three fiducials are required to define a full spatial transformation in all six degrees of target translation and rotation. An extra fiducial is placed to allow for a margin of error in case one fiducial cannot be properly imaged or perhaps migrates after placement. Fiducial migration has rarely occurred in our experience.

The fiducials may be placed literally anywhere near or around the target. The principle is that their position must be fixed relative to the target location.

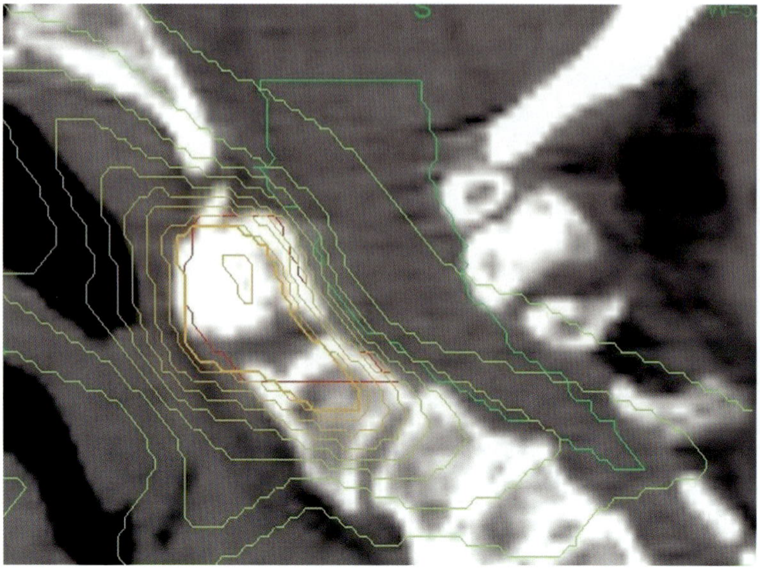

Fig. 5. Sagittal projection of the treatment plan of a 79-year-old man with a C_2 squamous cell carcinoma metastasis. The treatment plan was designed to treat the tumor with a prescribed dose of 1,600 cGy that was calculated to the 80% isodose line. The maximum tumor dose was 2,000 cGy, and the volume was 6.8 cm^3. The spinal cord received a maximum dose of 882 cGy.

For fiducials in the same vertebral body, it is preferential for them to be placed as closely as possible in the same coronal plane so that overlap in an orthogonal projection during X-ray imaging acquisition is minimized. For patients with lesions in nonadjacent vertebral bodies, fiducials are sometimes placed between the two lesions. For example, for two distinct lesions at T_{11} and L_3, fiducials may be placed at T_{12}, L_1, and L_2 without compromising target accuracy.

Treatment Planning

The patient returns as an outpatient for the treatment planning CT. The patient is placed in a supine position in a conformal alpha cradle during CT imaging as well as during treatment. CT images are acquired using 1.25-mm-thick slices to include the lesion of interest as well as all fiducials.

Each spinal radiosurgical treatment plan is devised jointly by a team composed of a neurosurgeon, a radiation oncologist, and a radiation physicist. In each case, the radiosurgical treatment plan is designed based on tumor geometry, proximity to the spinal cord, and location (fig. 5). The tumor dose is determined based upon the histology of the tumor, spinal cord tolerance, and previous radiation quantity to normal tissue, especially the spinal cord. The lesion is outlined based upon CT imaging or from an MR fusion capability. An 'inverse treatment planning' technique is utilized such that the tumor receives the maximum dose allowable with the restriction of the maximum spinal cord tolerance dose, as well as other critical structures such as small bowel and kidneys (figs. 6 and 7). In our experience, the mean tumor volume has been approximately 30 (range 0.16–298) cm^3. This is approximately ten times the average volume of intracranial lesions treated by radiosurgery.

For each case, the spinal cord and/or cauda equina is outlined as a critical structure. At the level of the cauda equina, the spinal canal is outlined. Therefore, at the level of the cauda equina, the critical volume is the entire spinal canal and not actual neural tissue. A limit of 800 cGy is set as the maximum spinal cord dose for treatment planning calculations. A limit of 200 cGy is set as the maximal dose to each of the kidneys. This especially becomes important in the treatment of lower thoracic and lumbar vertebrae, even more so if the patient has undergone a nephrectomy or received nephrotoxic chemotherapy.

Dose Prescriptions

There is no large experience to date with spinal radiosurgery or hypofractionated radiotherapy that has previously developed optimal doses for these treatment techniques. Other centers, using intensity-modulated, near-simultaneous, computed tomographic image-guided stereotactic radiotherapy techniques have used doses of 600–3,000 cGy in one to five fractions [8, 13, 14]. The dose to the tumor margin is based on tumor histology, location, and history of prior fractionated radiotherapy. Records regarding previous spinal cord irradiation are carefully considered. Many lesions have received prior external beam irradiation with maximum spinal cord doses. Published reports from the Stanford CyberKnife experience indicate that spinal lesions received total treatment doses of 1,100–2,500 cGy in one to five fractions [3].

At our institution, the tumor dose is prescribed to the 80% isodose line. Tumor dose is maintained at 1,200–2,000 cGy to the 80% isodose line contoured at the edge of the target volume (mean 1,700 cGy). The maximum intratumoral dose (measured at the center of the target) ranges from 1,500 to 2,500 cGy (mean 2,100 cGy). The higher doses were delivered to lesions further away from critical structures.

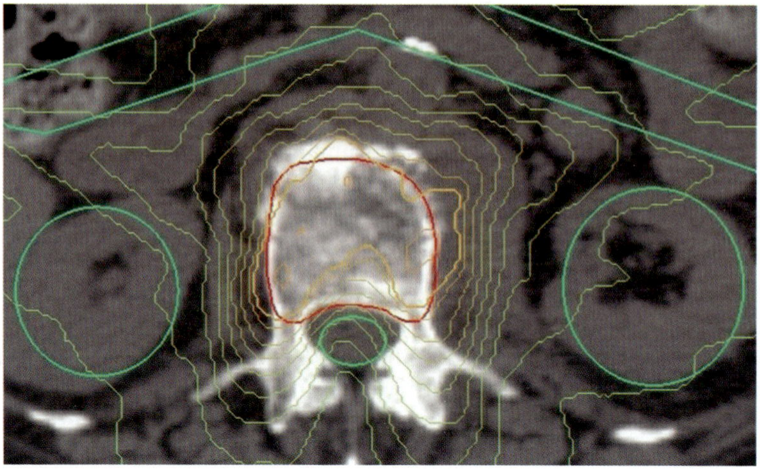

Fig. 6. Treatment plan of 63-year-old woman with an L_2 lung carcinoma metastasis. The treatment plan was designed to treat the tumor with a prescribed dose of 1,600 cGy that was calculated to the 80% isodose line. The maximum tumor dose was 2,000 cGy, and the tumor volume was 26.1 cm^3. The spinal cord received a maximum dose of 1,124 cGy and 0.64 cm^3 of the spinal canal received greater than 800 cGy. Notice the conformality of the treated tumor between the kidneys, the spinal canal, and the bowel.

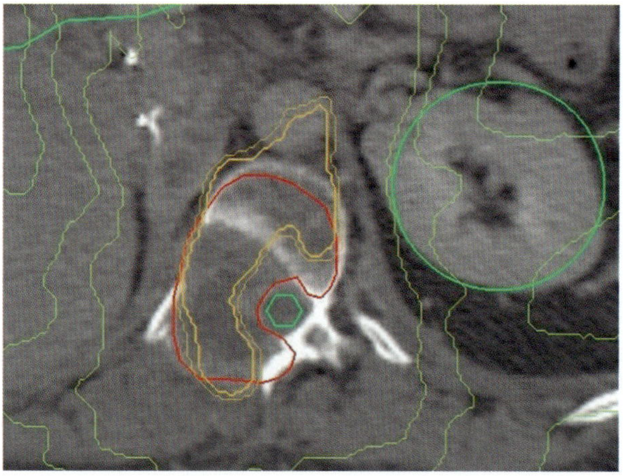

Fig. 7. Isodose lines of the treatment plan of a 41-year-old woman with a T_{12} renal cell metastasis. She had previously received external beam irradiation to the lesion with temporary improvement of symptoms. The treatment plan was designed to treat the tumor with a prescribed dose of 1,600 cGy that was calculated to the 80% isodose line. The maximum tumor dose was 2,000 cGy, and the tumor volume was 56.7 cm^3. The maximum dose to the remaining kidney was 200 cGy. Notice how the tumor encircles the spinal cord.

Unlike conventional radiation therapy that delivers a full dose to both the vertebral body and the spinal cord, the CyberKnife can deliver a single high-dose fraction of radiation to the target tissue while sparing most of the adjacent spinal cord. The treatment plan can create a high gradient dose falloff to the target tissue that should significantly reduce the possibility of radiation-induced myelopathy. This is the main advantage of using stereotactic radiosurgery for treatment of spinal tumors.

There is little experience regarding the tolerance of the human spinal cord to single-fraction doses, and the tolerance of the spinal cord to a single dose of radiation has not been defined well [8]. Spinal cord tolerance related to IMRT techniques has also not yet been addressed. One must still rely upon clinical data derived from external beam irradiation series in which the entire thickness of the spinal cord was irradiated. In a review evaluating 172 patients treated with fractionated radiotherapy to the cervical and thoracic spine at the University of California, San Francisco (total dose of 4,000–7,000 cGy fractionated over 2- to 3-week period), Wara et al. [32] reported 9 cases of radiation-induced myelopathy. Three out of 9 patients had mild cervical cord neurological deficits without any significant long-term symptoms. The length of the spinal cord that was exposed to radiation averaged from 4 to 22 cm. Hatlevoll et al. [33] reported a series of 387 patients with bronchial carcinoma treated with a split-course regimen using large single fractions. Seventeen patients developed radiation myelitis with average total dose of 3,800 cGy. Kim and Fayos [34] reported 7 patients with transverse myelopathy from a group of 109 patients treated with definitive radiotherapy for head and neck cancers to a total dose of 5,700–6,200 cGy with an average field size of 10 by 10 cm. Abbatucci et al. [35] reported 8/203 cases of radiation-induced myelopathy with a total radiation dose of 5,400–6,000 cGy to the cervical and thoracic spine. McCunniff and Liang [36] reported only 1 case or radiation myelopathy out of 652 patients who had received greater than 6,000 cGy using standard fractionation. Phillips and Buschke [37] reported 3 cases of transverse myelitis in 350 patients treated with tumors to the chest to a total radiation dose of 3,300–4,350 cGy. Based upon the above literature reviewed, the incidence of radiation-induced myelopathy using conventionally fractionated radiotherapy to the cervical and thoracic spine ranged from 0.2 to 5%.

CyberKnife spinal radiosurgery has been found to be safe at doses comparable to those used for intracranial radiosurgery without the occurrence of radiation-induced neural injury. There have been no cases at our institution of radiation-induced toxicity with a follow-up period long enough to have seen such events were they to occur [32–38]. This lack of adverse effect likely derives from a combination of the steep gradient dose falloff and high conformality of the CyberKnife.

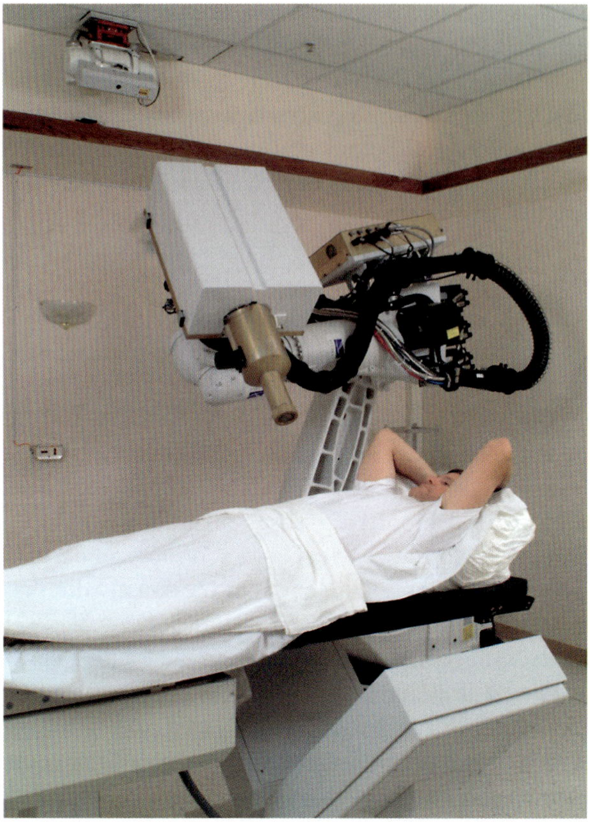

Fig. 8. Patient setup on the CyberKnife treatment couch. The patient is positioned supine with legs in an alpha cradle for comfort and to limit motion. The couch will move rostrally to place the fiducials between the amorphous silicon detectors.

Treatment Delivery

The third component of the CyberKnife treatment is the actual treatment delivery [24]. Treatments may be performed using either a single or multiple fractions in an outpatient setting. We prefer a single fraction technique. The patients are placed on the CyberKnife treatment couch in a supine position with the appropriate immobilization device (fig. 8). Some patients with thoracic or lumbar lesions localized with fiducials are actually more comfortable without the alpha cradle, and only pillows are used. During the treatment, real time digital X-ray images of the patient are obtained in order to track either skull bony landmarks or implanted fiducials (fig. 9). The location of the vertebral body

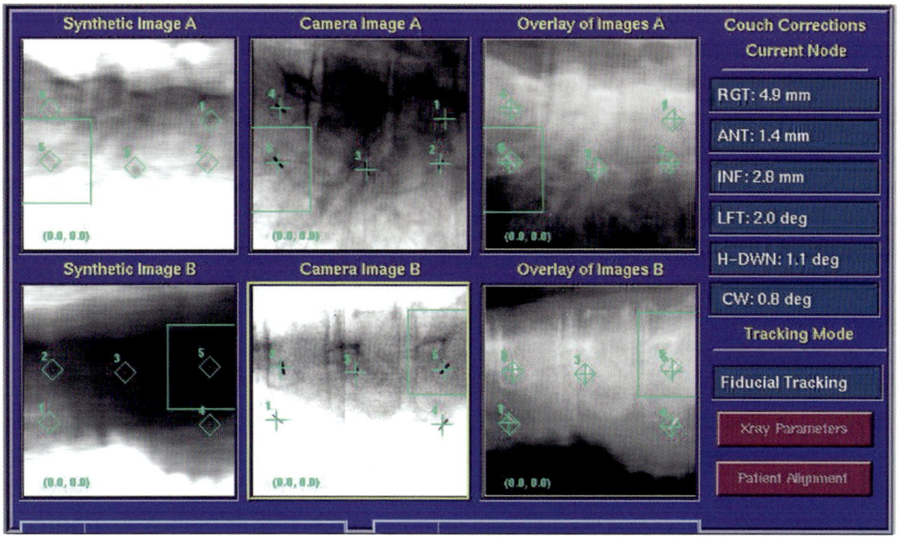

Fig. 9. All five fiducials are tracked for thoracic and lumbar lesions using real-time image guidance. Orthogonal digitally reconstructed radiographs are generated from the original CT. Throughout the treatment, the system correlates the original digitally reconstructed radiographs to the live images from the amorphous silicone detectors. The measured position as seen by both cameras is communicated through a real-time control loop to a robotic manipulator that redirects the beam to the precise intended target.

being treated is established from these images and is used to determine tumor location as previously described.

The CyberKnife delivery treatment follows a sequential format [28]. Once the patient is on the treatment couch, the imaging system acquires a pair of alignment radiographs and determines the initial location of the treatment site within the robotic coordinate system. This information allows initial positioning of the LINAC. The robotic arm then moves the LINAC through a sequence of preset points surrounding the patient. At each point, the LINAC stops and a new pair of images is acquired, from which the position of the target is redetermined. The position of the target is delivered to the robotic arm, which adapts beam pointing to compensate for small amounts of patient movement. The LINAC then delivers the preplanned dose of radiation for that direction. The complete process is repeated at each point, for a total of approximately 150 points, or nodes.

The patient is observed throughout the treatment by closed circuit television. No pulse oximetry or other monitoring is used during the treatment. The patient is asked to wave his/her hand or speak if he/she would like to temporarily halt the treatment. The duration of the treatment is approximately 1–2 h. Intravenous sedation is not required. Some patients are in significant pain and are uncomfortable in the supine position for prolonged periods of time. Treatments may be delivered under intravenous sedation or even a general anesthetic if necessary with the patient being monitored by the anesthetist from outside the treatment room. For the majority of cases, it is very easy to pause the treatment at any time for the patient to sit up. After a brief rest, the patient returns to the supine position on the treatment couch and the treatment resumes. Mild and transient nausea may be experienced by patients undergoing treatment to lesions of the lumbar spine. For these cases, patients are pretreated with antiemetics.

Conclusions

Tumors of the spine affect a large number of patients each year, resulting in significant pain, destruction of the spinal column causing mechanical instability, and neurological deficits. Standard therapeutic options include surgery and fractionated external beam radiotherapy. The first option can be associated with significant morbidity and limited local tumor control. Radiotherapy may provide less than optimal clinical response since the total dose is limited by the tolerance of the spinal cord. The CyberKnife treatment represents a logical extension of the current state-of-the-art radiation therapy. It has the potential to significantly improve local control of cancer of the spine, which could translate into better palliation. Another advantage to the patient is that irradiation can be completed in a single day rather than over several weeks, something that is not inconsequential for patients with a limited life expectancy. In addition, cancer patients may have difficulty with access to a radiation treatment facility for prolonged, daily fractionated therapy. Finally, the procedure is minimally invasive and can be performed in an outpatient setting.

Similar to intracranial radiosurgery, stereotactic radiosurgery now has a feasible and safe delivery system available for the treatment of spinal lesions. The major potential benefits of radiosurgical ablation of spinal lesions are relatively short treatment time in an outpatient setting combined with potentially better local control of the tumor with minimal risk of side effects. CyberKnife spinal radiosurgery offers a new and important alternative therapeutic modality for the treatment of spinal metastases in medically inoperable patients, previously irradiated sites, and for lesions not amenable to open surgical techniques or as an adjunct to surgery. Spinal radiosurgery is likely to become an essential part of any neurosurgical spine center that treats a large number of patients with spinal tumors.

References

1 Gerszten PC, Welch WC: Current surgical management of metastatic spinal disease. Oncology 2000;14:1013–1036; discussion 1024.

2 Faul C, Flickinger J: The use of radiation in the management of spinal metastases. J Neuro oncol 1995;23:149–161.

3 Ryu SI, Chang SD, Kim DH, et al: Image-guided hypo-fractionated stereotactic radiosurgery to spinal lesions. Neurosurgery 2001;49:838–846.

4 Loblaw DA, Laperriere NJ: Emergency treatment of malignant extradural spinal cord compression: an evidence-based guideline. J Clin Oncol 1998;16:1613–1624.

5 Gerszten PC, Ozhasoglu C, Burton S, et al: CyberKnfe frameless stereotactic radiosurgery for spinal lesions: clinical experience in 125 cases. Neurosurgery 2004;55:89–99.

6 Leksell L: The stereotaxic method and radiosurgery of the brain. Acta Chir Scand 1951;102:316–319.

7 Luxton G, Petrovich Z, Jozsef G, et al: Stereptactoc radiosurgery: principles and comparison of treatment methods. Neurosurgery 1993;32:241–259.

8 Ryu S, Yin FF, Rock J, et al: Image-guided and intensity-modulated radiosurgery for patients with spinal metastasis. Cancer 2003;97:2013–2018.

9 Hamilton A, Lulu B, Fosmire H, et al: Preliminary clinical experience with linear accelerator-based spinal stereotactic radiosurgery. Neurosurgery 1995;36:311–319.

10 Kuriyama K, Onishi H, Sano N, et al: A new irradiation unit constructed of self-moving gantry-CT and linac. Int J Radiat Oncol Biol Phys 2003;55:428–435.

11 Colombo F, Pozza F, Chierego G: Linear accelerator radiosurgery of cerebral arteriovenous malformations: an update. Neurosurgery 1994;34:14–21.

12 Hitchcock E, Kitchen G, Dalton E, et al: Stereotactic linac radiosurgery. Br J Neurosurg 1989;3: 305–312.

13 Bilsky MH, Yamada Y, Yenice K, et al: Intensity-modulated stereotactic radiotherapy of paraspinal tumors: a preliminary report. Neurosurgery 2004;54:823–830.

14 Chang EL, Shiu AS, Lii M-F, et al: Phase I clinical evaluation of near-simultaneous computed tomographic image-guided stereotactic body radiotherapy for spinal metastases. Int J Radiat Oncol Biol Phys 2004;59:1288–1294.

15 Milker-Zabel S, Zabel A, Thilmann C, et al: Clinical results of retreatment of vertebral bone metastases by stereotactic conformal radiotherapy and intensity-modulated radiotherapy. Int J Radiat Oncol Biol Phys 2003;55:162–167.

16 Pirzkall A, Lohr F, Rhein B, et al: Conformal radiotherapy of challenging paraspinal tumors using a multiple arc segment technique. Int J Radiat Oncol Biol Phys 2000;48:1197–1204.

17 Isacsson U, Hagberg H, Johansson K, et al: Potential advantages of protons over conventional radiation beams for paraspinal tumours. Radiother Oncol 1997;45:63–70.

18 Colombo F, Benedetti A, Pozza F, et al: Stereotactic radiosurgery utilizing a linear accelerator. Appl Neurophysiol 1985;48:133–145.

19 Kuo JS, Yu C, Petrovich Z, et al: The cyberKnife stereotactic radiosurgery system: description, installation, an initial evaluation of use and functionality. Neurosurgery 2003;53:1235–1239.

20 Adler J Jr, Chang S, Murphy M, et al: The CyberKnife: a frameless robotic system for radiosurgery. Sterotact Funct Neurosurg 1997;69:124–128.

21 Adler J, Murphy M, Chang S, et al: Image-guided robotic radiosurgery. Neurosurgery 1999;44: 1299–1307.

22 Gerszten PC, Ozhasoglu C, Burton S, et al: Feasibility of frameless single-fraction stereotactic radiosurgery for spinal lesions. Neurosurg Focus 2002;13:1–6.

23 Murphy M, Cox R: The accuracy of dose localization for an image-guided frameless radiosurgery system. Med Phys 1996;23:2043–2049.

24 Gerszten PC, Welch WC: CyberKnife radiosurgery for the spine. Tech Neurosurg 2003;9: 232–241.

25 Gerszten PC, Ozhasoglu C, Burton SA, et al: CyberKnife frameless single-fraction stereotactic radiosurgery for benign tumors of the spine. Neurosurg Focus 2003;14:1–5.

26 Chang S, Adler J: Current status and optimal use of radiosurgery. Oncology 2001;15:209–221.

27 Yu C, Jozsef G, Apuzzo ML, et al: Dosimetric comparison of cyberKnife with other radiosurgical modalities for an ellipsoidal target. Neurosurgery 2003;53:1155–1163.
28 Romanelli P, Chang SD, Koong A, et al: Extracranial radiosurgery using the cyberKnife. Tech Neurosurg 2003;9:226–231.
29 Adler J, Cox R, Kaplan I, et al: Stereotactic radiosurgical treatment of brain metastases. J Neurosurg 1992;76:444–449.
30 Guthrie B, Adler J: Computer-assisted preoperative planning, interactive surgery, and frameless stereotaxy. Clin Neurosurg 1991;38:112–131.
31 Chang SD, Main W, Martin DP, et al: An analysis of the accuracy of the cyberKnife: a robotic frameless stereotactic radiosurgical system. Neurosurgery 2003;52:140–147.
32 Wara W, Phillips T, Sheline G, et al: Radiation tolerance of the spinal cord. Cancer 1975;35: 1558–1562.
33 Hatlevoll R, Host H, Kaalhus O: Myelopathy following radiotherapy of bronchial carcinoma with large single fractions: a retrospective study. Int J Radiat Oncol Biol Phys 1983;9:41–44.
34 Kim Y, Fayos J: Radiation tolerance of the cervical spinal cord. Ther Radiol 1981;139:473–478.
35 Abbatucci JS, Delozier T, Quint R, et al: Radiation myelopathy of the cervical spinal cord: time, dose and volume factors. Int J Radiat Oncol Biol Phys 1978;4:239–248.
36 McCuniff A, Liang M: Radiation tolerance of the cervical spinal cord. Int J Radiat Oncol Biol Phys 1989;16:675–678.
37 Phillips T, Buschke F: Radiation tolerance of the thoracic spinal cord. Am J Radiol 1969;105: 659–664.
38 Boden G: Radiation myelitis of the cervical spinal cord. Br J Radiol 1948;21:464–469.

Peter C. Gerszten, MD, MPH
Department of Neurological Surgery, Presbyterian University Hospital
Suite B-400, 200 Lothrop St
Pittsburgh, PA 15213 (USA)
Tel. +1 412 647 0958, Fax +1 412 647 0989, E-Mail gersztenpc@upmc.edu

Szeifert GT, Kondziolka D, Levivier M, Lunsford LD (eds): Radiosurgery and Pathological Fundamentals. Prog Neurol Surg. Basel, Karger, 2007, vol 20, pp 359–374

15.1. Heritage of Radiosurgical Research, Current Trends and Future Perspective

Ajay Niranjan, Glenn T. Gobbel, Douglas Kondziolka, L. Dade Lunsford

Department of Neurological Surgery, The University of Pittsburgh, and Center for Image-Guided Neurosurgery, University of Pittsburgh Medical Center, Pittsburgh, Pa., USA

Abstract

Advances in neuroimaging, stereotactic techniques, and robotic technology in the last decade have significantly expanded the applications of radiosurgery. Radiosurgery has become a preferred management modality for many intracranial tumors such as schwannomas, menigiomas and metastatic tumors. While indications of radiosurgery continue to expand, further investigations are critical to understand the mechanism of biological response of CNS tissues to radiation as well as the potential of long-term adverse effects. The effects and the pathogenesis of biologic effects following radiosurgery may be unique. The need for basic research concerning the radiobiology of high-dose single-fraction ionizing radiation on nervous system tissue is crucial. The development of future applications of radiosurgery will depend upon our understanding of radiobiology of radiosurgery. The present review examines the state of radiobiological investigations into the nature of CNS effects, the newer techniques developed, and the use of radiosurgery as a tool for understanding basic CNS biology.

The field of stereotactic radiosurgery represents one of the fundamental shifts in the neurological surgery over the last 2 decades. Compared to conventional invasive surgery techniques, radiosurgery is minimally invasive and relies on biological response of tissues in order to eradicate or inactivate them. Radiosurgery is conceptually different from the fractionated radiation therapy. The efficacy of large-field fractionated radiotherapy to treat brain tumors is dependent on biologic differences between normal and tumor cells. Fractionated radiotherapy exploits these differences to limit the risk of normal tissue injury in patients with malignant brain tumors, thus it can increase the therapeutic ratio, which is equivalent to the rate of tumor control, divided by the rate of complications.

Radiosurgery, in contrast to conventional radiotherapy, uses a single high dose of radiation. Normal tissue effects are limited by the highly focused nature of the radiosurgical beams. In addition, unlike radiotherapy, radiosurgery treats small volume targets using much higher doses. Finally, whereas fractionated radiotherapy is generally most effective in killing rapidly dividing cells, radiosurgery induces biological response irrespective of the mitotic activity, oxygenation, and inherent radiosensitivity of target cells. Considering the unique biological response of tissues to radiosurgery, it is important to study the biological effects of radiosurgery in both normal and pathological nervous system tissues in animal models. Information gained from radiosurgical research studies would be useful in devising strategies to avoid, prevent, or ameliorate damage to normal tissue without compromising treatment efficacy. As radiosurgery evolves from a treatment specifically for brain tumors into a widely available treatment modality for a variety of intracranial lesions, understanding of biological responses using animal investigations becomes crucial.

Investigations Seeking to Explore Focused Radiation as a Neurosurgical Tool

In one of the initial studies, Larsson et al. [1] investigated the use of the high-energy proton beam (185-MeV proton beam from 230-cm synchrocyclotron) as a neurosurgical tool. The early histological results (3rd–8th day) showed complete transection of the rabbit spinal cord using 40,000 rad (400 Gy) with 1.5-mm beam diameter and 20,000 rad (200 Gy) with 10-mm beam diameter. Using 20,000 rad of stereotactic multiple port proton beam radiation, these investigators documented sharply defined lesions in deep parts of the goat brain within 4–7 weeks. Rexed et al. [2] studied the long-term effects (2–56 weeks) of proton beam irradiation on the rabbit brain. Using a 1.5-mm collimator, 20,000 rad (200 Gy) was delivered to the anterior part of the rabbit brain. Serial histology revealed a well-demarcated lesion in the path of beam up to 3 months. After 3 months, a lesion broader than the beam size was noted. Leksell et al. [3] investigated the features of a radiolesion in the depth of the brain produced by cross-fired irradiation with a narrow beam of high energy. Their results showed that with 20,000 rad (200-Gy central dose) well-circumscribed intracerebral lesions of appropriate size and shape could be created.

Andersson et al. [4] studied the late histologic effects of the cross-fired beams of 185-MeV protons on the goat brain. No late untoward changes in or around the lesion (e.g. elements resembling neoplasm, hemorrhage, or teleangiectasis) were seen 1.5–4 years after 20,000-rad (200-Gy) radiosurgery. Nilsson et al. [5] irradiated (100–300 Gy) the basilar artery of cats by stereotactic technique using 179-source cobalt-60 prototype gamma unit. Histology demonstrated vascular lesions such as vacuolization, degeneration and desquamation of the endothelium, and hyalinization and necrosis of the muscular coat. The reparatory reactions were relatively sparse and thrombosis was completely absent. These investigations demonstrated that radiosurgery could be potentially used to create lesions in deep parts of the brain (table 1).

Investigations into Effects of Dose and Time Latency of Normal Brain Radiosurgery

The effect of fractionated radiation therapy on the nervous system depends on both the radiation dose and the time elapsed after irradiation [6–8]. The radiation response tends to be most severe in white matter regions, although all regions of the brain may be affected [9–11]. A dose-related variable latency period after irradiation can last from months to years [6–8]. A single radiation dose of 20 Gy to the rat brain creates lesions that are primarily confined to the vasculature at latencies of more than 12 months [12, 13]. Radiation-induced vascular changes in the CNS include perivascular fibrosis and fibrinoid necrosis of vessel walls, hyaline degeneration, edema, telangectasia, thrombosis, and hemorrhage [14]. At higher doses of around 25 Gy, white-matter lesions predominate in irradiated rat brain at latencies of less than 12 months. Radiation-induced lesions in the white matter can range from demyelination to malacia [14]. Investigations seeking to study the biologic response of radiosurgery on the CNS are listed in table 1.

In one of the initial studies, Lunsford et al. [15] developed a baboon model to determine the in vivo radiobiological effects of stereotactic radiosurgery. Using an 8-mm collimator, a central dose of 150 Gy was delivered to the caudate, thalamus, or pons using the Gamma Knife. There were no changes visible by CT or by T_1-weighted, T_2-weighted, and gadolinium-enhanced MRI images at 4 weeks after irradiation. A circumscribed, contrast-enhanced lesion was visible by 6–8 weeks, and edema was first evident at 8 weeks. At 6 weeks after irradiation, there was a lesion at the focus of irradiation, which was characterized by demyelination, microvascular damage and hemorrhage, and astrocytosis. The irradiated region had undergone frank necrosis by 24 weeks.

Subsequent studies on the effects of radiation on normal brain have extended our understanding of the radiosurgical dose response. Kondziolka et al. [16]

Table 1. Radiosurgery as a neurosurgical tool

First author	Maximum dose, krad	Region(s) irradiated	Irradiation technique	Animal model	Results
Larsson, 1958 [1]	20	internal capsule	proton beam	rabbit, goat	stereotactic proton beam radiation can produce restricted brain and spinal cord lesions in 4–6 weeks
Rexed, 1960 [2]	20	forebrain	proton beam	rabbit	high-energy proton irradiation can cause a well-defined lesion in 2–56 weeks
Leksell, 1960 [3]	20–38	internal capsule	proton beam	goat	well circumscribed radiolesions of appropriate size and shape can be produced with a suitable dose (20 krad)
Andersson, 1970 [4]	15–20	basal ganglia, internal capsule, optic chiasm, optic tract	proton beam	goat	no untoward late effects (neoplasia, teleangiectasis, hemorrhage) were noted 1.5–4 years after proton beam radiosurgery

studied the histologic changes in the rat brain 90 days after radiosurgery. The frontal lobe of rats was irradiated with maximal doses of 30–200 Gy using a 4 mm collimator. Doses of more than 70 Gy induced detectable histologic alterations. Necrosis was seen only in tissues irradiated with more than 100 Gy. Blatt et al. [17], evaluated serial tissue changes after 125-Gy LINAC radiosurgery of internal capsule of cats. MRI and histopathological evaluations were performed serially for 1 year starting at 3.5 weeks after irradiation. Tissue necrosis was evident in the cat brain by 3.5 weeks and was accompanied by vascular proliferation and edema. Unlike the previously cited baboon study, where the focal lesion in one baboon became progressively larger from 8 to 24 weeks after irradiation, the lesions in the cat study showed increased vascularity, microglia and infiltration that resolved by 12–29 weeks. Because of differences in irradiation protocol, dose, species, and time point of evaluation, it is difficult to determine the exact cause of the dissimilar results. Certainly, the potential for resolution is important because progressive radionecrosis would generally have severe clinical consequences.

In a study evaluating the effects of radiation dose and time after treatment on the radiosensitivity of the brain, rats were irradiated with maximum doses of 50, 75, or 120 Gy and analyzed for histologic changes and blood-brain barrier integrity up to 12 months later [18]. Whereas 120 Gy induced alterations in astrocytic morphology by just 3 days after treatment, such changes were not observed until 3 months after 50 Gy. Blood-brain barrier breakdown as assessed by Evans Blue leakage was evident within 3 weeks of 120 Gy irradiation but was not seen across 12 months after 50 Gy. These findings indicate that the latent period between irradiation and detection of pathologic alterations is dependent on both the dose and the biological end point used. Such findings are consistent with the results of studies using a more conventional radiation source (^{60}Co) to irradiate the rat spinal cord. In this model of radiation-induced CNS injury, latency to paralysis following irradiation of 8- or 16-mm segment of the cervical spinal cord decreased as dose increased [19]. Also, the ED50 for paralysis following 4 mm of spinal cord irradiation was 51 Gy, whereas the ED50 for vascular damage was only 25.6 Gy. The impact of dose and biological end points on latency was also reported by Karger et al. [20], who evaluated the rat brain using T_1- and T_2-weighted, gadolinium-enhanced MRI at 15, 17, or 20 months after treatment with 26–50 Gy after linear accelerator-based radiosurgery. A 3-mm collimator was employed to deliver the radiosurgical dose using a convergent arc technique and resulted in an 80% isodose distribution of 4.7 mm in diameter. No radiation-induced affect on MRI was noted after at any time point for doses less than 30 Gy. After 40 Gy, the latency of detectable MRI changes was approximately 19–20 weeks, whereas the latency after 50 Gy was 15–16 weeks. In addition, T_1-weighted changes in the MRI signal had a shorter latency than T_2-weighted changes. Considering that the changes in T_1-weighted images are due to leakage of gadolinium-DTPA across the blood-brain barrier, the results of this study point to the likely role of vascular damage in radiation-induced injury. The importance of the vasculature in radiation-induced brain injury is well recognized; a prevalent hypothesis regarding the pathogenesis following conventional radiotherapy is that damage to capillary endothelium and/or supporting cells ultimately interrupts blood flow resulting in secondary ischemic necrosis. In a report focusing on vascular changes after a maximal dose of 75 Gy delivered to the rat brain using the Gamma Knife, it was noted that vascular changes, specifically alterations in the basement membrane, preceded changes in necrosis [21]. This finding suggests that vascular damage is also an important component in biologic response following radiosurgery.

Although radiosurgery generally involves the use of higher single doses and smaller treatment volumes than conventional irradiation, the histologic effects of these two methodologies appear similar. The biggest differences are that the latency period following radiosurgery is shorter and the major histologic finding is vascular damage (table 2).

Investigations into Strategies Enhancing the Efficacy of Radiosurgery

Although benign tumor radiosurgery is associated with high tumor control rates, malignant glial tumors almost invariably recur. Additional strategies to improve cell kill of malignant brain tumors and to protect normal surrounding brain are needed. A few strategies for radioprotection of normal tissue and radiosensitization of tumor tissue have already been explored.

Radiation Protection and Repair

The initial strategies included use of cerebral protective agents while delivering a high dose to tumor cells. Oldfield et al. [22] noted protection from radiation-induced brain injury using pentobarbital. The 21-aminosteroids (21-AS) have been evaluated as potential radioprotecive agents. The 21-AS commonly known as lazaroids, have been advocated as cerebral protective agents in patients with head trauma or subarachnoid hemorrhage [23]. The 21-AS act as antioxidants [24], and much of the damage from radiation is due to the production of oxygen free radicals, which can induce DNA modifications and strand breaks and initiate lipid peroxidation of vascular membranes, ultimately leading to membrane lysis and cell death. As a lipid antioxidant and free radical scavenger, 21-AS inhibits oxygen radical-initiated peroxidation of vascular membrane. 21-AS also blocks the release of free arachidonic acid from cell membrane,

Table 2. Dose and latency effects of radiosurgery on the normal nervous system

First Author	Maximum dose, Gy	Region(s) irradiated	Irradiation technique	Animal model	Results
Lunsford, 1990 [15]	150	caudate, thalamus, pons	Gamma Knife, 8-mm collimator	baboon	MRI and histology showed lesion 45–60 days after treatment
Kondziolka, 1992 [16]	30–200	r. frontal lobe	Gamma Knife, 4-mm collimator	rat	histopathology at 90 days showed tissue changes at doses lower than 60 Gy, necrosis at 100-Gy doses
Blatt, 1994 [17]	149	internal capsule	LINAC, 10-mm collimator	cat	MRI and serial histopathology showed mass effect and neurologic deficits at 3.5–5.5 weeks, some necrosis 12–29 weeks, and late resorption of necrosis
Kamiryo, 2001 [21]	75	parietal cortex	Gamma Knife, 4-mm collimator	rat	electron microscopy at 3.5 months showed decreased vascularity and increased capillary diameter in irradiated regions; basement membrane changes precede vascular damage
Karger, 2002 [20]	26–50	parietal cortex	LINAC, 3-mm collimator	rat	MRI showed contrast enhancement at 15 weeks after 50-Gy, and 19 weeks after 40-Gy radiosurgery

thereby inhibiting activation of the proinflammatory cyclo-oxygenase pathway. These properties of 21-AS are thought to protect cerebral vessels from injury and prevent cerebral edema. The effects of the 21-AS known as U-74389G on radiation injury have been evaluated in both rat and cat models. Bernstein et al. [25] reported that U-74389G reduced brachytherapy-induced brain injury in the rat. Buatti et al. [26] found that this same agent also protected the cat brain from injury due to radiosurgery and was significantly more effective than corticosteroids [26]. In our own studies, 15 mg/kg but not 5 mg/kg of U-74389G was effective at reducing injury in the rat when administered 1 h before radiosurgery. U-74389G ameliorated vasculopathy and regional edema and delayed the onset of necrosis, while gliosis was unaffected [27]. Preliminary results suggest that this agent may be acting through reduction of the cytokines induced by brain irradiation.

Alternative strategy for radiation protection seeks to repair radiation-induced brain damage. At present, the cellular target that is primarily responsible for radiation-induced breakdown of normal tissue is unclear. The white matter and the cerebral vasculature appear to be particularly susceptible to radiation, which suggests that oligodendrocytes and endothelial cells may be critical targets of radiation. Recent studies have also implicated a potential role for neural progenitors in radiation-induced brain injury [28, 29]. We hypothesize that radiation-induced damage to these cell types can be repaired by neural stem cells. Neural stem cells can be isolated from normal adult mammalian brain and can be induced to differentiate into neurons or glia. The role of neural and endothelial precursors in repairing radiation-induced brain damage is being evaluated. In the future, if implanted neural stem cells could prevent or repair radiation-induced damage to normal brain, then the tumor could be targeted with higher radiosurgery doses. These higher doses may prove lethal to tumor cells while stem cells will prevent damage to surrounding normal tissue.

Radiation Potentiation

We studied the synergistic effect of tumor necrosis factor alpha (TNF-α) on enhancing the tumor response to radiosurgery. TNF-α can act as a tumoricidal agent with direct cytotoxicity mediated through binding to its cognate cell-surface receptors and a variety of activities triggering a multifaceted immune attack on tumors [30–35]. In addition, locally produced TNF-α has been reported to enhance the sensitivity of tumors to radiation in nude mice [30]. We employed a replication defective herpes simplex virus (HSV) as a vector to deliver thymidine kinase (TK) and/or TNF-α genes to U-87 MG tumors in nude mice. Gene transfer was followed by radiosurgery using 15 Gy to the tumor margin (21.4 Gy to the center) after 48 h and daily ganciclovir therapy (GCV) for 10 days. The combination of radiosurgery with TNF-α or with HSV-TK-GCV (suicide gene therapy, SGT) and TNF-α significantly improved median survival of animals [36]. In additional experiments, the connexin-43 gene was added to enhance the formation of gap junctions between tumor cells, which should facilitate the intercellular spread of TK-activated GCV from virus-infected cells to noninfected surrounding cells. This creates a bystander effect that can improve tumor cell killing [37]. Addition of connexin-43 gene to this paradigm (TK-GCV + TNF-α + radiosurgery) further improved survival (90% survival in tumor-bearing mice). We studied this strategy in a 9L rat glioma model and found that addition of radiosurgery to SGT significantly improved animal survival compared to SGT alone. The combination of HSV-based SGT (TK-GCV), TNF-α gene transfer and radiosurgery was more effective than SGT or radiosurgery alone. The combination of SGT with radiosurgery was also more effective than SGT or radiosurgery alone. Gene therapy seems to be an effective strategy for enhancing radiosurgery. However, the exact mechanism of this effect is unclear and the subject of future investigations. In other studies, tumor sensitization to radiation was apparently mediated by extracellular TNF-α promoting the destruction of tumor vessels, whereas HSV vector-mediated TNF-α-enhanced killing of malignant glioma cell cultures is presumably a consequence of an intracellular TNF-α activity [35, 38] (table 3).

Investigations into Effects of Functional Radiosurgery

Radiosurgery is rapidly expanding beyond its use as a treatment of brain tumors and arteriovenous malformations. It has been found effective for other neurologic disorders, such as epilepsy, movement disorder, and trigeminal neuralgia. The promise of 'functional' radiosurgery has led to a need to investigate its efficacy, limitations, and potential drawbacks.

Hippocampal Radiosurgery

The potential efficacy of radiosurgery for the treatment of epilepsy has been evaluated using rat models. Kainic acid reproducibly induces epilepsy in the rat when injected into the hippocampus. Mori et al. [39] treated kainic acid-induced epilepsy in rats with doses of 20–100 Gy using the Gamma Knife. The efficacy of the treatment on epilepsy was evaluated by direct observation and scalp EEG for 42 days. Even 20 Gy significantly reduced the number of seizures, and the efficacy improved with increasing dose. Only doses >60 Gy induced histologic changes. Maesawa et al. [40] treated epileptic rats with a single dose of 30 or 60 Gy. Both doses significantly reduced EEG-defined seizures, and this effect occurred sooner after the higher dose (5–9 weeks for 60 Gy versus 7–9 weeks for 30 Gy). While kainic acid injection alone reduced

Table 3. Effects of radiosurgery on malignant brain tumors and strategies to enhance the effect

First author	Tumor margin dose, Gy	Tumor model	Animal model	Irradiation technique	Experimental treatment	Results
Kondziolka, 1992 [45]	15–50	C6 glioma	rat	Gamma Knife, 4-mm collimator	radiosurgery	treated animals survived 39 days (control 29 days); treated tumors had hypocellular appearance with cellular edema
Kondziolka, 1999 [46]	35	C6 glioma	rat	Gamma Knife, 4-mm collimator	radiosurgery + 21-aminosteroid	21-aminosteroid exhibited a radioprotectant effect on normal brain tissue, but did not protect the tumor
Niranjan, 2000 [36]	15	U87 MG	nude mouse	Gamma Knife, 4-mm collimator	radiosurgery + HSV TK-GCV + TNF	the combination treatment enhanced median survival (75 days) with 89% animals surviving
Nakahara, 2001 [47]	16	MADB 106 cells	rat	Gamma Knife, 4-mm collimator	radiosurgery + cytokine transduced tumor cell vaccine	the combination treatment significantly prolonged animal survival and protected animals from a subsequent challenge by parental tumor cells placed in the CNS
Niranjan, 2003 [48]	15	9L gliosarcoma	rat	Gamma Knife, 4-mm collimator	radiosurgery + HSV TK-GCV + TNF + connexin	the combination of radiosurgery and multigene therapy enhanced median animal survival (150 days) with 75% animals surviving

performance of rats on the water maze task, the performance of rats that were treated by radiosurgery after kainic acid administration was not different from controls.

Liscak et al. [41] evaluated the effects of radiosurgery on normal hippocampus in an effort to identify potential normal tissue complications and determine dose limits for hippocampal radiosurgery. This study employed 4 separate 4-mm isocenters to irradiate the entire hippocampus with 25–100 Gy. Doses <50 Gy did not cause any perceptible changes based on histology, MRI, and Morris water maze testing. In contrast, after doses >50 Gy, performance on the Morris water maze was significantly worse than that of controls. These investigations support the concept that radiosurgery may be an effective method for treating epilepsy, but they also suggest that doses to the hippocampus should be limited to reduce potential effects on learning and memory.

Movement Disorders

The effect of radiosurgery on potential targets for the treatment of movement disorders has been evaluated. De Salles et al. [42] used a linear accelerator and 3-mm collimator to deliver a maximal dose of 150 Gy to the subthalamic nucleus of one vervet monkey and to the substantia nigra of another. Follow-up MRI detected a 3-mm lesion that did not increase in size throughout the course of the study. Kondziolka et al. [43] examined the effect of thalamic radiosurgery in the baboon model, and reported that a dose of 100 Gy (central dose using a 4-mm collimator) was sufficient to induce contrast enhancement of MR images and coagulative necrosis as evaluated by histology.

Trigeminal Neuralgia

Radiosurgery has a significant potential as an effective, noninvasive method for treatment of trigeminal neuralgia, and the effect of Gamma Knife irradiation on the trigeminal nerve has been evaluated in the baboon [44]. The proximal trigeminal nerve was irradiated with 80 or 100 Gy using a 4-mm collimator. A 4-mm region of contrast enhancement was visible by MRI at 6 months after treatment. Both large and small fibers were affected with axonal degeneration occurring after 80 Gy and necrosis after 100 Gy. Neither dose was effective at selectively damaging fibers responsible for transmission of pain while maintaining those responsible for other sensations, which would be optimal for effective treatment of trigeminal neuralgia. Nevertheless, this study does demonstrate that it is possible to noninvasively and precisely affect specific nerves using the Gamma Knife. Whether other dose regimens might cause selective damage to pain fibers will require further investigation (table 4).

Table 4. Biologic response to functional radiosurgery

First author	Maximum dose, Gy	Region(s) irradiated	Irradiation technique	Animal model	Results
Ishikawa, 1999 [49]	200	medial temporal lobe	Gamma Knife, 4-mm collimator	rat	sequential MRI and histopathology showed consistent necrosis at 2 weeks after 200-Gy radiosurgery
Mori, 2000 [39]	20–100	hippocampus	Gamma Knife, 4-mm collimator	rat	seizure frequency decreased after ≥20-Gy radiosurgery
Maesawa, 2000 [40]	30–60	hippocampus	Gamma Knife, 4-mm collimator	rat	seizure frequency decreased after 30- to 60-Gy radiosurgery, shorter latency after higher dose, learning and memory unaffected
Kondziolka, 2000 [44]	80–100	trigeminal nerve	Gamma Knife, 4-mm collimator	baboon	MRI, histology at 6 months showed axonal degeneration at all doses
Chen, 2001	20–40	hippocampus	Gamma Knife, 4-mm collimator	rat	subnecrotic (20- to 40-Gy) radiosurgery substantially reduces seizure frequency and duration
De Salles, 2001 [42]	150	subthalamic nucleus, substantia nigra	LINAC, 3-mm collimator	monkey	MRI and histology showed that necrotic lesion remained at <3-mm size.
Kondziolka, 2002 [43]	100	thalamus	Gamma Knife, 4-mm collimator	baboon	MRI, histology showed necrosis at 6 months
Liscak, 2002 [41]	25–150	hippocampus	Gamma Knife, 4-mm collimator	rat	more than 50 altered memory performance
Zerris, 2002	140	caudate-putamen complex	Gamma Knife, 4-mm collimator	rat	6-OHDA-induced hemiparkinsonian behavior was significantly reduced; necrotic lesions were surrounded by regions that were highly positive for GDNF
Brisman, 2003 [50]	5–130 CGE	hippocampus	proton beam	rat	doses 90 CGE or higher resulted in adverse behavioral effects and necrosis in 3 months; 30- or 60-CGE radiosurgery led to marked increase in HSP-72 staining but no necrosis

Future Direction of Radiosurgery Investigations

Rapid developments in neuroimaging, stereotactic techniques, and robotic technology in the last decade have contributed to improved results and wider applications of radiosurgery. The role of radiosurgery has expanded well beyond its initial application for functional neurosurgery, pain management, arteriovenous malformations, and selected skull base tumors. The clinical spectrum now includes a wide variety of rare skull base neoplasms, serves as the primary treatment of metastatic brain cancer, and provides adjuvant management of malignant primary brain tumors. Although radiosurgery provides survival benefits in diffuse malignant brain tumors, cure is still not possible. Microscopic tumor infiltration into surrounding normal tissue is the main cause of recurrence. Additional strategies are needed to specifically target tumor cells. In the future, gene transfer to sensitize malignant tumor cells to radiosurgery may provide enhanced tumor cell kill while radioprotective agents will prevent damage to surrounding normal tissue.

Although the nature of brain injury following radiosurgery appears similar to that following conventional radiation treatments, there remain a number of questions concerning the effects and the pathogenesis of such effects following both forms of radiotherapy. Further research to answer these questions is needed to maximize the effectiveness of treatment on target regions and minimize injury to other areas. While radiosurgery usage continues to expand as we sort out the roles of precision radiation, we must strive to understand the mechanism of biological response of CNS tissues to radiation as well as the potential of long-term adverse effects including the risk of delayed oncogenesis.

References

1 Larsson B, Leksell L, Rexed B, Sourander P, Mair W, Anderson B: The high-energy proton beam as neurosurgical tool. Nature 1958;182:1222–1223.

2 Rexed B, Mair W, Sourander P, Larsson B, Leksell L: Effect of high-energy protons on the rabbit. Acta Radiol Oncol Radiat Phys Biol 1960;53:289–299.

3 Leksell L, Larsson B, Anderson B, Rexed B, Sourander P, Mair W: Lesions in the depth of the brain produced by a beam of high-energy protons. Acta Radiol Ther Phys Biol 1960;53:251–264.

4 Andersson B, Larsson B, Leksell L, Mair W, Rexed B, Sourander P, Wennerstrand J: Histopathology of late local radiolesions in the goat brain. Acta Radiol Ther Phys Biol 1970;9: 385–394.

5 Nilsson A, Wennerstrand J, Leksell D, Backlund EO: Stereotactic gamma irradiation of basilar artery in cat. Preliminary experiences. Acta Radiol Oncol Radiat Phys Biol 1978;17:150–160.

6 Calvo W, Hopewell JW, Reinhold HS, Yeung TK: Time- and dose-related changes in the white matter of the rat brain after single doses of X rays. Br J Radiol 1988;61:1043–1052.

7 Fike J, Gobbel G: Central nervous system radiation injury in large animal models; in Gutin P, Leibel S, Sheline G (eds): Radiation Injury to the Nervous System. New York, Raven Press, 1991, pp 113–135.

8 van der Kogel A: Central nervous system radiation injury in small animal models; in Gutin P, Leibel S, Sheline G (eds): Radiation Injury to the Nervous System. New York, Raven Press, 1991, pp 113–135.
9 Calvo W, Hopewell J, Reinhold H, van den Berg A, Yeung T: Dose-dependent and time-dependent changes in the choroid plexus of the irradiated rat brain. Br J Radiol 1987;60:1109–1117.
10 Hopewell J, Calvo W, Campling D, Lauk S, Reinhold H, Reyners H, Rezvani M, Yeung T: The role of the vasculature in normal tissue responsesq; in Fielden E, Fowler J, Hendry J, Scott D (eds): Radiation Research, Proceedings of the 8th International Congress of Radiation Research. London, Taylor & Francis, 1987, vol 2, pp 789–794.
11 Zeman W, Samorajski T: Effects of irradiation on the nervous system; in Berdjis CC (ed): Pathology of Irradiation. Baltimore, Williams & Wilkins, 1971, pp 213–277.
12 Hopewell JW, Wright EA: The nature of latent cerebral irradiation damage and it modification by hypertension. Br J Radiol 1970;43:161–167.
13 Reinhold H, Hopewell J: Late changes in the architecture of blood vessesls of the rat brain after irradiation. Br J Radiol 1980;53:693–696.
14 Schultheiss T, Stephens L: Permanent radiation myelopathy. Br J Radiol 1992;65:737–753.
15 Lunsford LD, Altschuler EM, Flickinger JC, Wu A, Martinez AJ: In vivo biological effects of stereotactic radiosurgery: a primate model. Neurosurgery 1990;27:373–382.
16 Kondziolka D, Lunsford LD, Claassen D, Maitz AH, Flickinger JC: Radiobiology of radiosurgery: Part I. The normal rat brain model. Neurosurgery 1992;31:271–279.
17 Blatt DR, Friedman WA, Bova FJ, Theele DP, Mickle JP: Temporal characteristics of radiosurgical lesions in an animal model. J Neurosurg 1994;80:1046–1055.
18 Kamiryo T, Kassell NF, Thai QA, Lopes MB, Lee KS, Steiner L: Histological changes in the normal rat brain after gamma irradiation. Acta Neurochir (Wien) 1996;138:451–459.
19 Hopewell JW, Wright EA: The effects of dose and field size on late radiation damage to the rat spinal cord. Int J Radiat Biol Relat Stud Phys Chem Med 1975;28:325–333.
20 Karger CP, Munter MW, Heiland S, Peschke P, Debus J, Hartmann GH: Dose-response curves and tolerance doses for late functional changes in the normal rat brain after stereotactic radiosurgery evaluated by magnetic resonance imaging: influence of end points and follow-up time. Radiat Res 2002;157:617–625.
21 Kamiryo T, Lopes MB, Kassell NF, Steiner L, Lee KS: Radiosurgery-induced microvascular alterations precede necrosis of the brain neuropil. Neurosurgery 2001;49:409–414.
22 Oldfield EH, Friedman R, Kinsella T, Moquin R, Olson JJ, Orr K, DeLuca AM: Reduction in radiation-induced brain injury by use of pentobarbital or lidocaine protection. J Neurosurg 1990;72: 737–744.
23 Smith SL, Scherch HM, Hall ED: Protective effects of tirilazad mesylate and metabolite U-89678 against blood-brain barrier damage after subarachnoid hemorrhage and lipid peroxidative neuronal injury. J Neurosurg 1996;84:229–233.
24 Braughler JM: Lipid peroxidation-induced inhibition of gamma-aminobutyric acid uptake in rat brain synaptosomes: protection by glucocorticoids. J Neurochem 1985;44:1282–1288.
25 Bernstein M, Ginsberg H, Glen J: Protection of iodine-125 brachytherapy brain injury in the rat with the 21-aminosteroid U-74389F. Neurosurgery 1992;31:923–927.
26 Buatti JM, Friedman WA, Theele DP, Bova FJ, Mendenhall WM: The lazaroid U74389G protects normal brain from stereotactic radiosurgery-induced radiation injury. Int J Radiat Oncol Biol Phys 1996;34:591–597.
27 Kondziolka D, Somaza S, Martinez AJ, Jacobsohn J, Maitz A, Lunsford LD, Flickinger JC: Radioprotective effects of the 21-aminosteroid U-74389G for stereotactic radiosurgery. Neurosurgery 1997;41:203–208.
28 Tada E, Yang C, Gobbel GT, Lamborn KR, Fike JR: Long-term impairment of subependymal repopulation following damage by ionizing irradiation. Exp Neurol 1999;160:66–77.
29 Tada E, Parent JM, Lowenstein DH, Fike JR: X-irradiation causes a prolonged reduction in cell proliferation in the dentate gyrus of adult rats. Neuroscience 2000;99:33–41.
30 Staba MJ, Mauceri HJ, Kufe DW, Hallahan DE, Weichselbaum RR: Adenoviral TNF-alpha gene therapy and radiation damage tumor vasculature in a human malignant glioma xenograft. Gene Ther 1998;5:293–300.

31 Cao G, Kuriyama S, Du P, Sakamoto T, Kong X, Masui K, Qi Z: Complete regression of established murine hepatocellular carcinoma by in vivo tumor necrosis factor alpha gene transfer. Gastroenterology 1997;112:501–510.
32 Han SK, Brody SL, Crystal RG: Suppression of in vivo tumorigenicity of human lung cancer cells by retrovirus-mediated transfer of the human tumor necrosis factor-alpha cDNA. Am J Respir Cell Mol Biol 1994;11:270–278.
33 Ostensen ME, Thiele DL, Lipsky PE: Enhancement of human natural killer cell function by the combined effects of tumor necrosis factor alpha or interleukin-1 and interferon-alpha or interleukin-2. J Biol Resp Mod 1989;8:53–61.
34 Owen-Schaub LB, Gutterman JU, Grimm EA: Synergy of tumor necrosis factor and interleukin 2 in the activation of human cytotoxic lymphocytes: effect of tumor necrosis factor alpha and interleukin 2 in the generation of human lymphokine-activated killer cell cytotoxicity. Cancer Res 1988;48:788–792.
35 Gridley DS, Archambeau JO, Andres MA, Mao XW, Wright K, Slater JM: Tumor necrosis factor-alpha enhances antitumor effects of radiation against glioma xenografts. Oncol Res 1997;9: 217–227.
36 Niranjan A, Moriuchi S, Lunsford LD, Kondziolka D, Flickinger JC, Fellows W, Rajendiran S, Tamura M, Cohen JB, Glorioso JC: Effective treatment of experimental glioblastoma by HSV vector-mediated TNF alpha and HSV-tk gene transfer in combination with radiosurgery and ganciclovir administration. Mol Ther 2000;2:114–120.
37 Marconi P, Tamura M, Moriuchi S, Krisky DM, Niranjan A, Goins WF, Cohen JB, Glorioso JC: Connexin 43-enhanced suicide gene therapy using herpesviral vectors. Mol Ther 2000;1: 71–81.
38 Moriuchi S, Oligino T, Krisky D, Marconi P, Fink D, Cohen J, Glorioso JC: Enhanced tumor cell killing in the presence of ganciclovir by herpes simplex virus type 1 vector-directed coexpression of human tumor necrosis factor-alpha and herpes simplex virus thymidine kinase. Cancer Res 1998;58:5731–5737.
39 Mori Y, Kondziolka D, Balzer J, Fellows W, Flickinger JC, Lunsford LD, Thulborn KR: Effects of stereotactic radiosurgery on an animal model of hippocampal epilepsy. Neurosurgery 2000;46: 157–165.
40 Maesawa S, Kondziolka D, Dixon CE, Balzer J, Fellows W, Lunsford LD: Subnecrotic stereotactic radiosurgery controlling epilepsy produced by kainic acid injection in rats. J Neurosurg 2000;93: 1033–1040.
41 Liscak R, Vladyka V, Novotny J Jr, Brozek G, Namestkova K, Mares V, Herynek V, Jirak D, Hajek M, Sykova E: Leksell gamma knife lesioning of the rat hippocampus: the relationship between radiation dose and functional and structural damage. J Neurosurg 2002;97(suppl): 666–673.
42 De Salles AA, Melega WP, Lacan G, Steele LJ, Solberg TD: Radiosurgery performed with the aid of a 3-mm collimator in the subthalamic nucleus and substantia nigra of the vervet monkey. J Neurosurg 2001;95:990–997.
43 Kondziolka D, Conce M, Niranjan A, Maesawa S, Fellows W: Histology of the 100 Gy thalomotomy in the baboon. Radiosurgery 2002;4:279–284.
44 Kondziolka D, Lacomis D, Niranjan A, Mori Y, Maesawa S, Fellows W, Lunsford LD: Histological effects of trigeminal nerve radiosurgery in a primate model: implications for trigeminal neuralgia radiosurgery. Neurosurgery 2000;46:971–976.
45 Kondziolka D, Lunsford LD, Claassen D, Pandalai S, Maitz AH, Flickinger JC: Radiobiology of radiosurgery: Part II. The rat C6 glioma model. Neurosurgery 1992;31:280–287.
46 Kondziolka D, Mori Y, Martinez AJ, McLaughlin MR, Flickinger JC, Lunsford LD: Beneficial effects of the radioprotectant 21-aminosteroid U-74389G in a radiosurgery rat malignant glioma model. Int J Radiat Oncol Biol Phys 1999;44:179–184.
47 Nakahara N, Okada H, Witham TF, Attanucci J, Fellows WK, Chambers WH, Niranjan A, Kondziolka D, Pollack IF: Combination of stereotactic radiosurgery and cytokine gene-transduced tumor cell vaccination: a new strategy against metastatic brain tumors. J Neurosurg 2001;95:984–989.
48 Niranjan A, Wolfe D, Tamura M, Lunsford LD, Fellows W, Cohen JB, Glorioso JC: Treatment of rat gliosarcoma brain tumors by HSV-based multigene therapy combined with radiosurgery. Mol Ther 2003;8:530–542.

49 Ishikawa S, Otsuki T, Kaneki M, Jokura H, Yoshimoto T: Dose-related effects of single focal irradiation in the medial temporal lobe structures in rats–magnetic resonance imaging and histological study. Neurol Med Chir (Tokyo) 1999;39:1–7.
50 Brisman JL, Cole AJ, Cosgrove GR, Thornton AF, Rabinov J, Bussiere M, Bradley-Moore M, Hedley-Whyte T, Chapman PH: Radiosurgery of the rat hippocampus: magnetic resonance imaging, neurophysiological, histological, and behavioral studies. Neurosurgery 2003;53:951–961.

Ajay Niranjan, MD
Department of Neurological Surgery, Suite B-400
University of Pittsburgh Medical Center, 200 Lothrop Street
Pittsburgh, PA 15213 (USA)
Tel. +1 412 647 9699, Fax +1 412 647 8447, E-Mail niranjana@upmc.edu

Szeifert GT, Kondziolka D, Levivier M, Lunsford LD (eds): Radiosurgery and Pathological Fundamentals. Prog Neurol Surg. Basel, Karger, 2007, vol 20, pp 375–387

15.2. Physiological and Pathological Observations on Rat Middle Cerebral Arteries and Human AVM Tissue Cultures following Single High-Dose Gamma Irradiation

Ottó Major[a], *György T. Szeifert*[a], *Andras A. Kemeny*[b]

[a]National Institute of Neurosurgery and Department of Neurological Surgery, Semmelweis University, Budapest, Hungary; [b]Royal Hallamshire Hospital, Sheffield, UK

Abstract

In vitro isometric myograph and histopathological studies were performed on rat middle cerebral arteries (MCAs) to explore changes in contractile capacity following experimental Gamma Knife radiosurgery. Right MCAs were treated with 25 Gy and 50 Gy at the 50% isodose line, while contralateral vessels received 15 Gy and 20 Gy at the 20% isodose region. Survival period varied from 3 to 18 months. Reduction in contractile capacity of irradiated normal rat MCAs was detected but their lumina remained patent. In another study, we investigated human AVM tissue cultures in order to detect genetic and phenotypic modifications contributing to vessel occlusion after irradiation. In culture, the proliferation index decreased considerably following 15-, 20-, 25- or 50-Gy irradiation at the 5th posttreatment day and remained depressed during the observation period of 14 days. P53, p21Waf-1 and mdm-2 mRNA contents were elevated significantly after irradiation, indicating enhanced apoptosis. Immunohistochemistry revealed vigorous vimentin positivity in the nonirradiated control AVM cultures, which gradually decreased by the time in the irradiated specimens. Smooth muscle α-actin positivity was prominent in the irradiated cultivated samples, suggesting transformation of resting fibroblasts onto activated myofibroblastic elements with contractile capacity. This transformation process was confirmed by the appearance of TGF-β in the irradiated AVM cell lines also. These data support the hypothesis that one of the contributing factors to AVM shrinkage and obliteration after radiosurgery might be fibrocyte-myofibroblastic cell transformation in the vessel wall.

Table 1. Groups and treatments

Group name	Treatment	Timing after treatment	Viable vessels
Normal	None	Acute	68
Denuded	Removal of endothelium	Acute	12
12w20 Gy	20 Gy	12 weeks	8
12w50 Gy	50 Gy	12 weeks	8
1y20 Gy	20 Gy	1 year	4
1y50 Gy	50 Gy	1 year	4
18m15 Gy	15 Gy	18 months	3
18m20 Gy	20 Gy	18 months	3
18m25 Gy	25 Gy	18 months	3
18m50 Gy	50 Gy	18 months	3

It is supposed that late radiation-induced alterations in the CNS are related to apoptotic and vascular changes, especially in benign lesions and normal brain tissue. Cerebral AVMs were among the first pathologies that were treated by stereotactic radiosurgery in 1970. According to the literature, 65–85% of AVMs undergo obliteration during a 2-year period after irradiation. As the time course of the obliterative process is slow, one of the most intriguing features of radiation-induced AVM occlusion is the latency period with a hemorrhage risk corresponding to the natural history of the disease [1–4].

The aim of this study was to analyze late changes in cerebral vessels' function and morphology following single high-dose gamma irradiation. To understand better the postirradiation changes in human pathological vessels, an AVM tissue culture model was also established to perform histological and genetic investigations following focused irradiation.

Materials and Methods

Thirty-four Wistar rats were used as normal controls, providing 68 middle cerebral arteries (MCAs). Stereotactic radiosurgery was performed in 18 rats (table 1).

Irradiation Procedure

According to Paxino's rat stereotactic atlas, 8-mm collimator field was defined by Leksell GammaPlan® (Elekta, Sweden) onto the right MCA. In 15 animals, 50 Gy was delivered to the 50% isodose line, allowing 20 Gy to the contralateral MCA located at the 20% isodose region, and 3 more rats received 25 Gy to the ipsilateral and 15 Gy to the contralateral vessel. The lower doses fell into the range of those that are therapeutically employed in the treatment of AVMs, while reactions to higher doses are comparable with other experimental results [5–7].

Myograph Studies

After exsanguination, the most proximal 3-mm section of the MCA was cut and mounted into an automated small vessel myograph (Cambustion, Cambridge, UK) [5, 8, 9]. Concentration-response curves were obtained by adding KCl solution or prostaglandin F2α (PGF; Prostin F2 Alpha, Upjohn) to the bath in a stepwise cumulative manner. The maximal contractions were recorded. Next, various relaxants were tested. After preconstriction with 50 μM of PGF, solutions of histamine, papaverine, L-arginine (L-arg) or sodium nitroprusside were added to the bath in a cumulative fashion to record relaxation dose-response curves.

Endothelial Lesion

The endothelial layer of the MCA was mechanically traumatized in 12 of the nonirradiated vessels.

Diameter-Tension Graph

At the end of the myograph experiments, diameter-tension graphs were recorded. The irradiated vessels and normal controls were also compared with vessels incubated with 100 μM papaverine for 1 h in order to achieve maximal dilatation. The latter reveals the normal vessel wall elasticity without internal muscle activity.

Histological Investigations

Hematoxylin-eosin staining was performed on 5-μm paraffin sections for light microscopy at the end of myograph experiments.

Tissue Cultures and Genetic Studies

Human AVM tissue samples removed by operation were cultured to 75–80% of shading, and irradiated with a single 15-, 20-, 25- or 50-Gy dose of gamma rays from ^{60}Co isotope sources. Cell proliferation index and changes in gene activation of p53, p21Waf-1, mdm-2 and HSP were determined. Immunohistochemical reactions were carried out for vimentin, desmin, smooth muscle α-actin, GFAP, factor VIII, cytokeratin, S-100 and TGF-β to disclose phenotypic changes.

Data Processing

All data are expressed as mean ± standard deviation. The differences between the various treatment groups were analyzed using Student's t test.

Results

Maximal Potassium Response

The maximal potassium contraction decreased in the 20-Gy-irradiated vessels 12 weeks after the Gamma Knife treatment and remained in the same range in the 1 year and the 18 months groups as well. In the 50 Gy groups, the potassium

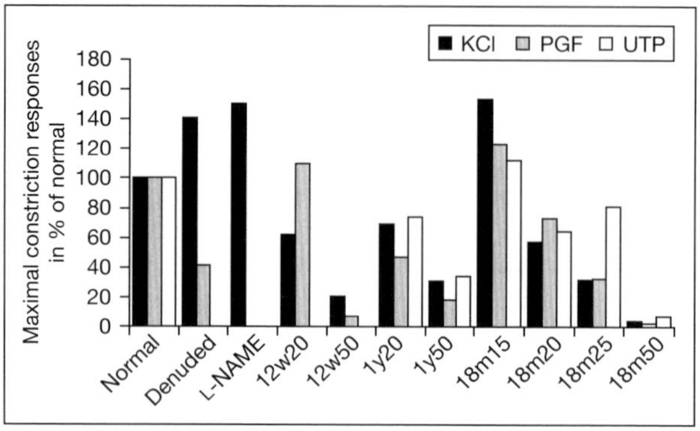

Fig. 1. Constriction responses to KCl, PGF and UTP. We can observe the difference in radiosensitivity among the different constriction mechanisms.

response was significantly diminished at 1 year, and abolished at 18 months. We have found an increased reaction in the 15 Gy group (fig. 1).

Maximal PGF Response

This test showed time and dose dependency. The tendencies were similar as in the case of potassium response in all but the 12 week 20-Gy-irradiated group, where the PGF reaction has remained near normal while after a 1 year it dropped to 50%. In the 50-Gy-irradiated groups, the PGF responses were abolished (fig. 1).

UTP Response

Contractions at 200 μM concentration were considered as maximal responses. The tendencies are very similar to the potassium or PGF responses with the exception of the good response in the 18 months 25 Gy group, indicating that the UTP response is possibly more radioresistant than potassium or PGF response for 25-Gy radiation dose (fig. 1).

Potassium Dose Response Studies

In the low K^+ concentration range (12 and 15 mM KCl), a reproducible relaxation was observed in the normal group. The relaxation was abolished in the 24 h groups. In the 12 weeks groups, this function seemed to be gradually recovered; however, the reaction was smaller than in the normal group. In the 1 year groups, the relaxation was almost normal, while the 18 months 15-Gy-irradiated vessels showed normal relaxation for KCl. In the 18 months 50 Gy group, this reaction was missing (table 2).

Table 2. Vessel relaxation response to KCl and its alteration after irradiation

Group name	12 mM	15 mM (bath concentration)
Normal	−8.6 ± 7.9	−9.2 ± 7.24
Denuded	1.7 ± 2.05*	2.3 ± 2.93
12w20 Gy	−7.06 ± 8.65	−8.79 ± 8.77
12w50 Gy	−6.71 ± 1.85	−6.41 ± 19.17
1y20 Gy	−13.88 ± 11.07	−11.58 ± 12.43
1y50 Gy	−18.32 ± 20.64	−17.65 ± 16.58
18m15 Gy	−9.85 ± 6.29	−9.79 ± 7.73
18m20 Gy	−18.99 ± 14.12	−19.27 ± 13.73
18m25 Gy	−41.37 ± 36.33	−41.95 ± 34.46
18m50 Gy	1.33 ± 2.51*	1.66 ± 2.88

Data are expressed in % of maximal response to 124 mM KCl. *$p<0.05$.

Relaxation Experiments

In the 50-Gy-irradiated groups, the PGF responses were so weak that we could not generate dose-response curves of elicit relaxation studies (fig. 1).

L-Arginine

We could demonstrate a significant overrelaxation in the response to L-arg in the 12 weeks 20 Gy group ($p < 0.05$). In all the others, the reaction for L-arg was remarkably smaller, in the 25 Gy group it was similar to vessels with mechanically damaged endothelium. However, according to constriction responses of the 'denuded vessels' the contractile apparatus remained intact (fig. 2).

Diameter-Tension Graph

The 50-Gy-irradiated group showed remarkably steeper lines (more rigid walls), while the others were between the maximally relaxed (as a reference) and the normal group (fig. 3).

Pathological Observations

There were some early degenerative changes in the 12 weeks 50-Gy-irradiated animals. On the right frontobasal surface, 3- to 4-mm yellowish discoloration plaques were noticed within the 90% isodose curve. In the 1 year and 18 months 50-Gy-irradiated groups, 5- to 6-mm cystic, bowl-shaped lesions in the brain tissue were observed by macroscopic examination, near the

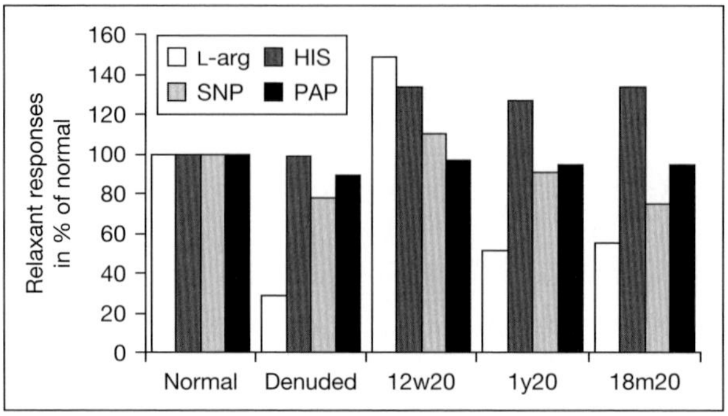

Fig. 2. Changes in vessel relaxation responses to various stimuli. The endothelium-dependent relaxation to L-arg is abolished when the endothelium is removed ('denuded'). Though there seems to be a transient regeneration at 12 weeks, 20-Gy irradiation eventually reduces the response by 1 year with only moderate restoration later. HIS = Histamine; PAP = papaverine; SNP = sodium nitroprusside.

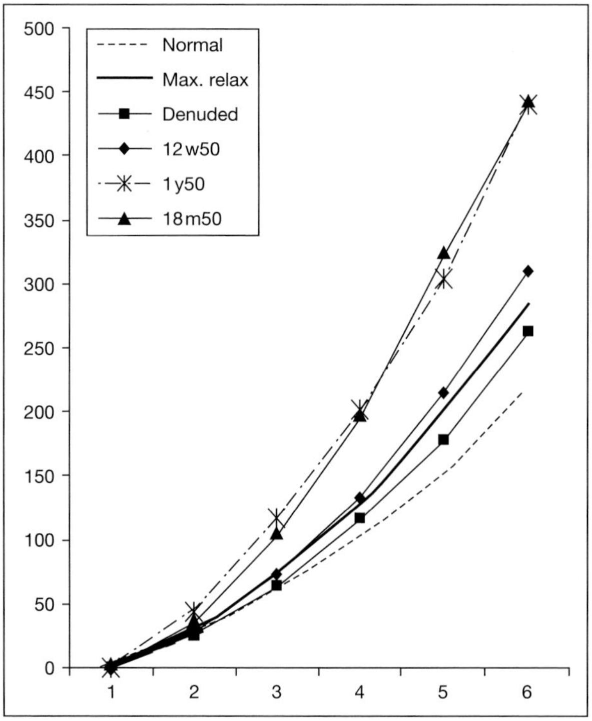

Fig. 3. The steepness of the lines represent 'stiffness' in the vessel wall. This figure demonstrates that in the late stages after irradiation, the vessel is rigid, fibrotic.

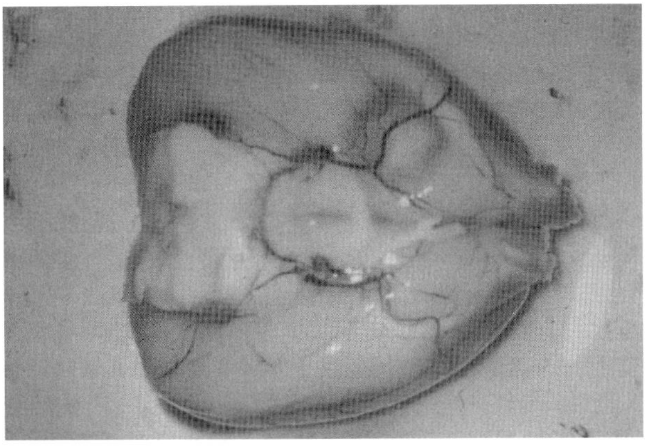

Fig. 4. The bowl-shaped necrotic cavity at the base of the right cerebral hemisphere.

targeted MCA, approximately corresponding to the 80% isodose curve (fig. 4).

Light Microscopy

Dilated subarachnoid spaces and moderate subarachnoid fibrosis was found around the irradiated MCA after the 3rd month following radiosurgery. Endothelial damage was shown by undulating endothelial lining, or even by complete destruction of the endothelial layer in vessels receiving 50-Gy irradiation. Nevertheless, subendothelial proliferation, intimal or medial wall thickening has not occurred in these experiments. Even in groups which developed late radiation injury at 12 or 18 months in the form of radiation necrotic cyst around the MCA, vessels still persisted, and the lumen was patent.

Human AVM Tissue Cultures

The proliferation index dramatically decreased at the 5th day, and remained depressed over the observed period in the irradiated AVM cultures (8 and 14 days). P53, p21Waf-1 and mdm-2 mRNA measurements showed considerable elevation in human AVM cultures after 15-Gy irradiation, indicating apoptosis.

Immunohistochemistry revealed strong vimentin positivity in the nonirradiated control cultures, which gradually decreased by the time in the irradiated samples. Smooth muscle α-actin positivity was detected in the irradiated specimens, indicating fibroblast transformation onto myofibroblastic elements. This transformation was confirmed by expressing TGF-β as well in the radiation-treated cell population (table 3).

Table 3. Immunohistological investigations of cultured and irradiated human AVM tissue

	Vimentin	Desmin	α-actin	Factor VIII	Cyto-keratin	GFAP	S-100	TGF-β
Control	++++	–	+/–	–	–	–	–	–
15 Gy	++	–	+	–	–	–	–	+/–
20 Gy	++	–	+	–	–	–	–	+
25 Gy	–	–	+++	–	–	–	–	++
50 Gy	–/+	–	+++	–	–	–	–	++

Discussion

The animal studies indicated radiosensitivity of the endothelial cell to an irradiation dose as small as 15 Gy. Six to 12 weeks after irradiation, there were some regenerative processes in the endothelial tissue as shown by blood-brain barrier studies. It was noteworthy, that in the late stages the sensitivity of vessels to pharmacological stimuli has increased, as shown by the considerable left shift of the dose-response curves, possibly by a new generation of prostanoid receptors. The adenylate cyclase system, involved in the UTP contraction, and the voltage-dependent calcium channels were probably more radioresistant than the other functions.

According to previous studies, the potassium-induced relaxation is a marker of Na^+/K^+ ATP-ase activity. Radiosensitivity of this enzyme had been shown before. The sodium/potassium pump-dependent potassium relaxation returned in 12 weeks, indicating regenerative processes in the involved enzymatic functions [5, 10, 13].

The endothelium-dependent relaxation responses showed time- and dose-dependent reduction after radiation. Relaxation of vessels after 25-Gy irradiation at 18 months was comparable to vessels with the endothelium physically removed, indicating that irradiation can abolish this endothelial function even in a radioresistant species such as rat [7–17]. Endothelial control mechanisms (relaxant effects) are more radiosensitive than the contractile functions of the smooth muscle cells [5, 12, 18–20].

In our experiments, no vessel occlusion was observed. This is contrary to the results of Nilsson et al. [21], who reported thrombo-obliterative changes in the basilar artery of the cat. In the recent literature, there are several reports of radiation-induced cerebrovasculopathies. These controversies could be explained on the basis of interspecies radiosensitivity differences, and the different irradiation doses, size and structure of the irradiated vessels [7, 11, 14, 16, 22–24]. The necrotic lesions in the 50 Gy groups, appearing 1 year after irradiation, are in good concordance with the literature [14].

The physiological changes to radiation are accompanied by morphological alterations. In a previous study, we presented the findings in human cerebral AVMs after Gamma Knife radiosurgery [4]. Light microscopy revealed spindle-shaped cell proliferation in the connective tissue stroma and in the subendothelial region of the vessels in the irradiated AVMs. Ultrastructural and immunohistochemical characteristics of these spindle-shaped cells were identical to those designated as myofibroblasts in wound healing processes and pathological fibromatoses [25]. Whereas in non-treated control specimens of AVMs, similar cells expressed vimentin and desmin positivity, in the Gamma Knife surgery-treated cases α-smooth muscle actin activity was also observed. In that study, we have suggested that radiosurgery stimulates proliferation of myofibroblasts in the stroma and vessels wall of AVMs and raised the potential role of these cells in the obliteration process of vessels and shrinkage of the lesion following radiosurgery. Other studies highlighted the endothelial damage and subendothelial proliferation of intimal spindle-shaped cells expressing smooth-muscle actin in the vessel wall [2, 3]. Both reports emphasized that in addition to cellular proliferation, there is a progressive deposition of collagenous matrix that contributes to luminal stenosis and ultimate obliteration.

On the cellular level, cytotoxicity of ionizing radiation closely related to the arrest of cell cycle and apoptosis mediated either by the p53 pathway or DNA mismatch repair. In our experiments, gamma irradiation caused induction of the p53 gene expression, indicating that even in those tissues where primary changes are phenotypic transformation some of the cells are going to suffer apoptosis. As the p21WAF-1, a cyclin-dependent kinase inhibitor, and the mdm-2 oncogene both were unregulated, one can state that gamma irradiation-induced apoptosis was specific and p53 dependent in our experiment. HSP plays an important role in radioresistance by modulating the metabolism of glutathione. We have not found any upregulation of this protein, indicating the lack of this mechanism in human AVM tissues. These observations are in good concordance with the immunohistochemical studies.

The most radiosensitive part of vessels appears to be the endothelial cell layer, and this is in good concordance with the literature [5, 11, 12, 24, 26]. Radiation injury to endothelial cells does not necessarily result in cell death but leads to demonstrable alterations in endothelial cell functions including depression of prostaglandin or amino-acid production [6, 12, 13, 18, 27–29]. Radiation effects on endothelial cells are the leading events in the pathogenesis of late irradiation changes in normal tissues. As the endothelial cell has several mechanisms to control the vessel tone [6, 12, 19, 24, 28], these functions could be damaged by the irradiation in different ways, by different doses or in different time scales [20, 26]. Table 4 shows the sequelae of the physiological

Table 4. Time & Dose relationship

Time Dose	1	42	84	360	540 days
200	reduced KCl response; reduced relaxations; no KCl relaxation				
80	reduced KCl response; increased relaxations; no KCl relaxations				
50	no KCl relaxation	reduced KCl and UTP response; small PGF response	reduced KCl and UTP response; small PGF response	minimal KCl and PGF and UTP response; rigid wall dilated	no reactions; maximally dilated rigid wall
25					reduced UTP response; minimal KCL and PGF response; minimal L-arginine; reaction maximal relaxations
20	no KCl relaxation	decreased KCl relaxation; reduced constrictor response; increased Relaxations	reappearance of KCl relaxation; reduced KCl and UTP response; increased PGF response; increased relaxations	reduced constrictions; increased relaxations; increased sensitivity for constrictors	further reduction in constrictions; decreased L-arginine reaction; remarkably increased relaxations
15	Gy				increased constrictions; increased sensitivity for constrictors; decreased L-arginine reaction; increased relaxations; normal sensitivity for relaxants

changes of the vessel wall after a single-dose gamma irradiation. Even smaller doses resulted in marked changes, only slower. Small radiation dose caused marked regulation error in the contractility, while higher doses showed dose-dependent reduction of vascular response in addition to progressive changes of the physical properties of the vessel wall.

The difference in radiosensitivity between the abnormal channels of an AVM and normal feeding arteries remains unexplained. Our experimental results and human pathological studies raise the following hypothesis. Normal cerebral arteries do not have connective tissue stroma and they are surrounded by subarachnoidal spaces (Virchow-Robin spaces). In spite of the damage to the endothelial cell layer of normal vessels, subendothelial cell proliferation does not develop. Perivascular fibrosis without narrowing of the vessel lumen does occur in subarachnoid spaces. It might originate either from the adventitial layer of the vascular channels, or from meningeal sheets. These observations draw our attention to the significance of connective tissue stroma in AVMs. Its existence is the most striking difference between the pathological and physiological vascular morphological conditions, and would suggest that myofibroblasts originate from this connective tissue stroma of AVMs following radiosurgery.

Conclusion

According to our experiments, different vessel wall functions appear to have different radiosensitivity, time course and capability for regeneration. Different radiosensitivity of various enzyme systems and related functions may suggest possible clinical implications. By the better understanding of the involved physiological systems and processes, and their response to irradiation, it may become possible to tailor radiation to individual enzyme systems which could open new indications for stereotactic radiosurgery [30–32].

References

1 Dandy WE: Arteriovenous aneurysm of the brain. Arch Surg 1928;17:190–213.

2 Gevirtz RJ, Sterinberg GK, Crowley R, Levy RP: Pathological changes in surgically resected angiographically occult vascular malformations after radiation. Neurosurgery 1998;42:738–742.

3 Schndeider BP, Eberhard DA, Steiner LE: Histopathology of arteriovenous malformations after gamma knife radiosurgery. J Neurosurg 1997;87:352–357.

4 Szeifert GT, Kemeny AA, Timperly WR, Forster DMC: The potential role of myofibroblasts in the obliteration of arteriovenous malformations after gamma knife radiosurgery. Neurosurgery 1997;40:61–65.

5 Major O, Kemeny AA, Forster DM, Jakubowski J, Morice AH: In vitro contractility studies of the rat middle cerebral artery after stereotactic gamma knife radiosurgery. Stereotact Funct Neurosurg 1996;66(suppl 1):17–28.

6 Bourlier V, Deserbo M, Joyeux M, Kibout D, Multon E, Gourmelon P, Verdetti J: Early effects of acute gamma-radiation on vascular arterial tone. Br J Pharmacol 1998;123:1168–1172.
7 Spiegelmann R, Friedman WA, Bova FJ, Theele DP, Mickle JP: LINAC radiosurgery: an animal model. J Neurosurg 1993;78:638–644.
8 Mulvany MJ, Halpern W. Mechanical properties of vascular smooth muscle cell in situ. Nature 1976;260:617–619.
9 Mulvany MJ, Warshaw DM: The active tension-length curve of vascular smooth muscle related to its cellular components. J Gen Physiol 1979;74:85–104.
10 Dvoretskii AI, Shainskaia AM, Anan'eva TV, Kulikova IA, Annenkova SV: Postradiation changes of active iontransport systems of the CNS: the effect of superlethal doses of ionizing radiation on the Na, K pump in surviving brain slices. Radiobiologia 1989;29:477–480.
11 Fajardo LF: The unique physiology of endothelial cells and its implications in radiobiology. Front Radiat Ther Oncol 1989;23:96–112.
12 Menendez JC, Casanova D, Amado JA, Salas C, Garcia-Unzueta MT, Fernandez F, de la Lastra LP, Berrazueta JR: Effect of radiation on endothelial function. Int J Radiat Oncol Biol Phys 1998;41: 905–913.
13 Shainskaia AM, Dvoretskii AI, Valetova O: Postradiation changes of the active ion transport systems of the CNS: Na, K-ATPase of neurons and neuroglia. Radiologia 1989;29:481–484.
14 Kondziolka D, Lunsford LD, Claassen D, Maitz AH, Flickinger JC: Radiobiology of radiosurgery: Part I. The normal rat brain model. Neurosurgery 1992;31:271–279.
15 Moustafa HF, Phil D, Hopewell JW: Late functional changes in the vasculature of the rat brain after local X-irradiation. Br J Radiol 1980;53:21–25.
16 Reinhold HS, Hopewell JW: Late changes in the architecture of blood vessels of the rat brain after irradiation. Br J Radiol 1980;53:693–696.
17 Shimotakahara S, Mayberg MR: Gamma irradiation inhibits neointimal hyperplasia in rats after arterial injury. Stroke 1994;25:424–428.
18 Kantak SS, Diglio CA, Onoda JM: Low dose radiation-induced endothelial cell retraction. Int J Radiat Biol 1993;64:319–328.
19 Speidel MT, Holmquist B, Kassis AI, Humm JL, Berman RM, Atcher RW, Hines JJ, Macklis RM: Morphological, biochemical and molecular changes in endothelial cells after alpha-particle irradiation. Radiat Res 1993;136:373–381.
20 Zhou Q, Zhao Y, Li p, Bai X and Ruan C: Thrombomodulin as a marker of radiation-induced endothelial cell injury. Radiat Res 1992;131:285–289.
21 Nilsson A, Wennerstrand J, Leksell D, Backlund EO: Stereotactic gamma irradiation of basilar artery in cat. Acta Radiol Oncol 1978;17:150–160.
22 Lundsford LD, Altschuler EM, Flickinger JF, Wu A, Martinez AJ: In vivo biological effects of stereotactic radiosurgery: a primate model. Neurosurgery 1990;27:373–382.
23 Nakagaki H, Brunhart G, Kemper TL, Caveness WF: Monkey brain damage from radiation in the therapeutic range. Neurosurgery 1976;44:3–11.
24 Qi F, Sugihara T, Hattori Y, Yamamoto Y, Kannio M, Abe K: Functional and morphological damage of endothelium in rabbit ear artery following irradiation with cobalt 60. Br J Pharmacol 1998;123:653–660.
25 Gabbiani G, Ryan GB, Majno C: Presence of modified fibroblasts in granulation tissue and their possible role in wound contraction. Experientia 1971;27:549–550.
26 Pearson JD: Endothelial cell biology. Radiology 1991;179:9–14.
27 Allan DJ: Radiation-induced apoptosis: its role in a MACDCaT (mitosis-apotosis-differenctiation-calcium toxicity) scheme of cytotoxicity mechanisms. Int J Radiat Biol 1992;62:145.
28 Allen JB, Sagerman RH, Stuart MJ: Irradiation decreases vascular prostacyclin formation with no concomitant effect on platelet thromboxane production. Lancet 1981;2:1193–1196.
29 Haimovitz-Friedman A, Kan CC, Ehleiter D, Persaud RS, McLoughlin M, Fuks Z, Kolesnick RN: Ionizing radiation acts on cellular membranes to generate ceramide and initiate apoptosis. J Exp Med 1994;180:525–535.
30 Leksell L: Cerebral radiosurgery. Acta Chir Scand 1968;134:585–595.

31 Lunsford LD: Stereotactic radiosurgery: at the threshold or at the crossroads? Neurosurgery 1993;33:799–804.
32 Major O, Szeifert GT, Radatz MWR, Walton L, Kemeny AA: Experimental stereotactic gamma knife radiosurgery: vascular contractility studies of the rat middle cerebral artery after chronic survival. Neurol Res 2002;24:191–198.

Ottó Major, MD, PhD
National Institute of Neurosurgery
Amerikai ut 57
HU–1145 Budapest (Hungary)
Tel. +36 1 2512 999, Fax +361 2515 678, E-Mail majoott@freestart.hu

Szeifert GT, Kondziolka D, Levivier M, Lunsford LD (eds): Radiosurgery and Pathological Fundamentals. Prog Neurol Surg. Basel, Karger, 2007, vol 20, pp 388–391

The Future of Radiosurgery

Dan Leksell

This volume of *Progress in Neurological Surgery* concerns a field of medicine, radiosurgery, which in itself is a worthy example of the meaning of the word 'progress'.

The title of the book and the subject it reviews are quite suitably matched.

I remember in the early years, 40 years ago, when we literally knew nothing about what to expect. We knew nothing about the histopathology of radiosurgery and what we thought could be gleaned from past experience in radiation therapy, proved to be less than enlightening. Dose planning was primitive, executed as it was, on the basis of a hand-drawn nomogram. The accuracy of the nomogram, with its wavy lines, was such, that had it been today, we probably would have had to report every case we did to the Swedish radiation protection institute, for overdosing or for underdosing.

However, since we did not know what would be the right dose for any particular target or disorder, none of all these deficiencies really mattered. Every procedure was a 'shot in the dark' and we were learning. I should say that we were fortunate then, that the research environment allowed this kind of 'hands-on' slow learning process. And we are fortunate today, all of us working with radiosurgery in one capacity or another, and the hundreds of thousands of patients that have come to benefit from the methodology, that in the early years in Stockholm we were allowed to test the waters the way we did!

I remember trips to numerous congresses where I talked about what we did in Stockholm, oftentimes only to be regarded as a 'charlatan' and sometimes only to be physically removed from a meeting. Fundamentally, this incredulity remained until 1987 when, with the installation of the first U.S. Gamma Knife, an increasing acceptance began to emerge. This was due to the dedication and innovative hard work performed by some of the new, non-Swedish, researchers in North America and later in Asia and in Europe.

The radiosurgical method was originally intended only for the treatment of a few functional disorders, mainly trigeminal neuralgia and movement disorders.

Today it has expanded and it is now a potential surgical option in almost all neurosurgical cases. Radiosurgery is an option in patients with all types of benign tumors and it is a well-proven treatment in vascular disorders, primarily arteriovenous malformations. It has contributed to a fantastic improvement in quality of life for patients with brain metastases, and it is increasingly explored also for primary brain malignancies, often in combination with other treatments. The functional field has seen a strong revival, as illustrated by the thousands of trigeminal neuralgia patients who have undergone radiosurgery over the last 10 years. At a time when patients are becoming better informed and more demanding, neurosurgeons can now offer alternative surgical strategies. These are not anymore just microsurgery or radiosurgery, but often also various combinations of the two. The words 'comprehensive management' now have real meaning when neurosurgeons strive to advise their patients.

The question now is – what lies ahead?

During the last 15 years, we have seen how radiosurgery, initially by many thought of as a temporary diversion, not only has taken a firm grip on the daily practice of brain surgery but also how it has begun to change the until now rather innovation-starved field of radiation therapy.

As far as the brain is concerned, there are several interesting areas which are being re-explored or explored de novo.

Movement disorders are the target of neuromodulation/stimulation and stem cell research but also of researchers believing that noninvasive radiation should be explored as an option, either with intent to lesion or with intent to modulate by the application of subthreshold doses of radiation.

Epilepsy in pharmacologically refractory epilepsy, many of them surgical candidates, constitutes a significant problem on all continents and the number of surgical candidates who never reach surgery is huge. A noninvasive radiosurgical alternative would be very attractive. If we could use magnetoencephalography for the preoperative work-up, carried out interictally and noninvasively in a few hours, then it may become possible to treat these patients with noninvasive radiosurgery. We would then have a wholly noninvasive treatment paradigm for epilepsy patients. The cost savings of such an approach would be considerable and would, together with time savings, provide relief for a much larger number of epileptics than what is currently possible. Several studies exploring magnetoencephalography for preoperative work-up will soon be underway, and the Gamma Knife is now being used for epilepsy under several research protocols. We will know more in the not too distant future.

Vestibular schwannomas have been operated with radiosurgery ever since we started with Gamma Knife surgery in Stockholm. The neuro-otology community for some time appeared oppositional to this innovative approach, often with arguments such as 'hearing is not a primary concern in these patients'.

Interesting when spoken by otologists! This is now changing and as patients increasingly demand to be offered radiosurgery, we are seeing the most vocal opponents from the past turning around and becoming involved. This is a very welcome change!

Ophthalmology is another closely related specialty. From this community, there never was any opposition. On the contrary, in recent years, with an increasing application of radiosurgery for ocular disorders, the ophthalmologists are becoming increasingly interested and involved. This will benefit patients with disorders such as uveal melanoma, macular degeneration, and, maybe most interestingly, glaucoma. The latter is like a functional disorder of the eye, and it has been shown that by irradiating the ciliary body, intraocular pressure can be brought down to within normal limits. This cures pain and allows patients to retain their eyes. Glaucoma, together with macular degeneration represent the single most prevalent causes of blindness among the elderly. A single non-invasive surgical procedure could possibly replace many years of medication. What a nice contribution this would be!

Finally, a few words about how radiosurgery, as practiced by neurosurgeons over the last almost 4 decades, has brought about significant change in the practice of radiation therapy.

While radiosurgery has made use of stereotaxy and sophisticated imaging all along, this has not been the case in radiation therapy, while radiosurgery has used finely collimated multiple beams all along, in radiation therapy they used crudely applied blocking patterns. I believe that the collective work done by all those – neurosurgeons, radiation oncologists, neuoradiologists, physicists and others – who were open-minded enough to engage in radiosurgery early on, has brought about the considerable changes that we have seen, transforming conventional radiotherapy (RT) into modern radiation therapy. Today, we speak about stereotactic RT, about image-guided RT, about intensity-modulated RT and other things which all have come from the practice of radiosurgery to fertilize and modernize cancer care.

Now, about 10 years later, we have seen a significant change in how radiation therapy treatment machines are designed. Not only do modern accelerators incorporate stereotactic localization and fixation, but radiation therapy dose planning is also based on these same prerequisites. In radiosurgery, we have understood the need for integrated imaging for a long time. Well, imaging is now also becoming an integral part of modern radiation therapy technology.

The advances we have seen in radiation medicine during the last 20 years have been astounding and have not been limited just to radiosurgery and radiation therapy. Specifically, and returning to the task at hand, our understanding of the fundamentals of radiosurgery today is amply illustrated by all of the important chapters making up this impressive volume. This book is a show-case example of how the perseverance and consistent contributions of the many brings progress, even in the most difficult fields of science. By joining forces neurosurgeons, radiation oncologists, neuroradiologists and physicists have brought about all of the changes mentioned above and have made possible the publication of this massive amount of new and updated information on radiosurgery.

Now it is time to bring the neurologist, the neurophysiologist, the neuro-otologist, the head & neck surgeon and the neuro-ophthalmologist into the fold! We will then see a new quantum leap in terms of clinical development and broadened clinical applications.

This book will be extensively used in radiosurgery training and I have already warmly recommended it to many colleagues in different parts of the world.

Dan Leksell, Stockholm, Sweden

Author Index

Subject Index